PEDIATRIC DIABETES

PEDIATRIC DIABETES

edited by

Ram K. Menon, M.D.
Division of Endocrinology, Metabolism & Diabetes
C.S. Mott Children's Hospital
University of Michigan Health System
Ann Arbor, MI

Mark A. Sperling, M.D.
Division of Endocrinology, Metabolism & Diabetes
Children's Hospital of Pittsburgh
University of Pittsburgh School of Medicine
Pittsburgh, PA

KLUWER ACADEMIC PUBLISHERS
Boston / New York / Dordrecht / London

Distributors for North, Central and South America:
Kluwer Academic Publishers
101 Philip Drive
Assinippi Park
Norwell, Massachusetts 02061 USA
Telephone (781) 871-6600
Fax (781) 681-9045
E-Mail: kluwer@wkap.com

Distributors for all other countries:
Kluwer Academic Publishers Group
Post Office Box 322
3300 AH Dordrecht, THE NETHERLANDS
Telephone 31 786 576 000
Fax 31 786 576 254
E-Mail: services@wkap.nl

Electronic Services <http://www.wkap.nl>

Library of Congress Cataloging-in-Publication Data

Pediatric diabetes / edited by Ram K. Menon and Mark A. Sperling
p. ; cm.
Includes bibliographical references and index.
ISBN 1-4020-7557-X (alk. paper)
1. Diabetes in children. 2. Diabetes in adolescence. I. Menon, Ram K. II. Sperling, Mark A.
[DNLM: 1. Diabetes Mellitus--Adolescent. 2. Diabetes Mellitus--Child. WK 810 P3715 2003]
RJ420.D5P44 2003
618.92'462--dc21 2003054607

Printed on acid-free paper.
Printed in the United States of America.

TABLE OF CONTENTS

Errata

The publisher regrets that the figures and tables from Chapter 10 from *Pediatric Diabetes*, edited by Ram K. Menon, M.D. and Mark A. Sperling, M.D., were inadvertently omitted when the book was first published. Please find the missing figures and tables on the following pages.

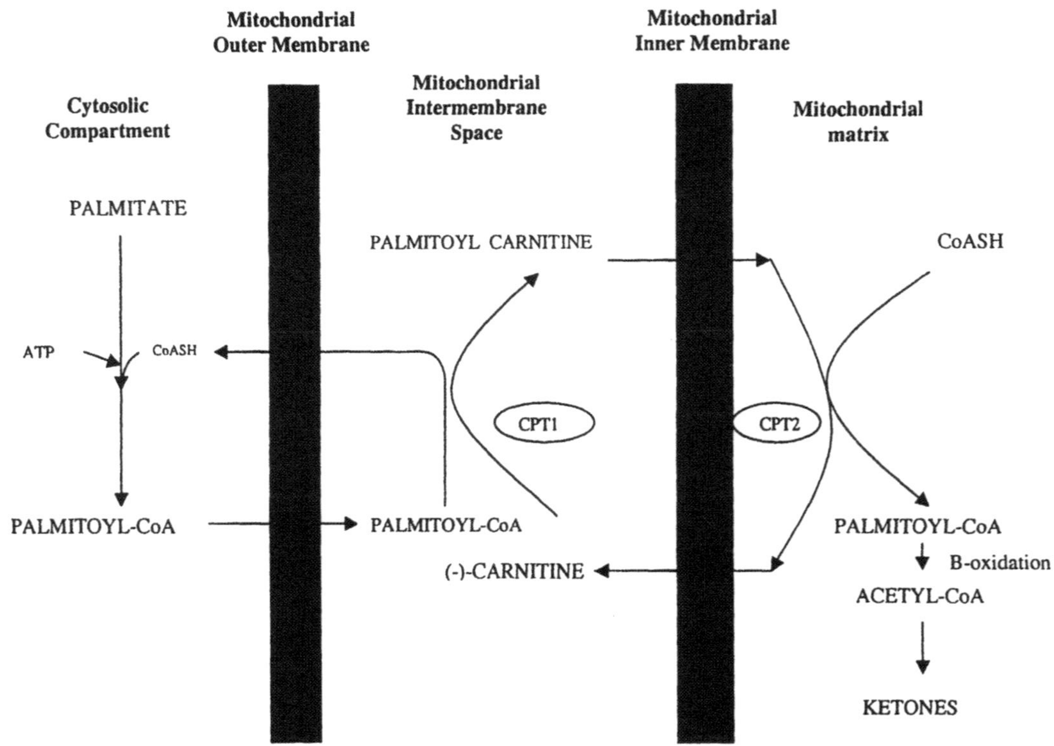

Fig 1 – Schematic representation of fatty acid oxidation system in liver. Formation of carnitine ester is catalyzed by carnitine palmitoyl transferase 1 (CPT1). The transesterification reaction is reversed inside the mitochondria by CPT2.

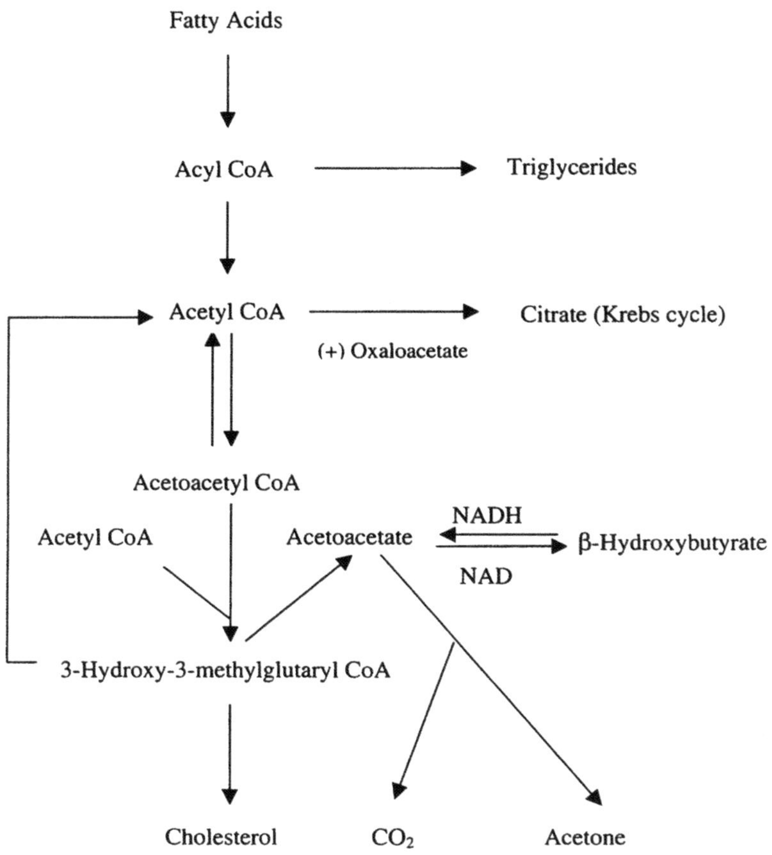

Fig 2 – Simplified schema of the formation of the major ketone bodies. The nitroprusside reaction commonly used to detect ketone bodies reacts strongly with AA, weakly with acetone, and not at all with BHOB. Acetoacetate (AA), beta-hydroxybutyrate (BHOB). See text for details.

Table 1 Influence of Feeding (High Insulin) or Fasting (Low Insulin) on Metabolic Processes in Liver, Muscle, and Adipose Tissue

	HIGH PLASMA INSULIN (postprandial state)	**LOW PLASMA INSULIN (fasted state)**
Liver	Glucose uptake Glycogen synthesis Absence of gluconeogenesis Lipogenesis Absence of ketogenesis	Glucose production Glycogenolysis Gluconeogenesis Absence of lipogenesis Ketogenesis
MUSCLE	Glucose uptake Glucose oxidation Glycogen synthesis Protein synthesis	Absence of glucose uptake Fatty acid and ketone oxidation Glycogenolysis Proteolysis and amino acid release
Adipose tissue	Glucose uptake Lipid synthesis Triglyceride uptake	Absence of glucose uptake Lipolysis and fatty acid release Absence of triglyceride uptake

Diabetes mellitus may be viewed as a permanent low-insulin state that if untreated results in exaggerated fasting.

Table 2 Fluid and Electrolyte Maintenance Requirements and Estimated Losses in Diabetic Ketoacidosis (assumed 10% dehydration).

APPROXIMATE DAILY MAINTENANCE REQUIREMENTS*		APPROXIMATE ACCUMULATED LOSSES**
Water	1500 mL/m^2	100 mL/kg (range, 60-100 mL/kg)
Sodium	45 mEq/m^2	6 mEq/kg (range, 5-13 mEq/kg)
Potassium	35 mEq/m^2	5 mEq/kg (range, 4-6 mEq/kg)
Chloride	30 mEq/m^2	4 mEq/kg (range, 3-9 mEq/kg)
Phosphate	10 mEq/m^2	3 mEq/kg (range, 2-5 mEq/kg)

*Maintenance is expressed in surface area to permit uniformity because fluid requirements change as weight increases.

**Losses are expressed per unit of body weight because the losses remain relatively constant in relation to total body weight.

Table 3 Fluid Electrolyte Therapy for Diabetic Ketoacidosis: Recommendations for Replacement of Fluid Losses and for Maintenance of a 30-kg (Surface Area, 1.0 m^2) Child with Assumed 10% Dehydration (Duration of Treatment, 36 Hours)

REPLACEMENT FLUIDS	APPROXIMATE ACCUMULATED LOSSES WITH 10% DEHYDRATION	APPROXIMATE REQUIREMENTS FOR MAINTENANCE (36 HR)	APPROXIMATE TOTALS FOR REPLACEMENT AND MAINTENANCE (36 HR)
Water (mL)	3000	2250	5500
Sodium (mEq)	180	65	250
Potassium (mEq)	150	50	200
Chloride (mEq)	120	45	165
Phosphate (mEq)	90	15	100

TABLE 4 Fluid and Electrolyte Replacement Schedule for Diabetic Ketoacidosis: Recommendations for Replacement of Fluid Losses and for Maintenance of a 30-kg (Surface Area, 1.0 m^2) Child with Assumed 10% Dehydration (Duration of Treatment, 36 Hours)

APPROXIMATE DURATION	FLUID (COMPOSITION)	Sodium (mEq)	Potassium (mEq)	Chloride (mEq)	Phosphate (mEq)
Hour 1	500 mL of 0.9% NaCl (isotonic saline)	75	–	75	–
Hour 2	500 mL of 0.45% NaCl (0.5 isotonic saline) plus 20 mEq of KCl	35	20	55	–
Hour 3-12 (200 mL/hr for 10 hr)	2000 mL of 0.45% NaCl with 30 mEq/L of potassium phosphate	150	60	150	40
Subtotal initial 12 hr	3000 mL	260	80	280	40
Next 24 hr 100 mL/hr	2400 mL of 5% glucose in 0.2% NaCl with 40 mEq/L of potassium phosphate	75	100	75	60
Total over 36 hours	5400 mL	335	180	355	100

All replacement values should be halved if dehydration is estimated to be 5%. Maintenance requirements remain the same.
Bicarbonate therapy: For pH >7.1, no therapy is necessary. For pH 7.00-7.10, 40 mEq/m^2 of bicarbonate over 2-4 hours may be considered. For pH<7.00, 80 mEq/m^2 of bicarbonate over 2-4 hours. After initial dose of bicarbonate, clinical and laboratory status should be reevaluated prior to making a decision for continuation of bicarbonate therapy. Bicarbonate should not be administered as a bolus.
Patients younger than 2 years with new-onset diabetes and diabetic ketoacidosis with 10% dehydration or any diabetic with pH<7.00, coma, or blood sugar >1000 mg/dl should be managed in an intensive care or equivalent setting.

Table 5. Continuous Low-Dose Intravenous Insulin Therapy for Diabetic Ketoacidosis

Priming dose: 0.1 Units/kg regular insulin, intravenously.

Continuous intravenous infusion: 0.1 Units/kg/hr regular insulin beginning with second hour.

Directions for making insulin infusion: Add 50 Units regular insulin to 500 ml of physiological saline solution. Flush 50 ml through the tubing to saturate insulin binding sites; initially infuse at a rate of 1 ml/kg/hr (for 30-kg patient, infuse at a rate of 30 ml/hr)

When the blood glucose concentration approaches 300 mg/dl add glucose (D_5 or D_{10}) to insulin infusion. Intravenous insulin therapy should be continued until *significant resolution of metabolic acidosis.* Upon discontinuation of the insulin infusion, subcutaneous injections of 0.2 - 0.4 Units/kg of regular insulin at 6-hour intervals should be initiated.

PREFACE

Type 1 diabetes mellitus is the most prevalent chronic disease in children in developed countries and has a major impact on the growth, development and emotional well being of the affected child. Worldwide there is an apparent increase in the incidence of this disease, especially in children under five years of age. In addition, this disease, if inadequately managed, increases the risk of developing microvascular and macrovascular complications. As a result, the economic impact of this disease on the global health care budget is enormous. Our motivation for bringing together a panel of experts in the field of childhood diabetes was the dearth of books that specifically address issues related to the care of children and adolescents with diabetes mellitus. The majority of available books dealing with practical issues of taking care of patients with diabetes mellitus are tailored to the needs of the adult patient. Our aim in undertaking the responsibility and privilege of editing this book was to provide a comprehensive description of the current state of the art management of diabetes mellitus in the pediatric population, based on contemporary developments in our scientific understanding of this entity.

The chapters on GENETICS and IMMUNITY describe the scientific basis for implicating autoimmunity in the causation of the most common form of disease process and explore its clinical implications. The epidemiology, clinical profile, and current strategies in the management of children with the syndrome of TYPE 2 Diabetes Mellitus, an increasing world-wide "epidemic" previously thought to only rarely affect children is discussed in a separate chapter. The genetic basis and clinical profiles of the newly described Maturity Onset Diabetes in Youth (MODY) syndromes is discussed, emphasizing that these are insulinopenic states due to transcriptional and other factors regulating insulin secretion. With the increasing longevity of patients with cystic fibrosis, diabetes mellitus is emerging as a significant clinical problem in this cohort; issues specific to the management of diabetes mellitus in these patients are discussed in the chapter on CYSTIC FIBROSIS RELATED DIABETES. Some of the societal, ethnic, and cultural issues in dealing with children with diabetes mellitus are described in the chapters on childhood diabetes in the DEVELOPING COUNTRIES and SOUTH EAST ASIA. Recent advances in the etiology, pathophysiology and management of patient with specific types of diabetes mellitus such as LIPOATROPHIC and NEONATAL diabetes are described in separate chapters. The chapters on clinical management include management of DIABETIC KETOACIDOSIS and OUTPATIENT treatment, a mainstay of routine management.The increasing use of insulin pumps in children has necessitated the formulation of guidelines and protocols tailored to children; this facet of care of a child with diabetes mellitus is addressed in the chapter on INSULIN PUMP therapy. The crucial and interrelated roles of patient education and that of nutrition are addressed in chapters on EDUCATION and NUTRITION. Special issues unique to the adolescent with diabetes mellitus are discussed in the chapter on THE ADOLESCENT with diabetes mellitus. The seminal findings of the Diabetes Control and Complications Trial (DCCT) and the role of the pediatrician / endocrinologist in the prevention and early detection of microvascular complication of diabetes mellitus are discussed in the chapters on the DCCT STUDY, NEPHROPATHY and RETINOPATHY. Recent advances in understanding the vulnerability to hypoglycemia and its long-term effects on cognitive function in children are addressed in the chapter on HYPOGLYCEMIA. In the day-to-day management of a child with diabetes mellitus the clinician is often confronted with issues related to the skin and integument; these issues pertinent to the care of a child with diabetes mellitus are discussed in the chapter on DERMATOLOGICAL manifestations. Related topics of the prevalence, significance, recognition, and the management of behavioral and psychological issues in children with diabetes mellitus are detailed in the chapter on PSYCHOLOGICAL problems. Thus, we have aimed to balance advances in scientific basis, practical developments and management issues to provide a comprehensive and contemporary approach to the child with diabetes mellitus.

We wish to acknowledge the contribution of all the authors who devoted their time and effort towards completion of this book. Ms. Michele Beckwith rendered invaluable secretarial assistance and we are indebted to the publishers, Kluwer, for their support and encouragement.

Chapter 1
GENETICS OF DIABETES IN CHILDHOOD

Paul R. Wraight *, Spiros Fourlanos †, Grant Morahan ‡ & Leonard C. Harrison †
† Autoimmunity & Transplantation Division, The Walter & Eliza Hall Institute of Medical Research, Royal Melbourne Hospital PO, Parkville 3050, Victoria, Australia
‡ Genetics & Bioinformatics Division, The Walter & Eliza Hall Institute of Medical Research, Royal Melbourne Hospital PO, Parkville 3050, Victoria, Australia
** Department of Diabetes & Endocrinology, The Royal Melbourne Hospital, Parkville 3050, Victoria, Australia*

INTRODUCTION

The syndrome of diabetes, centered on chronic hyperglycaemia, is categorised into two major clinical stereotypes: type 1 ('juvenile', insulin-dependent) and type 2 ('adult onset', non-insulin-dependent). Type 1 diabetes (T1D) is an autoimmune disease in which hyperglycaemia is secondary to insulin deficiency, following destruction of pancreatic islet β cells by cell-mediated autoimmunity[1,2]. T1D is one of the most common chronic diseases beginning in childhood and accounts for greater than 90% of cases of childhood diabetes, with an overall prevalence rate of 0.2-0.5% across Caucasoid populations[3]. The incidence of type 1 diabetes is increasing world-wide[4] and at least in several areas this increase is reported to be greater in the under 5-year olds[5,6]. In type 2 diabetes (T2D), hyperglycaemia can be attributed to defective glucose metabolism through pathways that are responsive to insulin ("insulin resistance"), a defect that appears to be present in many tissues including muscle, liver, fat and β cells. Although T2D is generally considered to be a polygenic 'inborn error of metabolism' disorder, its genetic and molecular basis in the vast majority of cases remains an enigma. In a minority of cases, presenting usually in childhood, monogenic defects are designated maturity onset diabetes of the young (MODY). A small but increasing proportion of childhood diabetes is T2D, related to the rising prevalence of childhood obesity in affluent young (MODY). A small but increasing proportion of childhood diabetes is T2D, related to the rising prevalence of childhood obesity in affluent societies[7]. Rare causes of diabetes in childhood include pancreatic fibrosis associated with cystic fibrosis or hemosiderosis, and extremely rarely genetic disorders affecting insulin receptors.

TYPE 1 DIABETES

T1D occurs in genetically-predisposed individuals, modulated by permissive and protective environmental factors. This is illustrated by data from family studies and by the incomplete penetrance in monozygotic twins in whom the concordance is at least 35 and possibly as high as 70%[8-10] (Table 1).

Table 1: Lifetime risks of type 1 diabetes in first-degree relatives (Proband diagnosed before 20 years of age)

Parents		2.2 ± 0.6%
Children		5.6 ± 2.8%
Siblings		6.9 ± 1.3%
Siblings		
	HLA non-identical sib	1.2%
	HLA haploidentical	4.9%
	HLA identical sib	15.9%
	Identical twin	30-70%

Refs: (Harrison, LC *et al.* 1999; Gale, EA *et al.* 2001)

These also reveal that the dominant genetic locus (*IDDM1*) is the major histocompatibility complex (MHC)[11]. The MHC accounts for at least 35% of familial clustering in T1D[12-14]. The difference between the concordance for T1D in monozygotic twins and that in HLA-identical siblings (Table 1) reflects the contribution of genes outside the MHC. Indeed, studies of the non-obese diabetic (NOD) mouse, the best experimental model of T1D, and linkage analysis studies of human populations clearly demonstrate the polygenic nature of autoimmune diabetes. At least 18 susceptibility loci for human T1D have been identified (Table 2). They have been conventionally named using the abbreviation *IDDM* and a number that reflects the order in which these loci were reported. Unravelling the complexity of human T1D remains a major challenge, due to the large number of minor genes involved and the heterogeneity of clinical phenotypes and environmental influences.

Table 2. T1D susceptibility loci

Association	Locus	Chromosome	Candidate gene	Reference
Confirmed (gene polymorphism demonstrated)	IDDM1	6p21.3	*HLA DR,DQ,DP*	(Concannon, P et al. 1998) (Davies, JL et al. 1994)
	IDDM2	11p15.5	*Insulin VNTR*	(Bennett, ST et al. 1995) (Davies, JL *et al.* 1994)
Confirmed (linkage analysis demonstrated)	IDDM4	11q13.3	*MDU1, ZFM1, RT6, ICE, LRP5, FADD, CD3*	(Davies, JL *et al.* 1994) (Field, LL et al. 1996) (Hashimoto, L et al. 1994)
	IDDM5	6q25	*MnSOD*	(Luo, DF et al. 1996)
	IDDM6	18q12-21	*JK/Kidd, ZNF236* ?	(Luo, DF *et al.* 1996) (Field, LL *et al.* 1996)
	IDDM8	6q25-27	*CTLA-4*	(Merriman, T et al. 1997) (Davies, JL *et al.* 1994)
	IDDM12	2q33		(Davies, JL *et al.* 1994) (Luo, DF et al. 1995) (Luo, DF *et al.* 1995) (Concannon, P *et al.* 1998)
Suggestive (less evidence)	IDDM3	15q26	?	(Field, LL *et al.* 1996)
	IDDM7	2q31-33	*NEUROD*	(Luo, DF *et al.* 1995)
	IDDM9	3q21-25	?	(Davies, JL *et al.* 1994)
	IDDM10	10p11.2-q11.2	?	
	IDDM11	14q24.3-q31	*ENSA, SE-IL*	(Davies, JL *et al.* 1994)
	IDDM13	2q34	*IGFBP2, IGFBP5, NEUROD, HOXD8*	(Field, LL *et al.* 1996) (Concannon, P *et al.* 1998)

	IDDM14 IDDM15 IDDM16 IDDM17 IDDM18	6q21 10q25 5q33-34	? ? *IL-12 p40*	(Owerbach, D et al. 1995) (Serreze, DV et al. 1998) (Concannon, P *et al.* 1998) (Podolin, PL et al. 1997) (Morahan, G *et al.* 2001)

Ref: (Pietropaolo, M, Trucco M 2000)

IDDM1
Major histocompatability complex (MHC)

Figure 1: The Major Histocompatibility Complex (6p21)

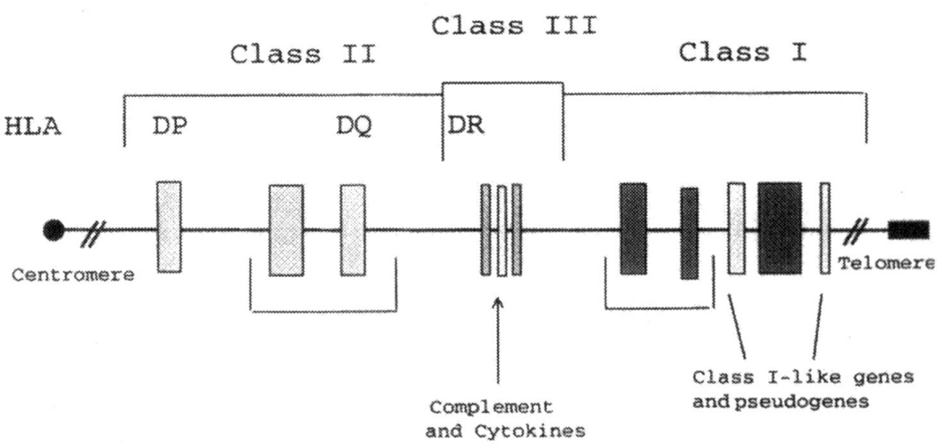

The MHC is located on human chromosome 6p21 and comprises class I, class II and class III regions (Figure 1). Class I and class II regions contain highly polymorphic genes that encode membrane-bound proteins and glycoproteins involved in immune function. Less is known about the class III region. The classical class I molecules are encoded by genes at the human leukocyte antigen (HLA)-A, -B and –C loci. When associated with β2-microglobulin they bind short (8- to 10-mer) cytoplasmic-derived peptides to be stably expressed on the cell surface and potentially recognisable by CD8 T-cell receptors. Class II molecules are heterodimers composed of α and β chains, encoded by genes at the DR, DQ and DP loci, that also bind short (9- to 15-mer) peptides for stable cell surface expression and potential recognition by CD4 T-cell receptors. Class I molecules are expressed by all nucleated cells while class II molecules are expressed by "professional" antigen-presenting cells, such as dendritic cells, monocyte-macrophages and B lymphocytes. Class II molecules are also constituitively expressed by intestinal epithelial cells and may also be induced on other epithelial cells by inflammatory mediators such as IFN-γ. The class I and II regions also contain other genes which encode proteins involved in antigen processing and transport. The interspersed class III region contains genes for tumour necrosis factor and complement factors and other genes whose functions remain unknown. The nomenclature for MHC (HLA) genes is shown in Table 3[15].

Table 3. HLA nomenclature (example forT1D susceptibility class II genes)

	Gene locus	*Gene allele*	*Serologic specificity*
Format	Class II	DRB1*0401 DQB1*0302	DR4 DQ8
Haplotype (single chromosome)	DRB1*0401- DQB1*0302		DR4-DQ8
Genotype	DRB1*0301*0401-DQB1*0201*0302		DR3,4-DQ2,8

The association of specific HLA genes with T1D was first recognised in 1974. Nerup[16] noted a higher frequency of HLA-B8 in T1D patients and Menser et al[17] a higher frequency of the HLA-A1-B8 haplotype in infants with congenital rubella who subsequently developed T1D. At that time, only these class I markers could be typed but they represented the A1-B8-DR3 risk haplotype.

HLA molecules play a key role in immune function by presenting peptide antigens to T cells. As T cells are thought to mediate the destruction of pancreatic β cells in T1D, the presentation of specific peptides by T1D-associated MHC class I and II molecules would appear to be an essential step in the disease process (Figure 2). The presence of specific amino acids comprising the peptide binding cleft of the class II susceptibility molecules, HLA-DQ8 (human) and I-Ag7 (NOD mouse), suggests that a distinct repertoire of peptides is bound and presented to T cells. Susceptibility HLA molecules could fail to negatively select and eliminate autoreactive T cells during their development in the thymus; alternatively, they could fail to positively select T cells that might have a regulatory function to prevent the activation of diabetogenic T cells.

Figure 2: Mechanisms of β-cell destruction in type 1 diabetes

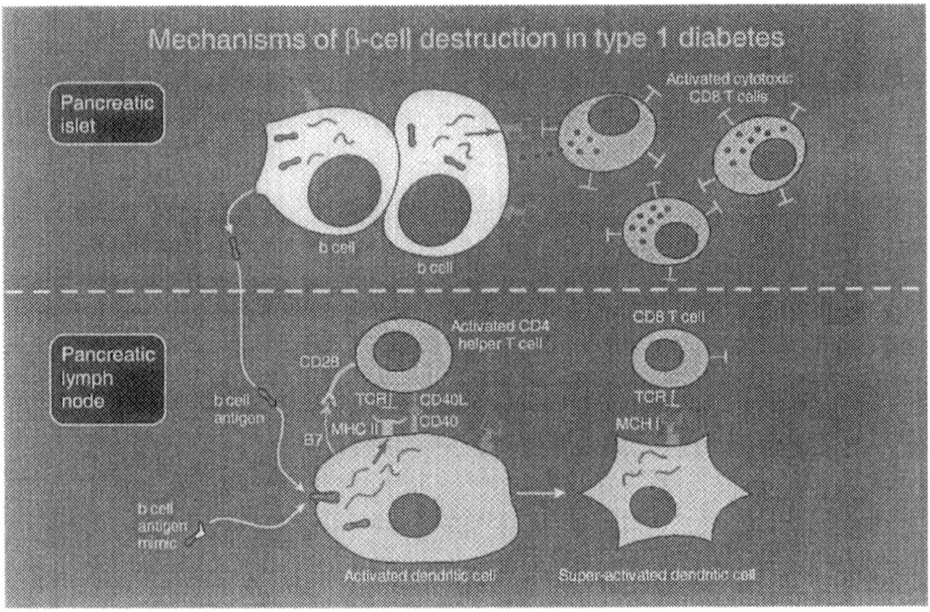

HLA class II associations

The strongest known association of the MHC with T1D is for HLA alleles at the class II loci, in particular DR3 and DR4, DQ2 and DQ8 (Table 4)[15,18]. 95% of Caucasoids with T1D have at least one DR3 or DR4 gene. After the DR3/DR4 genotype, the commonest associations are with DR4 and DR3 homozygosity, respectively. With the development of DNA-based sequencing the HLA-DQ locus has been found to be the most strongly associated with T1D susceptibility. In Caucasoids the highest risk DQ alleles for diabetes are DQ8 (DQA1*0301, DQB1*0302) and DQ2 (DQA1*0501,DQB1*0201)[19]. These alleles are in linkage disequilibrium with HLA DR4 and DR3, respectively. Most individuals with T1D and DR4 have the DQB1*0302 allele whereas in the general population the frequency of the DQB1*0302 and DQB1*0301 alleles is approximately equal. Individuals at highest risk for T1D are those with the HLA-DR3- DQ2 / DR4-DQ8 phenotype (DR3, DQA1 *0501, DQB1 *0201; DR4, DQA1 *0301, DQB1 *0302 genotype), whose risk is up to 25 times that of the general population[20.,21]. This genotype is present in 30-40% of Caucasoids with T1D compared with 2-3% of the background population and is associated with an earlier age at diagnosis[22]. DR4 has been shown to confer susceptibility independent of its linkage with DQ8[23,24]. Although the HLA-DP locus is in linkage disequilibrium with HLA DR-DQ alleles, DPB1 *0301 or *0202 may confer susceptibility independently in Caucasoids. In Finland, that has the highest incidence of T1D in the world (~ 40/100,000 per annum), the same HLA risk alleles apply. However, their frequency in the general population does not appear to be increased, implicating environmental factors. The absolute risk for T1D in Finland by age 15 conferred by the high-risk genotype (HLA DQB1*0201,*0302 is) ~ 6%, and by the moderate-risk genotype (HLA DQB1*0302, X, where X is not *0302, *0301 or *0602) is ~ 2%, compared to 0.6% in the background population[25]. Screening at birth for these genotypes identifies 60-80% of children who will develop T1D[25,26].

Table 4 . HLA class II haplotypes and lifetime risk of T1D in Caucasoids

Haplotype	Family	General population
DR3-DQ2/DR4-DQ8	1/5	1/25
DR4-DQ8/DR4-DQ8	1/10	1/60
DR4-DQ8/other	1/10	1/60
DR4-DQ8/DR2-DQ1	1/100	1/500
DR3-DQ2/DR3-DQ2	1/20	1/350
DR3-DQ2/other	1/40	1/400
Other	1/80	1/5000

HLA class II alleles can also be protective. HLA DR2 and DR5 alleles are negatively associated with T1D[27]. The haplotypes that confer protection to diabetes are DR2-DQ6 (DQB1*0602) (relative risk 0.12) and DR2-DQ1[15]. The DR2 negative association is dominant over the DR4 positive association because DR2/4 heterozygotes are disproportionately underrepresented in T1D patients[28]. DRB1 *0403 is also dominantly protective[29] and HLA-DPB1 *0402 appears to be protective[30].

HLA Class I and Class III associations

Following the original reports of their association with T1D, HLA class I alleles have received relatively little attention as risk markers independent of their linkage with class II alleles. There are several reasons for this. Class I alleles are more numerous and their comprehensive typing had to await the advent of molecular genotyping. Furthermore, they may have subtle effects that are not as easy to discern as those of class II alleles in cross-sectional population studies. For example, the relatively recent finding that A24 is associated with more rapid β-cell destruction depended on being able to monitor Japanese patients post-diagnosis[31] or Caucasoid subjects pre-diagnosis[32]. In addition, independent effects of specific HLA class I alleles such as A1, B8, B15 and B18 whose frequency is increased in T1D are difficult to discern because they are markers of susceptibility for DR3 or DR4 haplotypes with which they are in linkage disequilibrium. This also explains the decreased frequency of B7 compared to the background population[33].

HLA class III associations have not been clearly established. Candidate genes in the class III region include tumour necrosis factor[34], heat-shock protein (HSP) 70[35] and the MIC-A5[36] genes.

Age-related HLA associations

Studies of at-risk first-degree relatives suggest that those with 'mild' islet autoimmunity, reflected for example by the presence of a single islet autoantibody, usually to glutamic acid decarboxylase (GAD), have a slower rate of progression to clinical disease and a higher frequency of DR3, without DR4[37]. The first appearance of islet autoimmunity can occur later in childhood[38] and this may signify fewer HLA risk alleles and a slower rate of pre-clinical disease progression.

Although the classic textbook description of the presentation of childhood T1D is with symptoms of weight loss, lethargy, polyuria and polydipsia, sometimes culminating in ketoacidosis, over days to weeks, there is in fact a great deal of variation. Some of this is due to greater community awareness of diabetes and of the pre-clinical stage that may last from months to years[2,39] resulting in earlier presentation before severe metabolic decompensation. However, heterogeneity in the rate of progression to clinical disease and of the syndrome at diagnosis can also reflect the nature of genetic predisposition. Cross-sectional studies have shown that age at diagnosis is inversely related to the frequency of highest risk HLA genotypes[40-42]. The older the age of onset the greater the heterogeneity and lower the frequency of the highest risk DR3 and DR4 alleles/haplotypes.

IDDM2

The second T1D locus, identified by Bell and colleagues[43] in a case control study is a non-transcribed polymorphic minisatellite 5' of the human insulin (INS) gene on chromosome 11p15.5, a region which also contains genes for tyrosine hydroxylase (TH) and insulin-like growth factor II (*IGF2*). This locus was confirmed by both association and linkage studies and is now referred to as *IDDM2*[12]. Minisatellites are highly repetitive DNA sequences that may vary in length from a few to several thousand nucleotide base pairs and in complexity from simple di and tri-nucleotide repeats to more complex elements. Their function remains unknown. The minisatellites of *IDDM2*, which are unique in primates and highly polymorphic in human populations, are composed of a variable number of tandem repeats (VNTR) of 14- to 15-base pairs with the consensus sequence ACAGGGGTGTGGGG. Polymorphism is generated by variation in the number of tandem repeats within a given VNTR (changes the overall length) and also by minor nucleotide sequence heterogeneity within the individual repeats. Fourteen closely related repeats (a-n) have been described but not all repeats are found in every VNTR allele[44].

The INS VNTR has been subdivided into three class sizes of alleles. Class I, the most common, has an average of 40 tandem repeats (range 26-63) and is associated with T1D susceptibility. Class II, the least prevalent class size, has an average of 85 repeats (range 64-139), recorded in 6 of 300 chromosomes studied by Bell[43]. Class III, constituting approximately 25% of INS alleles, has an average of 157 repeats (range 140-210) and is associated with T1D resistance[45]. The frequency of the short class I alleles is significantly greater in people with T1D than in unrelated controls[43]. In Caucasoids, the class I homozygous genotype is associated with a relative risk of 1.9-5.0[46-50].

IDDM2 shows ethnic variation in T1D association. Awata et al[51] found that the majority (~95%) of Japanese were homozygous for Class I alleles, yet Japanese have a low prevalence of T1D. However, it was subsequently discovered that the Class I VNTR could be further divided into three sub-sizes: 1S with 25-38 repeat units, 1M with 39-41 repeat units and IL with 42-44 repeat units. In Japanese, the shortest (1S) alleles were significantly increased in T1D compared with control subjects (relative risk of 1S/1S genotype = 2.1). At least 40% of the alleles were smaller than 35 repeat units compared to ~20% in Caucasoids. Thus it has been postulated that a class I subset confers T1D susceptibility in Japanese[51].

The class III alleles can also be further subdivided into two size groups, each of which can be identified by linkage disequilibrium with neighbouring polymorphisms, one of which is more protective (very protective haplotype) than the other (protective haplotype).

Some studies have revealed preferential transmission of VNTR alleles at *IDDM2* from fathers to diabetic offspring, but others have not confirmed this[52]. Bennet et al[53] found that a particular class I allele did not predispose to T1D when paternally inherited, suggestive of imprinting (see below), but this effect was only observed when the father's untransmitted allele was class III. Paternally inherited 814 class I alleles did not predispose when the untransmitted paternal allele was class III, but were as predisposing as all other class I alleles when the untransmitted allele was class I[51]. This allelic interaction is reminiscent of epigenetic phenomena observed in plants and yeasts. It does not have a large effect on *IDDM2*-encoded susceptibility because only 5% of the individuals inherit an 814 allele from an 814/III father[53].

The molecular mechanisms by which *IDDM2* determines risk may be inferred. Since the VNTR is not transcribed, its allelic forms must exercise their effect by regulating gene transcription. Pugliese et al demonstrated not only INS gene expression in the thymus but also proinsulin protein in rare cells and Vafiadis et al [54,55] that the VNTR INS mRNA correlated with proinsulin expression. In the thymus, class III VNTR alleles are associated with 2-3 fold greater levels of INS mRNA than class I alleles[54]. Thus, it was proposed that because the protective class III VNTR is associated with higher steady state levels of INS mRNA expression it results in increased thymic expression of proinsulin, an autoantigen in T1D. In the NOD mouse model of autoimmune diabetes, transgenic expression of proinsulin in antigen-presenting cells in the thymus completely prevented disease[56]. Increased expression of proinsulin in the thymus could protect from T1D either by deletion of proinsulin-reactive T cells or by generation of regulatory T cells.

OTHER T1D SUSCEPTIBILITY LOCI

IDDM1 and *IDDM2* contribute approximately 40% and 10%, respectively, to the inheritance of T1D[57]. The remaining susceptibility loci have been mapped with varying degrees of support (Table 2). An interesting feature of *IDDM3* is that linkage is stronger in families with little evidence of HLA-associated predisposition (ie in whom affected siblings do not show increased sharing of HLA genes)[58]. This suggests that the *IDDM3* and the HLA region act in a complex, non-additive manner.

CTLA4

Several studies have shown evidence for a locus linked to diabetes susceptibility on chromosome 2q. A candidate for this locus was the gene encoding CTLA4 (CD152), a molecule on T cells involved in down-regulation of T cell activation. Inhibitory or stimulatory signals are delivered via the interaction of CTLA4 or CD28, respectively, with B7 family molecules on antigen-presenting cells. Genes encoding both CTLA4 and CD28 as well as another inducible co-stimulator (ICOS) are located adjacent to each other in a ~400kb segment on chromosome 2q.

Polymorphisms in the *CTLA4* gene were found to be transmitted preferentially to offspring with T1D. Further studies have shown a consistent effect for this locus not only in T1D but also in other autoimmune diseases[59]. Two different polymorphisms were shown to effect gene function: the position 49 (A->G) variant reduced the inhibitory effect of CTLA4 as did a dinucleotide repeat in the 3'UTR[60,61].

Different polymorphisms show effects in different ethnic groups. Marron et al[62] examined the 49 (A->G) and 3'UTR dinucleotide polymorphisms in multiple populations. Subjects from British, Sardinian and Chinese families showed no effect for the A/G variant; Caucasian-American families showed a weak effect. The strongest effects for CTLA4 involvement in T1D came from the other ethnic groups studied: Mediterranean-European populations (Italian, Spanish and French), Mexican-Americans and Koreans. The 49(A->G) polymorphism was subsequently found to show association in Chinese but not African subjects, while 159 (C->G) displayed the reverse association in these groups[63]. A further polymorphism in the *CTLA4* promoter showed significant association in Chinese subjects[64].

The association of different *CTLA4* alleles may be due to their being found in common haplotypes (ie they are in linkage disequilibrium)[65]. The extent of linkage disequilibrium around *CTLA4* would not only complicate the search for the causative polymorphism but also raise the possibility of *CD28* or *ICOS* contributing to disease susceptibility.

IL-12

Suggestive linkage to a locus on chromosome 5q was found in a study of Australian and British affected sib-pairs; this locus was named *IDDM18*[66]. This region contained an excellent candidate gene, *IL12B*, encoding the p40 subunit of interleukin (IL) -12. Several immune functions are mediated by IL-12[67], not least of which is the induction of uncommitted T lymphocytes into the Th1 subset, which is characterised by secretion of cytokines such as IFN-γ associated with cell mediated, immune inflammation characteristic of T1D. In the NOD mouse, administration of IL-12 precipitates diabetes whereas IL-12 antagonists are protective[68,69]. Similarly, Th1 cells induced diabetes in NOD mice while Th2 cells of the same specificity did not[70]. These and other indications prompted a detailed analysis of *IL12B* as a candidate susceptibility gene.

No commonly occurring polymorphism was found in the protein coding sequences of this gene, but there were common variants in its promoter, introns and 3'UTR region[71]. The 3'UTR polymorphism in particular showed preferential transmission to affected offspring, and the susceptibility allele had a higher level of gene expression. Other markers upstream or downstream of *IL12B* did not show preferential transmission. While its effects may not be observed in all ethnic groups, significant association of *IL12B* polymorphisms have since been reported in Danish and USA subjects[72]. Further evidence for effects of *IL12B* alleles on levels of gene expression was also reported by Davoodi-Semiromi et al., and this phenomenon extends to the mouse where there are also allelic differences in expression of the mouse homologue, *Il12b*[73]. Taken together, these results suggest that the *IL12B* gene itself is a type 1 diabetes susceptibility gene, and that the susceptibility allele mediates its effect via higher *IL12B* gene expression, in turn leading to increased levels of IL-12 which is known to promote diabetogenesis.

Parental Imprinting

Parental effects further complicate the genetics of T1D by influencing transmission and expression of genes. Several studies have shown that diabetes transmission risk is different in offspring of mothers versus fathers[74,75]. The risk of T1D is up to 5 times higher when the father has the disease (1 in 20-40) than when the mother is diabetic (1 in 40-80). Children with T1D inherit DR4 from DR4 heterozygote mothers less often than from DR4 heterozygote fathers and there are parental effects on the transmission of VNTR alleles at the *IDDM2* locus. Thus, parental effects may influence *IDDM1* and *IDDM2* transmission, but the evidence remains inconclusive[76,77].

TYPE 2 DIABETES

Type 2 diabetes (T2D) in children (described in detail in Chapter 3), including the relatively rare monogenic MODY forms described below and in Chapter 4, is relatively uncommon, accounting for 2-3% of childhood diabetes[78]. However, evidence is beginning to indicate that the prevalence of T2D is increasing steeply in childhood[79]. In Japan, where the prevalence of classic T1D is very low, T2D is the most common form of diabetes in childhood, being seven times more common than T1D with an incidence of 2.8 - 4.6 per 100,000 children per year[78]. The increase in the prevalence of T2D in childhood worldwide is associated with the increasing prevalence of obesity in childhood.

Twin, family and population studies demonstrate a major genetic contribution to T2D. These clearly demonstrate that the closer the genetic relationship between two individuals the more likely they are to have the same glucose tolerance[80]. T2D exhibits strong familial clustering. When one parent has T2D, the lifetime risk for offspring is 50%; if both parents are affected the risk is >90%. Further evidence to support the role of genetics in T2D is the marked difference in prevalence in different ethnic groups living in a similar environment or the similarity in the same ethnic groups living in different environments[81]. Nevertheless, non-genetic factors have an important permissive role in determining phenotypic expression of disease.

Although studies of the genetics of T2D have been performed almost exclusively in adults, there is no reason to think that childhood-onset T2D is different with regard to potential susceptibility loci (Table 5)[7]. A linkage analysis study of 330 Mexican American sibling pairs identified a major susceptibility locus on chromosome 2, termed *NIDDM1*, which accounted for 21% of the genetic susceptibility to T2D in this population[82,83]. The gene at the *NIDDM1* locus has not been identified. Other loci in adult T2D are associated with genes differentially expressed in β cells (eg. glucokinase, insulin, sulfonylurea receptor), insulin target cells (eg. insulin receptor, β 3 adrenergic receptor, muscle glycogen 1 synthase) and other cells (eg. growth hormone, cholecystokinin). Of the many loci that have been associated with diabetes only *IDDM2*, the INS VNTR, appears to influence susceptibility to both T1D and T2D.

Table 5. T2D potential susceptibility loci in adults

LOCUS	CHROMOSOME	REFERENCE
Unidentified		
NIDDM1	2	(Hanis, CL *et al.* 1996)
Beta cell		
Amylin	12p12.3-p12.1	(Gerbitz, KD et al. 1996)
Sulfonylurea receptor	11p15.1	(Inoue, H et al. 1997)
		(Hani, EH et al. 1997)
Glucokinase	7p15-p13	(Chiu, KC et al. 1992)
		(McCarthy, MI et al. 1993)
Target Cells		
Insulin receptor	19p13.2	(McClain, DA et al. 1988)
		(Raboudi, SH et al. 1989)
Insulin receptor substrate – 1	2q36-q37	(Stern, MP et al. 1996)
	19q13.3	
Muscle glycogen synthase	11q23	(Kuroyama, H et al. 1994)
	2p24	
Apolipoprotein A1, C3, A4	5q32-q34	(Xiang, KS et al. 1989)
Apolipoprotein B		(Xiang, KS *et al.* 1989)
β3-adrenergic receptor		(Walston, J et al. 1995)
Other Cells		
Growth hormone	17q22-q24	(Elbein, SC et al. 1995)
Cholecystokinin type B receptor	11p15.5-p15.4	(Vionnet, N et al. 1997)

MATURITY ONSET DIABETES OF THE YOUNG (MODY)

MODY encompasses monogenic forms of diabetes characterised by onset of non-ketotic diabetes before 25 years of age and an impaired insulin secretory response to glucose, inherited in an autosomal dominant manner, usually with a multi-generational family history[84]. MODY is uncommon and accounts for only 2-5% of cases of childhood-onset diabetes.

Since the initial description of MODY by Fajans and coworkers in the early 1960s, molecular genetic studies have shown that MODY is a clinically heterogenous disorder, five different genes being implicated thus far. Within any MODY family, diabetes results from a mutation in a single gene. The MODY genes identified to date include the glycolytic enzyme glucokinase (MODY2) as well as four transcription factors: hepatocyte nuclear factor-4α (HNF-4α) (MODY1), hepatocyte nuclear factor-1α (HNF-1α) (MODY3), insulin promoter factor-1 (IPF-1) (MODY4) and hepatocyte nuclear factor-1β (HNF-1β) (MODY5). MODY 1, 2 and 3 account for most cases of MODY in Caucasoids (Table 6).

Table 6. Maturity onset diabetes of the young (MODY)

MODY type	Gene location	Protein affected	% distribution among MODY British and French families respectively
MODY1	20q12-q13.1	Hepatocyte nuclear factor-4α	5%, -
MODY2	7p15-q13	Glucokinase	12.5% , 63%
MODY3	12q24.2	Hepatocyte nuclear factor-1α	65%, 21%
MODY4	13q12.1	Insulin promoter factor-1	uncommon
MODY5	17cen-q21.3	Hepatocyte nuclear factor-1β	uncommon

(Winter, WE et al. 1999)

The liver-enriched transcription factors HNF-1α, HNF-1β and HNF-4α were first identified through studies of tissue-specific regulation of gene expression. They act in concert with other liver transcription factors to regulate production of serum proteins and liver enzymes involved in carbohydrate, lipid and urea metabolism and detoxification. That mutations in these transcription factors are associated with MODY was first suggested by Bell and colleagues in 1991. They described linkage with a region of chromosome 20 (20q12-q13.1) near the adenosine deaminase gene in a large North American pedigree of European background[85]. This locus was termed MODY1, yet the gene wasn't identified for another five years until it was discovered that MODY3 was defined by a mutation in the HNF-1α gene. This lead investigators to the HNF-4α gene at the MODY1 locus on 20q. Several mutations in HNF-4α have subsequently been discovered, but overall they are an uncommon cause of MODY.

After exclusion of known MODY mutations in French MODY families, genome wide scanning revealed that half had linkage to another locus, MODY3, on chromosome 12q. The site was further mapped to a 3cM interval on 12q24.2 containing the HNF-1α gene. Over 65 independent mutations have now been identified in HNF-1α, the majority located in the DNA binding domain or transactivation domain. Yamagata et al[86] showed that some mutations produce a truncated HNF-1α protein still able to dimerize with wild-type HNF-1α. As it is essential for HNF-1α to dimerize to interact with DNA, dimerization of the truncated protein with the wild type HNF-1α produces a dominant negative effect, i.e. the normal function of HNF-1α is disrupted by the truncated HNF-1α protein. Other mutations have been identified in the promoter of the HNF-1α gene that result in reduced HNF-1α gene expression[87].

The identification of mutations in HNF-β in MODY5 was prompted by the finding of mutations in genes encoding other transcriptional factors in MODY 1, 3 and 4[88]. MODY5 is rare, only two cases so far reported[89].

After mapping of MODY1 to chromosome 20q, Froguel and colleagues[90] undertook a study of 16 French MODY families, 14 of which displayed linkage to chromosome 7p and to the glucokinase gene subsequently defined as MODY2. Over 100 molecular mutations have since been described in the glucokinase gene but clinical diabetes develops in only approximately 50% of these. The mutations in MODY2 reduce glucokinase activity, making β cells less sensitive to extracellular glucose and raising the set point for insulin secretion. Mutations have also been described that increase the activity of glucokinase, causing neonatal-onset familial hyperinsulinism and hypoglycaemia[91].

MODY4 results from mutations in the gene encoding the insulin promoter factor-1 (IPF-1) protein, also known as islet duodenal homeobox-1 (IDX-1) protein or or now more commonly as pancreatic duodenal homeobox-1 (PDX-1) protein. IPF-1 is central to the commitment of gut endoderm to pancreatic development, the specification of endocrine/exocrine function and the final definition of β-cell phenotype. Homozygous IPF-1 mutations lead to pancreatic agenesis[92]. In mature islets, increased glucose concentrations trigger phosphorylation of IPF-1 resulting in its nuclear translocation, binding to the insulin promoter and activation of insulin gene transcription. In the three IPF-1 mutations identified to date, there is reduced binding of the IPF-1 protein to the insulin gene promoter with consequent reduced insulin gene transcription in response to hyperglycaemia[93].

TRANSIENT NEONATAL DIABETES

Transient neonatal diabetes is due to inadequate insulin production and usually occurs in full-term infants with intrauterine growth retardation. It manifests with marked dehydration, fever, failure to thrive and wasting despite adequate colonic intake, and necessitates exogenous insulin therapy but usually remits by one year of age. Infants have no evidence of islet autoimmunity or HLA associations of T1D. Although rare, it represents 50-60% of all cases of neonatal diabetes, with a prevalence of 1 in 500,000 births.

About 2/3 of cases are sporadic and familial cases do not follow Mendelian inheritance[94,95]. It has been shown that 45% of cases have paternal disomy of chromosome 6 or a 6q23-24 duplication , which suggests that the disorder is due to increased gene dosage of a paternally inherited gene. The remaining cases may be due to another genetic defect but it is also possible that they may have 6q23-24 abnormalities that are below the resolution of the microsatellite typing and cytogenetics methods used.

OTHER RARE DISORDERS ASSOCIATED WITH HYPERGLYCAEMIA

Alstrom syndrome

Alstrom syndrome is a rare autosomal recessive disorder first described in 1959[96] characterized by atypical pigmentary retinal degeneration, neurogenic deafness, infantile obesity and insulin-resistant, non-insulin-dependent diabetes. Other features of the syndrome have since been identified including hypertriglyceridaemia, hepatic dysfunction, hyperuricaemia, slowly progressive chronic nephropathy, hypothyroidism, male hypogonadism, androgenic alopecia, growth retardation, scoliosis, hyperostosis frontalis interna, acanthosis nigricans, cataract and dilated cardiomyopathy. Genotyping has mapped the Alstrom's locus to a 6.1 cM region (between D2S2113 and D2S286) on chromosome 2p12-13.

Ataxia telangiectasia

Ataxia telangiectasia (A-T) is an autosomal recessive, multisystem disorder characterized by insulin resistance, cerebellar ataxia, telangiectasia in the conjunctivae, facial skin and flexor creases, cancer predisposition and immunodeficiency. A-T cells in culture have been shown to have a defect in DNA damage repair[97].

The identity of the A-T gene, ataxia-telangiectasia mutated gene (ATM), is now established and interacting proteins have been identified that further strengthen a role for ATM in DNA damage recognition and cell cycle checkpoint control[98,99]. The ATM gene has been mapped to chromosome 11q22-23, over 150kb of genomic DNA, and codes for a mRNA of approximately 13kb. A partial ATM cDNA clone of 5.9kb encodes a protein containing a domain related to that in the phosphatidyl inositol-3-kinase superfamily, involved in mitogenic signal transduction, meiotic recombination and cell cycle control.

Insulin receptor gene mutations

Mutations in the insulin receptor gene cause the severe insulin-resistant syndromes, leprechaunism and Rabson-Mendenhall syndrome, whose metabolic profiles include fasting hypoglycaemia, pastprandial hyperglycaemia, extremely elevated insulin levels (up to 1000 times greater than normal) and failure to respond to exogenous insulin[100]. These are autosomal recessive conditions in which both alleles for the insulin receptor are abnormal. Affected children have intrauterine and postnatal growth retardation (resulting from the defective mitogenic action of insulin), dysmorphic features, lack of subcutaneous fat, acanthosis nigricans, enlargement of genitalia and hirsutism.

Rabson-Mendenhall syndrome and leprechaunism have overlapping clinical features but different clinical courses. Rabson-Mendenhall syndrome differs in the presence of premature and dysplastic dentition, coarse facial features and pineal hyperplasia. Afflicted individuals live several years and develop severe and intractable diabetic ketoacidosis. Paradoxical fasting hypoglycaemia probably results from grossly elevated insulin levels, which decline with disease progression leading to severe ketoacidosis[101]. Children with leprechaunism, in contrast, usually die before one year of age and do not develop diabetic ketoacidosis. Because the insulin receptor mutation does not appear to fully account for the phenotype, it is hypothesized that additional factors, genetic and/or environmental, modulate the clinical characteristics of these syndromes.

CONCLUSION

T1D accounts for the vast majority of cases of diabetes in childhood, although the prevalence of T2D is increasing along with that of obesity in affluent societies. Genetic susceptibility plays the major aetiological role in both T1D and T2D. Typing for specific HLA genes and screening for islet antibody markers of sub-clinical islet autoimmunity identifies the majority of future cases of T1D. HLA genes also determine the natural history and age at diagnosis of T1D. The ability to identify children at-risk for T1D has set the stage for trials of intervention therapies that may one day prevent T1D.

REFERENCES

1. Harrison, L.C., Colman, P.G., Honeyman, M.C. and Kay, T.W.H. "Type 1 diabetes - from pathogenesis to prevention." In *Diabetes in the New Millenium,* K. T. Turtle JR, Osata S, ed. Sydney:Pot Still Press, 1999.

2. Bach, J.F. New concepts of the etiopathogenesis and treatment of insulin-dependent diabetes mellitus. Review. Clin Rev Allergy Immunol 2000; 19:217-225.
3. LaPorte, R.E., Matschushima, M. and Chang, Y.F., *Prevalence and incidence of Insulin-dependent diabetes*. Bethesda, Maryland:National Institute Health, 1995.
4. Onkamo, P., Vaananen, S., Karvonen, M. and Tuomilehto, J. Worldwide increase in incidence of Type I diabetes--the analysis of the data on published incidence trends. Diabetologia 1999; 42:1395-403.
5. Cinek, O., Lanska, V., Kolouskova, S., Sumnik, Z., Snajderova, M., Ronningen, K.S. and Vavrinec, J. Type 1 diabetes mellitus in Czech children diagnosed in 1990-1997: a significant increase in incidence and male predominance in the age group 0-4 years. Collaborators of the Czech Childhood Diabetes Registry. Diabet Med 2000; 17:64-69.
6. Zhao, H.X., Stenhouse, E., Demaine, A.G. and Millward, B.A. The average age at onset is decreasing in children with Type 1 diabetes in Devon and Cornwall, England. Diabet Med 2000; 17:877.
7. Rosenbloom, A.L., Joe, J.R., Young, R.S. and Winter, W.E. Emerging epidemic of type 2 diabetes in youth. Diabetes Care 1999; 22:345-54.
8. Barnett, A.H., Eff, C., Leslie, R.D. and Pyke, D.A. Diabetes in identical twins. A study of 200 pairs. Diabetologia 1981; 20:87-93.
9. Kumar, D., Gemayel, N.S., Deapen, D., Kapadia, D., Yamashita, P.H., Lee, M., Dwyer, J.H., Roy-Burman, P., Bray, G.A. and Mack, T.M. North-American twins with IDDM. Genetic, etiological, and clinical significance of disease concordance according to age, zygosity, and the interval after diagnosis in first twin. Diabetes 1993; 42:1351-1363.
10. Gale, E.A., Bingley, P.J., Eisenbarth, G.S., Redondo, M.J., Kyvik, K.O. and Petersen, J.S. Reanalysis of twin studies suggests that diabetes is mainly genetic. BMJ 2001; 323:997-998.
11. Merriman, T.R. and Todd, J.A. Genetics of autoimmune disease. Curr Opin Immunol 1995; 7:786-92.
12. Lucassen, A.M. and Bell, J.I., *Genetics of Insulin-dependent diabetes*. Cambridge:Cambridge University Press, 1995.
13. Todd, J.A. Genetic analysis of type 1 diabetes using whole genome approaches. Proc Natl Acad Sci U S A 1995; 92:8560-5.

14. Noble, J.A., Valdes, A.M., Cook, M., Klitz, W., Thomson, G. and Erlich, H.A. The role of HLA class II genes in insulin-dependent diabetes mellitus: molecular analysis of 180 Caucasian, multiplex families. Am J Hum Genet 1996; 59:1134-48.
15. Tait, B.D. and Harrison, L.C. Overview: the major histocompatibility complex and insulin dependent diabetes mellitus. Baillieres Clin Endocrinol Metab 1991; 5:211-28.
16. Nerup, J., Platz, P., Andersen, O.O., Christy, M., Lyngsoe, J., Poulsen, J.E., Ryder, L.P., Nielsen, L.S., Thomsen, M. and Svejgaard, A. HL-A antigens and diabetes mellitus. Lancet 1974; 2:864-6.
17. Menser, M.A., Forrest, J.M., Honeyman, M.C. and Burgess, J.A. Letter: Diabetes, HL-A antigens, and congenital rubella. Lancet 1974; 2:1508-9.
18. Pugliese, A. and Eisenbarth, G.S., *Type 1 Diabetes Mellitus of Man: Genetic Susceptibility and Resistance*Oxford, 2000.
19. Todd, J.A., Bell, J.I. and McDevitt, H.O. HLA-DQ beta gene contributes to susceptibility and resistance to insulin-dependent diabetes mellitus. Nature 1987; 329:599-604.
20. Erlich, H.A., Bugawan, T.L., Scharf, S., Nepom, G.T., Tait, B. and Griffith, R.L. HLA-DQ beta sequence polymorphism and genetic susceptibility to IDDM. Diabetes 1990; 39:96-103.
21. Ronningen, K.S.S.A., Tait BD. "HLA class II association in insulin-dependent diabetes mellitus among Blacks, Caucasoids and Japanese." In *HLA,* A. M. Tsui K, Sasazuki T, ed. Oxford:Oxford University Press, 1991.
22. Rewers, M., Bugawan, T.L., Norris, J.M., Blair, A., Beaty, B., Hoffman, M., McDuffie, R.S., Jr., Hamman, R.F., Klingensmith, G., Eisenbarth, G.S. and Erlich, H.A. Newborn screening for HLA markers associated with IDDM: diabetes autoimmunity study in the young (DAISY). Diabetologia 1996; 39:807-12.
23. Thorsby, E. and Ronningen, K.S. Particular HLA-DQ molecules play a dominant role in determining susceptibility or resistance to type 1 (insulin-dependent) diabetes mellitus. Diabetologia 1993; 36:371-7.
24. Tait, B.D., Drummond, B. and Harrison, L.C. DRB1*0401 is associated with susceptibility to insulin-dependent diabetes mellitus independently of the DQB1 locus. Europ J Immunogen 1995; 22:289-297.

25. Ilonen, J., Reijonen, H., Knip, M. and Simell, O. Population-based genetic screening for IDDM susceptibility as a source of HLA-genotyped control subjects. Diabetologia 1996; 39:123.
26. Kimpimaki, T., Kupila, A., Hamalainen, A.M., Kukko, M., Kulmala, P., Savola, K., Simell, T., Keskinen, P., Ilonen, J., Simell, O. and Knip, M. The first signs of beta-cell autoimmunity appear in infancy in genetically susceptible children from the general population: the Finnish Type 1 Diabetes Prediction and Prevention Study. J Clin Endocrinol Metab 2001; 86:4782-4788.
27. Nepom, G.T. A unified hypothesis for the complex genetics of HLA associations with IDDM. Diabetes 1990; 39:1153-7.
28. Thomson, G., Robinson, W.P., Kuhner, M.K., Joe, S., MacDonald, M.J., Gottschall, J.L., Barbosa, J., Rich, S.S., Bertrams, J., Baur, M.P. and et al. Genetic heterogeneity, modes of inheritance, and risk estimates for a joint study of Caucasians with insulin-dependent diabetes mellitus. Am J Hum Genet 1988; 43:799-816.
29. Roep, B.O., Schipper, R., Verduyn, W., Bruining, G.J., Schreuder, G.M. and de Vries, R.R. HLA-DRB1*0403 is associated with dominant protection against IDDM in the general Dutch population and subjects with high-risk DQA1*0301-DQB1*0302/DQA1*0501-DQB1*0201 genotype. Tissue Antigens 1999; 54:88-90.
30. Noble, J.A., Valdes, A.M., Thomson, G. and Erlich, H.A. The HLA class II locus DPB1 can influence susceptibility to type 1 diabetes. Diabetes 2000; 49:121-125.
31. Nakanishi, K., Kobayashi, T., Murase, T., Nakatsuji, T., Inoko, H., Tsuji, K. and Kosaka, K. Association of HLA-A24 with complete beta-cell destruction in IDDM. Diabetes 1993; 42:1086-93.
32. Honeyman, M.C., Harrison, L.C., Drummond, B., Colman, P.G. and Tait, B.D. Analysis of families at risk for insulin-dependent diabetes mellitus reveals that HLA antigens influence progression to clinical disease. Mol Med 1995; 1:576-82.
33. Robinson, W.P., Barbosa, J., Rich, S.S. and Thomson, G. Homozygous parent affected sib pair method for detecting disease predisposing variants: application to insulin dependent diabetes mellitus. Genet Epidemiol 1993; 10:273-88.
34. Obayashi, H., Nakamura, N., Fukui, M., Tegoshi, H., Fujii, M., Ogata, M., Hasegawa, G., Shigeta, H., Kitagawa, Y., Nakano, K., Kondo, M., Fukui, I., Maruya, E., Saji, H., Ohta, M. and Nishimura, M. Influence of TNF microsatellite polymorphisms (TNFa) on age-

at-onset of insulin-dependent diabetes mellitus. Hum Immunol 1999; 60:974-8.
35. Chuang, L.M., Jou, T.S., Wu, H.P., Tai, T.Y. and Lin, B.J. A rapid method to study heat shock protein 70-2 gene polymorphism in insulin-dependent diabetes mellitus. Pancreas 1996; 13:268-72.
36. Gambelunghe, G., Ghaderi, M., Cosentino, A., Falorni, A., Brunetti, P. and Sanjeevi, C.B. Association of MHC Class I chain-related A (MIC-A) gene polymorphism with Type I diabetes. Diabetologia 2000; 43:507-14.
37. Harrison, L.C., Honeyman, M.C., DeAizpurua, H.J., Schmidli, R.S., Tait, B.D., Cram, D.S. and Colman, P.G. Inverse relationship between humoral and cellular immunity to glutamic acid decarboxylase in humans at-risk for insulin-dependent diabetes. Lancet 1993; 341:1365-1369.
38. Colman, P.G., McNair, P.D., Gellert, S., Kewming, K., Schmidli, R.S., Steele, C.E. and Harrison, L.C. Development of autoantibodies to islet antigens is not restricted to early childhood: implications for pre-clinical type 1 diabetes screening. Pediatric Diabetes 2002; in press:
39. Harrison, L.C. Risk assessment, prediction and prevention of type 1 diabetes. Pediatric Diabetes 2001; 2:71-82.
40. Karjalainen, J., Salmela, P., Ilonen, J., Surcel, H.M. and Knip, M. A comparison of childhood and adult type I diabetes mellitus. N Engl J Med 1989; 320:881-6.
41. Caillat-Zucman, S., Garchon, H.J., Timsit, J., Assan, R., Boitard, C., Djilali-Saiah, I., Bougneres, P. and Bach, J.F. Age-dependent HLA genetic heterogeneity of type 1 insulin-dependent diabetes mellitus. J Clin Invest 1992; 90:2242-50.
42. Tait, B.D., Harrison, L.C., Drummond, B.P., Stewart, V., Varney, M.D. and Honeyman, M.C. HLA antigens and age at diagnosis of insulin-dependent diabetes mellitus. Hum Immunol 1995; 42:116-22.
43. Bell, G.I., Horita, S. and Karam, J.H. A polymorphic locus near the human insulin gene is associated with insulin-dependent diabetes mellitus. Diabetes 1984; 33:176-83.
44. Kennedy, G.C., German, M.S. and Rutter, W.J. The minisatellite in the diabetes susceptibility locus IDDM2 regulates insulin transcription. Nat Genet 1995; 9:293-8.

45. Bell, G.I., Selby, M.J. and Rutter, W.J. The highly polymorphic region near the human insulin gene is composed of simple tandemly repeating sequences. Nature 1982; 295:31-5.
46. Julier, C., Hyer, R.N., Davies, J., Merlin, F., Soularue, P., Briant, L., Cathelineau, G., Deschamps, I., Rotter, J.I. and Froguel, P. Insulin-IGF2 region on chromosome 11p encodes a gene implicated in HLA-DR4-dependent diabetes susceptibility. Nature 1991; 354:155-9.
47. Bain, S.C., Prins, J.B., Hearne, C.M., Rodrigues, N.R., Rowe, B.R., Pritchard, L.E., Ritchie, R.J., Hall, J.R., Undlien, D.E. and Ronningen, K.S. Insulin gene region-encoded susceptibility to type 1 diabetes is not restricted to HLA-DR4-positive individuals. Nature Genetics 1992; 2:212-5.
48. Lucassen, A.M., Julier, C., Beressi, J.P., Boitard, C., Froguel, P., Lathrop, M. and Bell, J.I. Susceptibility to insulin dependent diabetes mellitus maps to a 4.1 kb segment of DNA spanning the insulin gene and associated VNTR. Nat Genet 1993; 4:305-10.
49. Pugliese, A., Gianani, R., Eisenbarth, G.S., De Camilli, P. and Solimena, M. Genetics of susceptibility and resistance to insulin-dependent diabetes in stiff-man syndrome. Lancet 1994; 344:1027-8.
50. Owerbach, D. and Gabbay, K.H. The HOXD8 locus (2q31) is linked to type I diabetes. Interaction with chromosome 6 and 11 disease susceptibility genes. Diabetes 1995; 44:132-6.
51. Awata, T., Kurihara, S., Kikuchi, C., Takei, S., Inoue, I., Ishii, C., Takahashi, K., Negishi, K., Yoshida, Y., Hagura, R., Kanazawa, Y. and Katayama, S. Evidence for association between the class I subset of the insulin gene minisatellite (IDDM2 locus) and IDDM in the Japanese population. Diabetes 1997; 46:1637-42.
52. Vafiadis, P., Grabs, R., Goodyer, C.G., Colle, E. and Polychronakos, C. A functional analysis of the role of IGF2 in IDDM2-encoded susceptibility to type 1 diabetes. Diabetes 1998; 47:831-6.
53. Bennett, S.T., Wilson, A.J., Esposito, L., Bouzekri, N., Undlien, D.E., Cucca, F., Nistico, L., Buzzetti, R., Bosi, E., Pociot, F., Nerup, J., Cambon-Thomsen, A., Pugliese, A., Shield, J.P., McKinney, P.A., Bain, S.C., Polychronakos, C. and Todd, J.A. Insulin VNTR allele-specific effect in type 1 diabetes depends on identity of untransmitted paternal allele. The IMDIAB Group. Nature Genetics 1997; 17:350-2.

54. Pugliese, A., Zeller, M., Fernandez, A., Jr., Zalcberg, L.J., Bartlett, R.J., Ricordi, C., Pietropaolo, M., Eisenbarth, G.S., Bennett, S.T. and Patel, D.D. The insulin gene is transcribed in the human thymus and transcription levels correlated with allelic variation at the INS VNTR-IDDM2 susceptibility locus for type 1 diabetes. Nature Genetics 1997; 15:293-7.
55. Vafiadis, P., Bennett, S.T., Todd, J.A., Nadeau, J., Grabs, R., Goodyer, C.G., Wickramasinghe, S., Colle, E. and Polychronakos, C. Insulin expression in human thymus is modulated by INS VNTR alleles at the IDDM2 locus. Nat Genet 1997; 15:289-92.
56. French, M.B., Allison, J., Cram, D.S., Dempsey-Collier, M., Silva, A., Georgiou, H.M., Kay, T.W.H., Harrison, L.C. and Lew, A.M. Transgenic expression of mouse proinsulin II prevents diabetes in non-obese diabetic mice. Diabetes 1997; 46:34-39.
57. Bennett, S.T. and Todd, J.A. Human type 1 diabetes and the insulin gene: principles of mapping polygenes. Annu Rev Genet 1996; 30:343-370.
58. Field, L.L., Tobias, R. and Magnus, T. A locus on chromosome 15q26 (IDDM3) produces susceptibility to insulin-dependent diabetes mellitus. Nat Genet 1994; 8:189-94.
59. Kristiansen, O.P., Larsen, Z.M. and Pociot, F. CTLA-4 in autoimmune diseases--a general susceptibility gene to autoimmunity? Genes Immun 2000; 1:170-184.
60. Huang, D., Giscombe, R., Zhou, Y., Pirskanen, R. and Lefvert, A.K. Dinucleotide repeat expansion in the CTLA-4 gene leads to T cell hyper-reactivity via the CD28 pathway in myasthenia gravis. J Neuroimmunol 2000b; 105:69.
61. Kouki, T., Sawai, Y., Gardine, C., Fisfalen, M.-E., Alegre, M.-L. and DeGroot, L.J. CTLA-4 gene polymorphism at position 49 in exon 1 reduces the inhibitory function of CTLA-4 and contributes to the pathogenesis of Graves' disease. J Immunol 2000; 165:6606.
62. Marron, M.P., Raffel, L.J., Garchon, H.J., Jacob, C.O., Serrano-Rios, M., Martinez Larrad, M.T., Teng, W.P., Park, Y., Zhang, Z.X., Goldstein, D.R., Tao, Y.W., Beaurain, G., Bach, J.F., Huang, H.S., Luo, D.F., Zeidler, A., Rotter, J.I., Yang, M.C., Modilevsky, T., Maclaren, N.K. and She, J.X. Insulin-dependent diabetes mellitus (IDDM) is associated with CTLA4 polymorphisms in multiple ethnic groups. Hum Mol Genet 1997; 6:1275-1282.
63. Osei-Hyiaman, D., Hou, L., Zhiyin, R., Zhiming, Z., Yu, H., Amankwah, A.A. and Harada, S. Association of a novel point

mutation (C159G) of the CTLA4 gene with type 1 diabetes in West Africans but not in Chinese. Diabetes 2001; 50:2169-2171.

64. Lee, Y.J., Lo, F.S., Shu, S.G., Wang, C.H., Huang, C.Y., Liu, H.F., Wu, C.C., Yang, T.Y. and Chang, J.G. The promoter region of the CTLA4 gene is associated with type 1 diabetes mellitus. J Pediatr Endocrinol Metab 2001; 14:383-8.

65. Holopainen, P.M. and Partanen, J.A. Technical note: linkage disequilibrium and disease-associated CTLA4 gene polymorphisms. J Immunol 2001; 167:2457-2458.

66. Morahan, G., Huang, D., Ymer, S.I., Cancilla, M.R., Stephen, K., Dabadghao, P., Werther, G., Tait, B.D., Harrison, L.C. and Colman, P.G. Linkage disequilibrium of a type 1 diabetes susceptibility locus with a regulatory IL12B allele. Nat Genet 2001; 27:218 –221.

67. Gately, M.K., Renzetti, L.M., Magram, J., Stern, A.S., Gubler, U. and Presky, D.H. The interleukin-12/interleukin-12-receptor system: Role in normal and pathologic immune responses. Annual Review of Immunology 1998; 16:495-521.

68. Trembleau, S., Penna, G., Bosi, E., Mortara, A., Gately, M.K. and Adorini, L. Interleukin 12 administration induces T helper type 1 cells and accelerates autoimmune diabetes in NOD mice. J Exp Med 1995; 181:817-821.

69. Trembleau, S., Penna, G., Gregori, S., Gately, M.K. and Adorini, L. Deviation of pancreas-infiltrating cells to Th2 by interleukin-12 antagonist administration inhibits autoimmune diabetes. Eur J Immunol 1997; 27:2230–2239.

70. Katz, J.D., Benoist, C. and Mathis, D. T helper cell subsets in insulin-dependent diabetes. Science 1995; 268:1185-1188.

71. Huang, D., Cancilla, M.R. and Morahan, G. Complete primary structure, chromosomal localisation, and definition of polymorphisms of the gene encoding the human interleukin-12 p40 subuniT. Genes Immunity 2000a; 1:515-520.

72. Davoodi-Semiromi, A., Yang, J.J. and She, J.-X. IL-12p40 is associated with Type 1 Diabetes in Caucasian-American families. Diabetes 2002; 51:2334-2336.

73. Ymer, S.I., Huang, D., Penna, G., Gregori, S., Branson, K., Adorini, L. and Morahan, G. Polymorphisms in the Il12b gene affect structure and expression of IL-12 in NOD and other autoimmune-prone mouse strainS. Genes Immun 2002; 3:151-157.

74. Warram, J.H., Krolewski, A.S., Gottlieb, M.S. and Kahn, C.R. Differences in risk of insulin-dependent diabetes in offspring of

diabetic mothers and diabetic fathers. N Engl J Med 1984; 311:149-52.
75. Bleich, D., Polak, M., Eisenbarth, G.S. and Jackson, R.A. Decreased risk of type I diabetes in offspring of mothers who acquire diabetes during adrenarchy. Diabetes 1993; 42:1433-9.
76. Vadheim, C.M., Rotter, J.I., Maclaren, N.K., Riley, W.J. and Anderson, C.E. Preferential transmission of diabetic alleles within the HLA gene complex. N Engl J Med 1986; 315:1314-8.
77. Bain, S.C., Rowe, B.R., Barnett, A.H. and Todd, J.A. Parental origin of diabetes-associated HLA types in sibling pairs with type I diabetes. Diabetes 1994; 43:1462-8.
78. Pinhas-Hamiel, O., Dolan, L.M., Daniels, S.R., Standiford, D., Khoury, P.R. and Zeitler, P. Increased incidence of non-insulin-dependent diabetes mellitus among adolescents. J Pediatr Endocrinol Metab 1996; 128:608-615.
79. Laron, Z. Type 2 diabetes mellitus in childhood--a global perspective. J Pediatr Endocrinol Metab 2002; 15 S1:459-469.
80. McCarthy, M. and Menzel, S. The genetics of type 2 diabetes. Br J Clin Pharmacol 2001; 51:195-9.
81. Zimmet, P., Taylor, R., Ram, P., King, H., Sloman, G., Raper, L.R. and Hunt, D. Prevalence of diabetes and impaired glucose tolerance in the biracial (Melanesian and Indian) population of Fiji: a rural-urban comparison. Am J Epidemiol 1983; 118:673-88.
82. Hanis, C.L., Boerwinkle, E., Chakraborty, R., Ellsworth, D.L., Concannon, P., Stirling, B., Morrison, V.A., Wapelhorst, B., Spielman, R.S., Gogolin-Ewens, K.J., Shepard, J.M., Williams, S.R., Risch, N., Hinds, D., Iwasaki, N., Ogata, M., Omori, Y., Petzold, C., Rietzch, H., Schroder, H.E., Schulze, J., Cox, N.J., Menzel, S., Boriraj, V.V., Chen, X. and et al. A genome-wide search for human non-insulin-dependent (type 2) diabetes genes reveals a major susceptibility locus on chromosome 2. Nat Genet 1996; 13:161-6.
83. Cox, N.J., Frigge, M., Nicolae, D.L., Concannon, P., Hanis, C.L., Bell, G.I. and Kong, A. Loci on chromosomes 2 (NIDDM1) and 15 interact to increase susceptibility to diabetes in Mexican Americans. Nat Genet 1999; 21:213-215.
84. Fajans, S.S. Scope and heterogeneous nature of MODY. Diabetes Care 1990; 13:49-64.
85. Bell, G.I., Xiang, K.S., Newman, M.V., Wu, S.H., Wright, L.G., Fajans, S.S., Spielman, R.S. and Cox, N.J. Gene for non-insulin-

dependent diabetes mellitus (maturity-onset diabetes of the young subtype) is linked to DNA polymorphism on human chromosome 20q. Proc Natl Acad Sci U S A 1991; 88:1484-1488.

86. Yamagata, K., Yang, Q., Yamamoto, K., Iwahashi, H., Miyagawa, J., Okita, K., Yoshiuchi, I., Miyazaki, J., Noguchi, T., Nakajima, H., Namba, M., Hanafusa, T. and Matsuzawa, Y. Mutation P291fsinsC in the transcription factor hepatocyte nuclear factor-1alpha is dominant negative. Diabetes 1998; 47:1231-5.

87. Gragnoli, C., Lindner, T., Cockburn, B.N., Kaisaki, P.J., Gragnoli, F., Marozzi, G. and Bell, G.I. Maturity-onset diabetes of the young due to a mutation in the hepatocyte nuclear factor-4 alpha binding site in the promoter of the hepatocyte nuclear factor-1 alpha gene. Diabetes 1997; 46:1648-1651.

88. Horikawa, Y., Iwasaki, N., Hara, M., Furuta, H., Hinokio, Y., Cockburn, B.N., Lindner, T., Yamagata, K., Ogata, M., Tomonaga, O., Kuroki, H., Kasahara, T., Iwamoto, Y. and Bell, G.I. Mutation in hepatocyte nuclear factor-1 beta gene (TCF2) associated with MODY. Nature Genetics 1997; 17:384-5.

89. Nishigori, H., Yamada, S., Kohama, T., Tomura, H., Sho, K., Horikawa, Y., Bell, G.I., Takeuchi, T. and Takeda, J. Frameshift mutation, A263fsinsGG, in the hepatocyte nuclear factor-1beta gene associated with diabetes and renal dysfunction. Diabetes 1998; 47:1354-5.

90. Froguel, P., Vaxillaire, M., Sun, F., Velho, G., Zouali, H., Butel, M.O., Lesage, S., Vionnet, N., Clement, K. and Fougerousse, F. Close linkage of glucokinase locus on chromosome 7p to early-onset non-insulin-dependent diabetes mellitus. Nature 1992; 356:162-4.

91. Glaser, B., Thornton, P.S., Herold, K. and Stanley, C.A. Clinical and molecular heterogeneity of familial hyperinsulinism. J Pediatr Endocrinol Metab 1998; 133:801-802.

92. Stoffers, D.A., Zinkin, N.T., Stanojevic, V., Clarke, W.L. and Habener, J.F. Pancreatic agenesis attributable to a single nucleotide deletion in the human IPF1 gene coding sequence. Nature Genetics 1997; 15:106-10.

93. Macfarlane, W.M., Frayling, T.M., Ellard, S., Evans, J.C., Allen, L.I., Bulman, M.P., Ayres, S., Shepherd, M., Clark, P., Millward, A., Demaine, A., Wilkin, T., Docherty, K. and Hattersley, A.T. Missense mutations in the insulin promoter factor-1 gene predispose to type 2 diabetes. J Clin Invest 1999; 104:R33-39.

94. Gardner, R.J., Mungall, A.J., Shield, J.P.H., Robinson, D.O., Barber, J.C.K. and Temple, I.K. Further localisation of a gene for transient neonatal diagetes mellitus to chromosomal band 6q24. Am J Hum Genet 1998; 63 (Suppl.):A55.
95. Cave, H., Polak, M., Drunat, S., Denamur, E. and Czernichow, P. Refinement of the 6q chromosomal region implicated in transient neonatal diabetes. Diabetes 2000; 49:108-13.
96. Alstrom, C., Hallgren, B. and Nilsson, L. Retinal degeneration combined with obesity, diabetes mellitus and neurogenous deafness. A specific syndrome (not hitherto described) distinct from the Laurence-Moon-Bardet-Biedel syndrome: a clinical and genetic examination based on a large pedigree. Acta Psychiatr Scand 1959; Suppl 129:1-35.
97. Lavin, M.F. and Shiloh, Y. The genetic defect in ataxia-telangiectasia. Annu Rev Immunol 1997; 15:177-202.
98. Shafman, T., Khanna, K.K., Kedar, P., Spring, K., Kozlov, S., Yen, T., Hobson, K., Gatei, M., Zhang, N., Watters, D., Egerton, M., Shiloh, Y., Kharbanda, S., Kufe, D. and Lavin, M.F. Interaction between ATM protein and c-Abl in response to DNA damage. Nature 1997; 387:520-523.
99. Watters, D., Khanna, K.K., Beamish, H., Birrell, G., Spring, K., Kedar, P., Gatei, M., Stenzel, D., Hobson, K., Kozlov, S., Zhang, N., Farrell, A., Ramsay, J., Gatti, R. and Lavin, M. Cellular localisation of the ataxia-telangiectasia (ATM) gene product and discrimination between mutated and normal forms. Oncogene 1997; 14:1911-1121.
100. Taylor, S.I., Cama, A., Accili, D., Barbetti, F., Quon, M.J., de la Luz Sierra, M., Suzuki, Y., Koller, E.L.-T., R. and Wertheimer, E. Mutations in the insulin receptor gene. Endocr Rev 1992; 13:566-595.
101. Longo, N., Wang, Y. and Pasquali, M. Progressive decline in insulin levels in Rabson-Mendenhall syndrome. Journal of Clinical Endocrinology & Metabolism 1999; 84:2623-9.

Chapter 2
IMMUNOLOGY OF TYPE 1 DIABETES MELLITUS

Massimo Pietropaolo, Ying-Jian Zhang and Massimo Trucco
Department of Pediatrics, University of Pittsburgh School of Medicine, Children's Hospital of Pittsburgh, Pittsburgh, PA

Abstract

Type 1 diabetes mellitus (T1DM) is caused by autoimmune destruction of the insulin-secreting cells within the islets of Langerhans and Type 1 diabetic patients generally require exogenous insulin to survive. The autoimmune nature of this disease was elegantly demonstrated when a recipient affected by T1DM was transplanted with pancreatic tissue from a discordant monozygotic twin. In the absence of immunosuppression, the pancreatic β cells within the graft were destroyed by an autoimmune reaction. The fact that in both humans and animal models of autoimmune diabetes a number of immunosuppressive treatments can alter the disease course strengthens the latter observation. Pancreas or islet transplantation can reverse hyperglycemia, but unfortunately require lifelong immunosuppression and mechanisms controlling transplantation tolerance and autoimmunity may be potentially different. The association of certain human leukocyte antigen (HLA) alleles with T1DM is very strong, and this genetic locus is estimated to account for approximately 50% of genetic contributions to disease susceptibility. The search for non-HLA susceptibility genes has received great attention in recent years and genome wide scans yielded a stampede of data suggesting the association of numerous non-MHC loci with T1DM that still require careful follow-up examination.

Current evidence suggests that T1DM could be considered an immunoregulatory disorder with a relative excess of islet β-cell specific autoreactive T cells and a deficiency of regulatory (suppressor) T cells. A number of new therapeutic approaches may be directed at correcting the underlying immunoregulatory defects in T1DM.

INTRODUCTION

In support of the role of islet cell autoimmunity in Type 1 diabetes, it has been thoroughly documented that in T1DM there is a mononuclear cell infiltration in the pancreatic islets, predominantly $CD4^+$ $CD8^+$ cells, which are likely involved in the selective pancreatic β cell destruction [1, 2]. In addition, humoral abnormalities are generally present in individuals affected by T1DM, but organ dysfunction may also be absent or occurring subclinically in individuals carrying these immunologic abnormalities[3, 4]. Both genetic and environmental factors play a major role in the pathogenesis of the disease process.

Since T1DM is a chronic autoimmune disease with a long preclinical course[4], the identification of individuals during this preclinical phase of the disease process provides a real opportunity for predictive testing and therapeutic intervention. It has been well established that the presence of multiple islet autoantibodies to glutamic acid decarboxylase, 65 kDa isoform (GAD65), insulin, the neuroendocrine molecule IA-2 and cytoplasmic islet cell antibodies (ICA), is associated with high risk of Type 1 diabetes progression[5-8]. Intervention trials aimed at preserving endogenous insulin secretion mainly rely on islet autoantibody assessment to enroll in these trials both individuals at risk to develop T1DM and newly diagnosed Type1 diabetic patients[9, 10]. Prediction of T1DM by immunologic markers is now sufficiently accurate to allow the design of large clinical trials in individuals who are at risk of developing the disease for the prevention of the disease process and for a better understanding of disease pathogenesis.

GENETIC PREDISPOSITION

The overall risk for developing Type 1 diabetes in North American Caucasian siblings, parents and offspring of individuals with Type 1 diabetes, ranges from 1% to 15% (Table 1) compared to 0.12% in the general population.

Table 1. Empiric risk of Type 1 diabetes. These estimates are for North American Caucasian* and Scandinavian populations**

	Empiric Risk
First degree relatives of T1DM probands*	5-7%‡
Individuals without relatives with T1DM*	<1%
Children of affected father**	~6%
Children of affected mother**	~2%

‡ 1-15% range depending on the populations

However, over 80% of cases of Type 1 diabetes occur in individuals with no apparent family history of the disease. In the remaining 20%, this disease clusters in families[11].

The utilization of genome-wide scans has resulted in the identification of over eighteen putative loci but, for now, only linkage to HLA loci appears to be unambiguous[12-14]. Although excitement has been generated by the results of genome-wide scans for Type 1 diabetes, as well as many other polygenic disorders, careful and rigorous replication in many populations along with association studies must be conducted before any attempts are made by either positional cloning or the candidate gene approach to identify potentially elusive sequence variations that could influence genetic susceptibility[15-19].

There is convincing evidence that at least two chromosomal regions are associated with and linked to Type 1 diabetes. The HLA region on chromosome 6p21 (*IDDM1*) and the insulin gene region on chromosome 11p15 (*IDDM2*) confer susceptibility to Type 1 diabetes. The contribution of these two loci to familial inheritance is approximately 42% for *IDDM1* and 10% for *IDDM2*[11].

HLA complex and mechanisms of susceptibility or protection from Type 1 diabetes

Amino acid polymorphism at position 57 the HLA-DQβ-chain could influence the interaction between the class II molecule, the peptide antigen and the T cell receptor. This consequently influences the control of the specificity of the immune response to foreign and/or self-antigens. However, other residues in the DQβ-chain as well as the DQ α-chain also appear to be involved in the susceptibility to Type 1 diabetes. Genetic susceptibility to autoimmune diabetes appears to be strongly conferred by HLA-DQA1*0501-DQB1*0201, and -DQA1*0301-DQB1*0302 haplotypes. This concept is strengthened by recently published results obtained *in vivo* providing experimental evidence for the contribution of HLA-DQ molecules to autoimmune-related diabetes development. Using a unique "humanized" animal model of diabetes, the replacement of human HLA-DQ6 for human HLA-DQ8 molecules completely prevented the disease[20].

The importance of class II molecules in playing a role in the pathogenesis of Type 1 diabetes is also indicated by studies in a transgenic nonobese diabetes (NOD) mouse model, in which the expression of a modified I-Aβ chain (the equivalent to the human class II DQB1 locus) transgene carrying Asp 57 instead of Ser 57 prevents these mice from developing diabetes[21, 22]. Moreover, expression of Pro 56 instead of the normal His 56 in the I-A β chain has the same effect. Finally, expression of I-E transgenes (the equivalent of the human HLA-DR allele) appears to confer resistance to the disease[21, 23]. Of note, if NOD mice are treated with a monoclonal antibody reacting with the murine class II molecule, this also prevents the progression to overt diabetes[24]. These findings obtained in an animal model of Type 1 diabetes, certainly support the role of both HLA-DQ and HLA-DR in human Type 1 diabetes.

The mechanisms by which the class II genes can influence susceptibility to or protection from Type 1 diabetes are still the subject of discussion. Brown, et al.,[25] have characterized the structure of the crystallized HLA class II molecule. One hypothesis is that effective antigen binding depends on the conformation of the antigen binding site on the DQ dimer. The two critical residues, DQα Arg-52 and DQβ Asp-57 are located at opposite ends of the α-helices that form the antigen binding site of the DQ molecule. It has been postulated that a substitution of an amino acid residue at these positions of the DQ molecule leads to conformational changes of the antigen-binding site and consequently to a modification of the affinity of the class II molecule for the "diabetogenic" peptide(s). Using X-ray crystallography, Lee et. al have determined the three-dimensional structure of DQ8 complexed with the insulin B chain that represents an important T cell epitope for islet-infiltreting T cells in NOD mice[26].

We reported that *HLA-DQ* typing can identify a phenotype associated with 2 *HLA-DQ* high-risk haplotypes and insulin-requiring diabetes progression and the absence of conventional autoantibody markers for T1DM prediction, namely GAD65, IA-2, insulin and cytoplasmic islet cell antibodies (ICA) (Figure 1)[8]. Based on the presence of the alleles *DQA1*0501-DQB1*0201* and/or *DQA1*0301-DQB1*0302*, the number of *HLA-DQ* high-risk haplotypes was assigned as 0, 1 or 2. In support of our findings, preliminary results indicate that the distribution of *HLA* genotypes in patients with Type 1 diabetes diagnosed as having Type 1B diabetes, seems equivalent to that of Type 1A diabetic patients[27]. These observations raise the concept that the classification of autoimmune diabetes based on current conventional islet autoantibody testing alone, may not yet be satisfactory and should also include additional criteria such as HLA genotypes and potential novel immunologic markers.

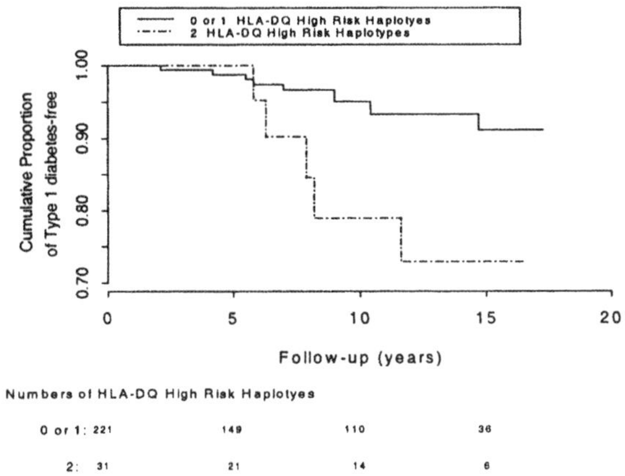

Figure 1
Cumulative risk to develop Type 1 diabetes in seronegative relatives (N=252) who carry 2 vs. 0 or 1 *HLA-DQ* high-risk haplotypes. Two *HLA-DQ* high-risk haplotypes conferred a cumulative risk to insulin-requiring diabetes of 27% after a follow-up of 12.5 years, compared to a risk of 6% for relatives who had 0 or 1 *HLA-DQ* high-risk haplotypes (log rank P = 0.01) (with permission from Pietropaolo M et al. Diabetologia 2002; 45:66-76).

There is still discussion as to whether DR molecules are also important in Type 1 diabetes susceptibility[28]. Whether some investigators have argued that DR alleles are not the primary factors in conferring disease susceptibility since they are in linkage disequilibrium with DQ alleles, others believe that the DR locus play a role in Type 1 diabetes susceptibility independently from DQ alleles.

The prevalence of HLA-DR2 is decreased[11] in patients with Type 1 diabetes, and the DQA1*0102/DQB1*0502/DRB1*1601 haplotype accounts for the most part of disease susceptibility in DR2-associated cases of Type 1 diabetes. In many populations, the frequency of the DQB1*0602 allele is rarely found among patients with IDDM. This suggests that this allele may play a protective role in the disease process. At present, carrying a "protective" DQB*0602 allele is considered as a criterion of exclusion for enrolling first degree relatives of diabetic patients in clinical trials, such as the Diabetes Prevention Trial 1 (DPT-1)[9], the TrialNet, which are being carried out in the U.S. These trials have been designed to delay and ultimately prevent by any effective treatment the progression to the clinical onset of Type 1 diabetes in individuals considered at high risk of developing the disease.

Environmental Triggers

In genetically predisposed individuals, environmental agents such as a virus, may play a role in the generation of autoimmunity[29-31]. For example, the incidence of both Type 1 diabetes and multiple sclerosis in a given population changes as these individuals migrate to different regions. Such observations, along with the lower than expected rate of concordance among monozygotic twins, suggest that an environmental factor could play a role in the development of autoimmune responses. In the case of Type 1 diabetes, the trigger could be identified as a virus[2], such as Coxsackie virus B virus[32].

Antigenic similarity between a foreign pathogen (*e.g.*, a virus) and an antigen normally present on or in the target tissue (e.g., an autoantigen) may be involved in triggering Type 1 diabetes onset. This concept is embodied in the term "molecular mimicry". A possible molecular mimicry-induced reaction involved in diabetes etiopathogenesis was reported by Atkinson and colleagues, in which an amino acid stretch of the P2-C protein of the Coxsackie virus B, the peptide PEVKEK, is shared by the glutamic acid decarboxylase (GAD65) and may activate T-cells to destroy GAD65-expressing cells[33]. What seems to primarily hamper the demonstration of a molecular mimicry involvement in Type 1 diabetes is the lack of recognition of an autoantigen causatively involved with the disease, or a virus directly able to trigger a diabetes-oriented autoimmune mechanism. In the case of enteroviruses like Coxsackie virus as well, molecular mimicry seems not to be the best hypothesis to explain the mechanisms involved in the etiopathogenesis of T1DM. A more convincing hypothesis which seems to explain the Coxsackie virus involvement in diabetes better than molecular mimicry, was recently proposed by the group of Nora Sarvetnick[34]. In this study conducted on the NOD mouse model, molecular mimicry evidence after Coxsackie virus exposure was compared with evidence supporting instead a bystander T-cell proliferation effect mediated by the virus[35].

To determine which of the two proposed hypotheses better explain the mechanism underlying CVB4-induced IDDM, Horwitz and collaborators[34] used CVB4 to infect BI0.H2^{g7} mice carrying the NOD MHC allele to which presentation of the cross-reactive epitope is restricted. They also used BDC2.5 mice harboring a diabetogenic T cell receptor as a transgene. The results showed that following CVB4 infection, the BIO.H2^{g7} mice generated a strong local immune response without any signs of pancreatic islet autoreactivity. On the basis of the molecular mimicry hypothesis, these mice, carrying the diabetogenic MHC restriction element, should instead promptly develop diabetes once exposed to CVB4. On the contrary, CVB4 infection in BDC2.5 mice generated a very quick diabetic response with all the signs of insulitis and a marked loss of insulin-producing β cells. These results were interpreted as evidence that in these mice, T1DM was the result of the activation of resting, islet-specific, memory lymphocytes through the bystander mechanism.

The bystander T-cell proliferation hypothesis is based on the evidence that although viral infections are in general able to induce vigorous immune responses, the increase in total T cell numbers is not due to the expansion of antigen-specific T cell clones[36, 37]. Actually, the number of antigen-specific T cells remains consistently low, while non-antigen-specific T cells seem to be stimulated solely because they are physically present in the area of infection. The bystander (i.e., non-antigen specific) reaction is then not TCR-dependent and can even be promoted by heterologous viruses as long as they are infectious and able to promote cytokine release. Among the cytokines most involved in this non-specific stimulation are the Type 1 interferons (IFN-1) which include IFN-α and IFN[35]. Although antigen-specific T cells are rapidly eliminated from the bloodstream, long-lived resting memory cells remain after receiving protective signals from the IFN-1 exposure.

The immunologic reaction of the BDC2.5 transgenic mice against CVB4 was considered an "exaggerated version" of the human preclinical situation in which, previously-inflicted, environmental insults could have caused an expansion of possibly cross-reactive T cell clones[34]. The viral infection seems to be able to indirectly activate autoreactive T cells that will then generate an initial pancreatic tissue damage. The first damaged β cells, in turn, will release previously "ignored" self-antigens, that once properly presented can now activate an autoimmune process able to rapidly proceed to the generation of insulitis and eventually overt diabetes. In their concluding remarks, the authors of this study[34] offer the explanation that in humans, enrichment or distortion of the T cell repertoire, similar to the one artificially created in the TCR transgenic BCD2.5 mice, could be due to a history of infections with pathogens expressing superantigens. This superantigen-mediated T-cell activation may render the patient over-represented for a particular variable segment of the TCR β-chain. Among the T-cells sharing this TCR Vβ segment, autoreactive T-cells able to attack specific pancreas structures can also be present[32].

Autoimmunity to islet antigens

A common characteristic of many autoimmune diseases, such as Type 1 diabetes, is that besides T cells a humoral response against multiple target antigens is commonly present[38, 39]. As autoimmunity in Type 1 diabetes progresses from initial activation to a chronic state, there is often an increase in the number of islet autoantigens targeted by T cells and antibodies. This condition is termed "epitope spreading" and also involves the overexpression of cytokines and other inflammatory mediators. This is a cascade process in that T cells activate additional autoreactive B cells, and B cells present additional epitopes from different proteins, until there is autoreactivity to numerous autoantigens. In a similar fashion, multiple novel peptides within the same molecule can activate T cells.

The immunological diagnosis of Type 1 diabetes relies essentially on the detection of autoantbodies to islet antigens in the serum of patients and on the presence of high risk HLADQ/DR alleles[40, 41]. Although their pathogenic significance is still unclear, they have the great advantage of serving as surrogate markers for specific autoimmune responses and they now represent major markers for the enrollment in primary intervention trails for Type 1 diabetes. The new radioimmunoassays for detecting antibodies to GAD65, insulin and IA-2 offer the practical advantage of reproducibility and ease standardization, otherwise not possible with techniques using indirect immunofluorescence, such as the methods to detect cytoplasmic ICA. During the past decade, a number of autoantibodies to islet antigens were molecularly characterized (Table 2). These antigens include insulin[42], glutamic acid decarboxylase (GAD)[43], ICA512/IA-2[44, 45], and I-A2β (phogrin)[46]. In addition, there are many other autoantigens in a variety of stages of characterization, including molecules with characterized sequences but without fully developed assays and proteins with known molecular masses 155, 52 and 37-38 kDa[47, 48]. Other molecules have been associated with Type 1 diabetes, such as anti-bovine serum albumin antibodies (anti-BSA)[49], antibodies reacting with ICA69[50, 51] anti-insulin receptor antibodies[52], antibodies to heat shock proteins[53-55], antibodies to jun-B,16[56], CD38[57], and glial fibrillary acidic protein (GFAP) [58]. Antibodies to a series of other autoantigens were identified by immunoscreening islet expression libraries[59, 60].

Table 2. Most characterized islet autoantigens associated with Type 1 diabetes.

	Localization	**Humoral Response**	**Cellular Response**
Insulin*	Secretory granules pancreatic β cells. Human thymus and PAE cells (Peripheral Antigen Expressing Cells)	Insulin autoantibodies are found in virtually 100% of young children (<5 years of age) before the onset of Type 1 diabetes. Correlation with younger age and fast rate of progression to insulin requirement in first-degree relatives of IDDM patients. Prophylactic subcutaneous injection of insulin, oral and intranasal administration prevent Type 1 diabetes in NOD mice.	PBLs from humans and NOD mice react with insulin β-chain.
GAD65* and GAD67	Synaptic-like microvesicles of neuroendocrine cells. Present in testis and ovary. Human thymus and PAE cells	A subset of 64-kDa autoantibodies recognize GAD. Autoantibodies to GAD65 are present in 70-80% of prediabetic subjects or newly diagnosed diabetic patients. GAD antibodies are also detected in patients with stiff man syndrome, and with autoimmunie thyroid disease. Radioimmunoassay of in vitro transcribed/translated GAD65 useful for large-scale screening.	PBL responses to GAD65 in newly diagnosed diabetic patients and in NOD mice
ICA512(IA-2)* and phogrin (IA-2β)	Neurosecretory granules (pancreatic β cells, CNS, pituitary, adrenal). Human thymus and PAE cells	Autoantibodies to ICA512(IA-2) are present in ~60% of prediabetics or newly diagnosed IDDM patients. Relationship between 37,000 and 40,000 Da tryptic fragments and ICA512(IA-2). Radioimmunoassay of in vitro transcribed/ translated ICA512(IA-2) useful for large-scale screening.	PBL responses in newly diagnosed diabetic patients.
Islet Cell Autoantigen 69 kDa (ICA69)	Neuroendocrine tissues (cytosol). Human, murine thymus and PAE cells	Autoantibodies to ICA69 can be detected in 43% of prediabetic subjects by Western blotting.	Association between HLA-DR3 and PBL responses in newly diagnosed diabetics. Regions of similarity with bovine serum albumin.

Carboxy peptidase H	Neurosecretory granules	Autoantibodies to carboxypeptidase H found in ~ 20% of prediabetics.	Present
Ganglioside GM2-1	Pancreatic islet cells	Autoantibodies to GM2-1 detected in -80% of prediabetic subjects and NOD mice.	?
Imogen 38 (38 kDa)	Mitochondria; widely distributed with variable levels of expression	Presence of circulating antibodies to 38-kDa proteins. Possible presence if antibodies to imogen 38.	PBLs from newly diagnosed diabetics proliferate to imogen 38
Glima 38	Amphiphilic N-Asp glycated β cell membrane protein that is expressed in islets and neuronal cell lines.	Autoantibodies to Glima 38 can be detected in 14-22.7% of newly diagnosed diabetics and prediabetics. The majority of these patients are negative for GAD65 and/or ICA512(IA-2) autoantibodies.	?
Peripherin	Neuronal cells	Autoantibody response against peripherin in NOD mice.	T cell responses against peripherin in NOD mice.
Heat-shock protein (Hsp60)	Ubiquitously inducible	Antibodies to Hsp60 in prediabetic NOD mice.	Hsp60-reactive T-cells can accelerate disease in prediabetic NOD mice.
SOX13 (ICA12)	SRY-type HMG box transcription factor family. Expressed in the nucleus and cytoplasm of most human tissues with the highest levels in the pancreas	Autoantibodies against SOX13 are detected in ~18% of Type 1 diabetics, the majority of whom are ICA negative. Anti-SOX13 Ab are more frequent in adults with Type 1 diabetes.	?

*Biochemical autoantibody assays readily available for large screening programs.

Several studies have suggested that using a combination of humoral immunological markers to these islet antigens rather than a single test, gives a higher predictive value for Type 1 diabetes, and greater sensitivity without significant loss of specificity[5, 6, 41]. These represent important prerequisites or the use of these radioimmunoassays in screening for individuals who are at risk for developing insulin requirement.

Thus far, insulin and proinsulin are considered the only candidate pancreatic β cell specific autoantigens[61-62-64]. Insulin autoantibodies (IAA) are among the earliest markers to appear in young children who eventually develop Type 1 diabetes[39]. This is particularly evident in infants younger than 1 year of age who begin to express these autoantibodies shortly after birth. High levels of IAA may be genetically influenced. An association was reported between high levels of IAA and HLA- DR4[65], and with other haplotypes, such as HLA-DQA1 alleles of lineage 2, DQA1*0102,0201,0301,0401[66].

Population studies suggest that this locus (i.e., *INS* VNTR or *IDDM2*) contributes approximately 10% of the genetic susceptibility to Type 1 diabetes[67]. Sequence analysis of the insulin gene region identified a polymorphic locus, which consists of a variable number of tandem repeats, or VNTR, present within the 5' regulatory region (promoter) adjacent to the coding sequence of the insulin gene. Each repeat element consists of a 14- to 15-bp DNA segment having the consensus nucleotide sequence A(C/T)AGGGGT(G/C)C(T/C/G)(G/A/T) (G/T/A)G(G/C/T). The number of repeats within sequenced alleles ranges from 26 to >200, with three classes of alleles identified on the basis of overall size: class I, class II and class III. Class I *INS* VNTR alleles consist of 26-63 repeats, averaging 570 bp in length, and are associated with IDDM susceptibility. Class III alleles consist of 140-200 or more repeats and are considered to be protective from diabetes. In size, class III alleles are the largest variants, averaging over 2.2 Kb in length. Class II alleles (1.2 kb average length) are too rare in the populations studied to draw any conclusion about their association with IDDM susceptibility[68].

Detailed analyses of the insulin region also indicate the presence of a number of additional polymorphism outside the VNTR region that are in strong linkage disequilibrium with the VNTR itself, which then appears to be the primary association with T1DM susceptibility. Bennet et al. reported that a 698-VNTR class I subtype is negatively associated with disease susceptibility, in contrast to other class I alleles which confer susceptibility to disease[68-70].

A number of studies have suggested that the INS VNTR may have a biological role in the genetic regulation of insulin expression[71-73]. The proximity of this polymorphism to the INS transcriptional start site (<400 bp upstream) makes this an attractive hypothesis. Furthermore, an association between VNTR polymorphisms and human disease is not unique. For example, the human HRAS1 gene, which encodes the H-ras protooncogene and is associated with a genetic susceptibility to certain cancers, is under the allelic effects of a VNTR polymorphism which lies downstream of the gene[74-76]. Expansions of nucleotide triplet repeat minisatellites have also been implicated in numerous progressive neurological diseases such as myotonic dystrophy[77].

A number of research groups have reported the expression of islet autoantigens within cells of the thymus[78-80] and in peripheral lymphoid organs[81], two tissues thought to be vital to the maintenance of immune self tolerance. In particular, the fact that T1DM-related autoantigens such as insulin, GAD65 and IA-2 appear to be expressed by the same thymic cell type suggest that these antigens can be manufactured by a common type of antigen presenting cell (APC) within lymphoid tissues[20]. Immunohistochemical and molecular analyses of these cells identify features of a dendritic cell (DC) phenotype[81-83], implicating these powerful APCs in the process of establishing and maintaining immune tolerance via de novo expression of self protein antigens.

Based on these observations, one may postulate that disruption of genetic elements regulating transcript and protein expression could short circuit mechanisms necessary for maintaining immune self-tolerance to autologous proteins. Functional DNA sequence polymorphisms in the promoter region of a given (autoantigen) gene would be likely candidates to mediate such an effect. For example, the structure of the insulin promoter region is well known, and a functional VNTR within this promoter does in fact correlate with variable levels of insulin expression[71, 72, 81]. Although the precise mechanism by which the insulin VNTR genetically predisposes to diabetes is unclear. In vitro evidence suggests that these genetic elements may exert a regulatory effect by strengthening nucleosome formation, thereby altering local chromatin structure and, consequently, decreasing the efficiency of transcription from nearby genes[77]. One conclusion from these data is that variation of *INS* promoter function conferred by the VNTR polymorphism relates to a failure to induce or to maintain self-tolerance to insulin because of impaired or altered *INS* expression within lymphoid tissues[78, 79]. In support of this conclusion, it has been recently reported that mice expressing low thymic insulin levels exhibit detectable peripheral reactivity to insulin, while mice with normal levels show no evidence of T cell reactivity to insulin[84].

In sum, the assessment of risk factors for the etiology of T1DM is very important for understanding the natural history of this disease. The new radioimmunoassays for detecting antibodies to islet autoantigens offer the practical advantage of reproducibility and ease standardization. GAD65 and IA-2 autoantibodies are now the most widely applied immunologic screening tests in major ongoing clinical trials, such as TrialNet, which is currently carried out in North America. The Centers for Disease Control (CDC) have evaluated filter paper collection of sera for determination of autoantibodies with the finding that autoantibodies can readily be measured following elution from such blood spots[85]. These results imply that screening for Type 1 diabetes risk with whole blood samples collected onto special filter paper, may represent a feasible solution to simplify collection and curtail the costs associated with diabetes screening programs.

If future studies validate the predictive value of screening strategies based on the use of multiple islel autoantibody testing, high throughput procedures could become an integral part of the routine medical examination.

Mechanisms of failure of immunologic tolerance to self-antigens

Tolerance to self-molecules is established and maintained through complex mechanisms taking place in both thymus (central tolerance) and peripheral lymphoid organs (peripheral tolerance). Because proteins with tissue-restricted or peripheral expression are traditionally thought to be unavailable for presentation in the thymus, it has been proposed that tolerance to such proteins can only be achieved through mechanisms of peripheral tolerance. Indeed, one attractive hypothesis is that Type 1 diabetes is essentially due to failure of negative selection of autoreactive T cells, either in the thymus or in the periphery, or because of a breakdown in tolerance to β-cell-specific antigens (Figure 2). This hypothesis has received support following thymic transplantation of islet antigens or expression of putative islet cell autoantigens resulting in prevention of diabetes in both NOD mouse and BB rat models[86, 87].

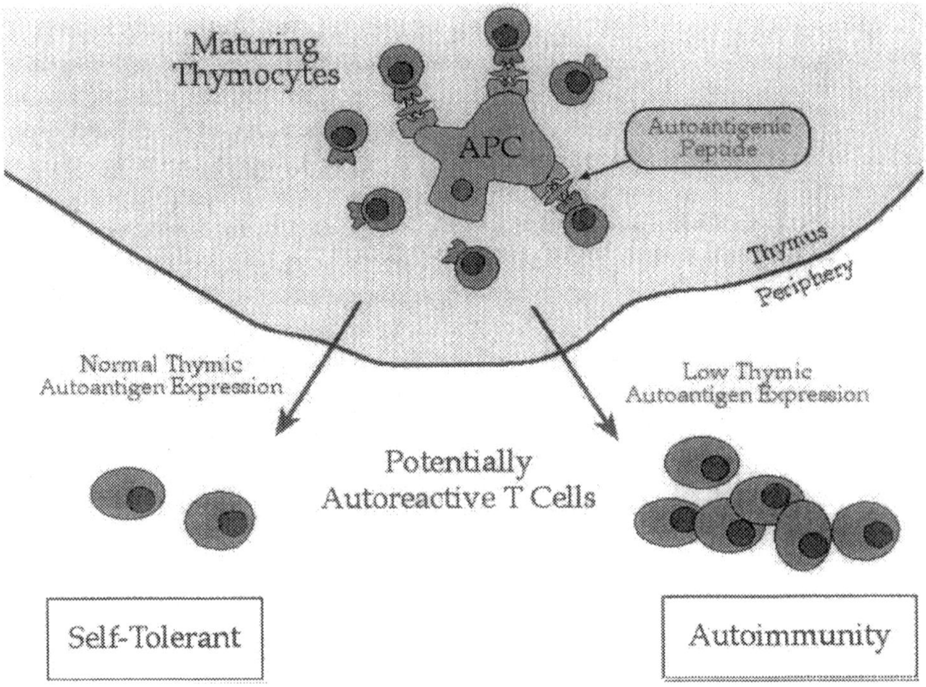

Figure 2
General hypothesis for the development of self-tolerance to endogenous proteins during thymic selection of T cells. According to this hypothesis, self-tolerance mechanisms are established centrally through the expression of peripheral tissue proteins by special antigen presenting cells (APCs) within the thymic medulla. Presentation of peptides derived from these self molecules to developing thymocytes provides a mechanism for negative selection of self-reactive T cells: cells that bind strongly to self peptides presented in the context of the appropriate MHC molecule (self-reactive) are deleted from the T cell repertoire, whereas those T cells not responding to the presented antigen (self-tolerant) may survive and pass out of the thymus to the peripheral circulation. Depending upon the activation state of a trafficking T cell and the nature of the co-stimulatory signals conveyed by an self-antigen-presenting APC, the response of the T cell may either be anergy with continued self-tolerance or autoimmunity.

Recent evidence suggests that molecules with tissue-restricted expression may also be expressed in the thymus[78]. Genes encoding the T1DM-related autoantigens insulin, IA-2, GAD, and the neuroendocrine antigen ICA69 are transcribed in human thymus throughout fetal life and childhood. Insulin gene transcription in human thymus was also reported by others and similarly insulin, glucagon, and GAD , ICA69 transcripts were detected in mouse and rat thymus[81, 83, 88]. Transcripts of several self-molecules have been detected in the thymus, such as pancreatic and thyroid hormones, neuroendocrine molecules, and other peripheral proteins, raising the concept that self-antigen expression in the thymus may be crucial for the development of self-tolerance. Studies in mice have shown that the thymus harbors cells (termed peripheral-antigen-expressing (PAE) cells) that express peripheral antigens such as insulin, and experiments in transgenic mice provide evidence that these PAE cells have a tolerogenic function[88]. Of note, several reports indicate that DCs can prevent diabetes in NOD mice as well as humans[89-91]. It remains to be determined whether self-antigen presenting DCs are fewer in number or less functionally competent in patients with T1DM.

Similar cells have recently been described in humans in both the thymus and peripheral lymphoid tissues, and were found to express islet cell antigens such as insulin/proinsulin, GAD, and IA-2. The subsequent phenotypic characterization of PAE cells in both mouse thymus and human lymphoid tissues indicates that these express phenotypic markers of antigen-presenting cells. Given their phenotype and the fact that they express self-antigens these cells have also been referred to as self-antigen-presenting (SAP) cells in humans.

Once a T cell expresses a functional T cell receptor (TCR) at the cell surface, it is subject to either positive or negative selection events. Both positive selection and negative selection depend on interactions between the TCR, MHC molecule, and antigenic self peptide. *Positive selection* occurs as thymic stromal cells bearing MHC molecules (containing self-peptide fragments) engage TCR molecules on the developing thymocytes and direct their continued maturation into functionally mature T cells. T cells with "useless" receptors (i.e., those that cannot bind the MHC molecule with sufficient affinity) are not driven to mature and expand, and these cells eventually die. *Negative selection* refers to the poorly understood set of events that specifically eliminates or, alternatively, "anergizes" potentially autoreactive cells, thereby inducing "tolerance" to self (*i.e.,* self-tolerance). During negative selection, factors such as affinity for self-antigen and antigen load likely influence the final outcome of cell death or clonal anergy. Thus, the peripheral T cell repertoire of each person (including identical twins) is unique and is a consequence of both the random generation of TCRs in the initial unselected thymocyte pool as well as of thymic positive and negative selection events.

Autoimmunity is thought to result from an imbalance between the two functionally opposite processes, *tolerance induction* and *immune responsiveness*, each dependent on the presence of class I and class II molecules with appropriate structures (dictated by the genes encoding them) that are able to present critical antigenic peptides. In genetically susceptible individuals, certain class II molecules may ineffectively present self-peptides, thereby leading to inadequate negative selection of T cell populations that could later become activated to manifest an autoimmune response. Nepom and Kwok explain the molecular basis of HLA-DQ associations with Type 1 diabetes exactly on this basis[92].

Recently published data generated in NOD, NOD *Idd* congenic, and (NOD x C57BL/6)F1 mice suggest that an autoimmune diabetes phenotype and a resistance to transplantation tolerance may be co-existing but may not be under identical genetic control[93]. The latter intriguing report indicates that autoimmune diabetes and transplantation tolerance induction may well have different genetic roots. If true, this would suggest the strategies aimed at treating autoimmune diabetes and preventing recurrent autoimmunity should be different from those required for inducing transplantation tolerance.

Dysfunction and/or deficiency of Regulatory Cells

Alterations in number and function of regulatory cells may contribute to the generation of an autoimmune state in Type 1 diabetes[94, 95]. Dysfunction and/or loss of CD1-restricted T cells, T cells with γ/δ receptors, CD4+/CD25+ T cells and NKT cells may all theoretically contribute to disease pathogenesis through inefficient suppression of pathogenic autoreactive T cells. For instance, in monozygotic twins who are discordant for diabetes, levels of CD1-restricted T cells appear to be diminished in the affected twin. The antigens that activate regulatory T cells are unknown, and the mechanisms in which these cells exert their effect on immune responses remains still unclear.

Results from a clinical trial of a humanized anti-CD3 monoclonal antibody in new onset Type 1 diabetes suggest that this treatment improves metabolic control beyond one year after treatment[10]. This monoclonal antibody, termed hOKT3γl(Ala-Ala) contains the binding region of OKT3 in which the C_H2 region has been modified by site-directed mutagenesis to alter FcR-binding activity (Figure 3). The outcome was the elimination T cell activation properties and to induce T cells with regulatory capabilities. Apparently this "humanized" hOKT3γl(Ala-Ala) monoclonal antibody treatment does not lead to major adverse effects due to release of cytokines by activated T cells, such as fever, headache, hypotension etc., which are common following anti-CD3 mAb treatment (OKT3)[10, 96]. The rationale for the clinical trial using the "humanized" hOKT3γl(Ala-Ala) monoclonal antibody is based on the observation that in NOD mice anti-CD3 mAb treatment reverses hyperglycemia in newly diagnosed NOD mice as a result of the induction of regulatory T cells[97].

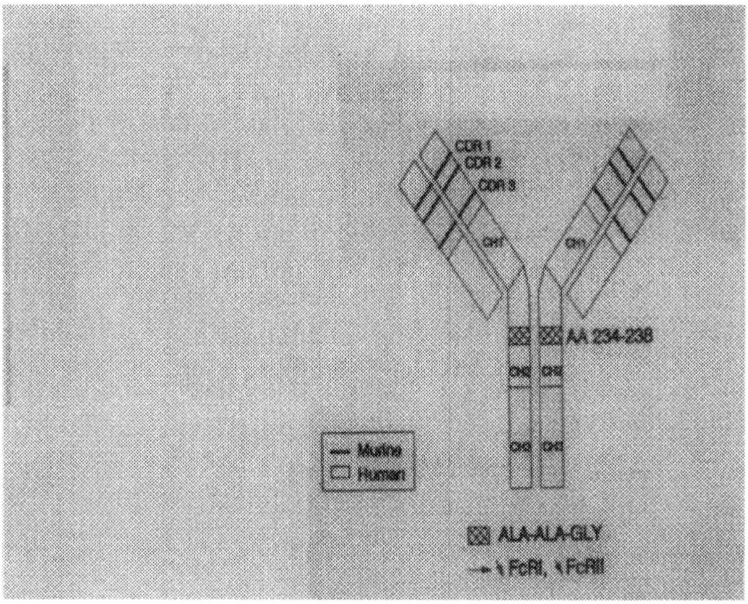

Figure 3
"Humanized" OKT3 Monoclonal Antibody (HU-IgG1) (with permission from Dr. Jeffrey Bluestone).

$CD4^+$ T cells appear to also be important in transplantation tolerance. In mice tolerized with donor-specific transfusion (DST) in addition to anti-CD154 mAb, depletion of $CD4^+$ T cells leads to rapid rejection of skin allografts[98, 99]. Mice genetically deficient in $CD4^+$ T cells are also resistant to costimulation blockade-based transplantation tolerance[98]. *In vitro* studies have demonstrated that alloantigen tolerance induced by costimulatory blockade is maintained by $CD4^+CD25^+$ T cells[100]. Furthermore, peripheral transplantation tolerance was shown to depend on a population of $CD4^+CD25^+$ T cells that regulate the activity of CD154-independent $CD8^+$ T cells[101]. The relationship of the $CD4^+$ T cells that regulate autoimmune diabetes and those that regulate transplantation tolerance is not known.

Interestingly, CD40L blockade completely prevents autoimmune diabetes in the RIP-LCMV model for virally induced T1DM by induction of a hybrid phenotype NK/DC regulatory cells[102].

NKT cells may also play a role in the pathogenesis of T1DM in both humans[103] and NOD mice[104]. NKT cells could have a general function of suppressing autoimmunity. For instance, reduced frequencies of these cells were reported in patients with T1DM[105], although others[106] did not confirm these results. NKT cell importance in NOD mice has been demonstrated by genetic disruption of CD1, which results in the absence of CD1-restricted invariant NKT cells[107]. In these mice, diabetes develops at an earlier age as well as an increased number of memory autoreactive and activated T cells. In addition, administration of the NKT agonist α galactosyl ceramide (αGalCer) dramatically reduces the frequency of diabetes in NOD mice[104] αGalCer also prevents autoimmune recurrence in spontaneously diabetic mice transplanted with syngeneic islet grafts. The proposed mechanism of action consists of a) NKT cell induction of tolerogenic dendritic cells in draining pancreatic lymph nodes; b) induction of regulatory cytokines;[104] and b) NKT cell induction of tolerogenic dendritic cells in draining pancreatic lymph nodes[108].

Of interest, NKT cells may also be important in transplantation tolerance. There is evidence that NKT cell deficient mice rapidly reject corneal allografts[109]. Mice deficient in NKT cells are also resistant to a transplantation tolerance induction protocol based on anti-LFA-1 and anti-B7.1/2 antibodies[110].

Other forms of autoimmune diabetes

Two syndromes have been described in which an autoimmune-mediated diabetes occurs as the result of a single gene defect. These syndromes are termed autoimmune polyglandular syndrome type I (APS-I) or autoimmune polyendocrinopathy-candidiasis-ectodermal dystrophy (APECED)[111,112], and X-linked poyendocrinopathy, immune dysfunction and diarrhea (XPID)[113]. These two syndromes are considered unique models to understand the mechanisms involved in the loss of tolerance to self-antigens in these two examples of autoimmune diabetes and its associated organ-specific autoimmune disorders.

APECED

This syndrome is rare in the majority of populations, except for the Finnish and Iranian Jews in which it is relatively more common. At least two of the three following disorders are required to diagnose APECED: primary hypoparathyroidism, Addison's disease and chronic mucocutaneous candidiasis. A response to immunosuppressive therapy could be achieved in severe cases[114,115]. Hypoparathyroidism, Addison's disease, autoimmune thyroid disease and other chronic organ-specific autoimmune disorders including insulin-requiring autoimmune diabetes can all develop in these patients during the natural course of the disease.

APECED is unique among well known autoimmune disorders in that it is caused by one single gene pair, homozygosity for defect in the *AIRE* (autoimmune regulator) gene, which is localized on chromosome 21q22.3. This disease has an autosomal recessive inheritance pattern. Over 31 different mutations within the *AIRE* locus have been described, being the most frequent a 13-bp deletion in exon 8 (1085-1097 deletion) among Norwegian patients[116]. There appears to be no relationship between the type of mutations at the *AIRE* locus and clinical phenotype[116].

The AIRE gene encodes a 57.5 kDa predicted protein carrying a conserved nuclear localization signal two putative plant homeodoain (PHD) zinc fingers, four LXXLL motifs or nuclear receptor interaction domains, and the SAND and HSR domains[117]. These nuclear localization signals and a putative DNA-binding SAND domain suggest that the *AIRE* gene product is indeed a transcription factor[117].

APECED is an example demonstrating that a mutation of a single gene can give rise to an array of autoimmune polyendocrine disorders, including insulin-requiring diabetes. The nature of the immune abnormalities remains still elusive, even though dysregulation of T cell function as well as cytokine patterns have been implicated in the pathogenesis of this polyendocrine disorder. Of note, similarly to Type 1 diabetes, autoantibodies to islet cell antigens, such as glutamic acid decarboxylase (GAD) and islet cell antibodies (ICA) can occur in patients affected by APECED.

The AIRE protein is expressed in a number of organs including the thymus. It has been postulated that *AIRE* could play a role in the thymic stromal organization and particularly in the induction of tolerance to self-antigens[118, 119]. Recently it has been reported that mice expressing a defective form of the *AIRE* gene develop a multiorgan autoimmune disease resembling that of APECED[119]. The latter findings underline the importance of central tolerance in controlling the generation of autoimmunity.

XIPD/XLAAD

This syndrome is an X-linked recessive immunologic disorder characterized by early onset of Type 1A diabetes mellitus, autoimmune thyroiditis, autoimmune enteropathy, hemolytic anemia, atopic dermatitis including food allergies, and immunodeficiency leading to fatal infections.

This syndrome is also known by X-linked autoimmunity-immunodeficiency syndrome (XLAAD).

The cause of the immunodeficiency is unclear as white blood counts as well as routine T cell proliferation tests are usually normal. However, there seems to be a markedly skewed cytokyne profile toward a Th2-like phenotype, with high levels of IL-4, IL-5, IL-13 and low levels of IFN gamma[113].

A number of mutations within the *JM2* gene, which is localized in the pericentrometric region of the X chromosome (Xp11.23-Xq13.3), have been documented in patients affected by XPID[113]. Recently it has been reported that different mutations of the human gene *FOXP3*, the ortholog of the gene mutated in scurfy mice (*Foxp3*) can cause this syndrome[120]. Although little is known about the mechanism of action of the *Fox3* protein product, scurfin, the phenotype of scurfy mice suggests a critical control switch for T cell activation. In particular, when scurfin is absent or inactive, T cell may become activated in an uncontrolled fashion or fail to undergo apoptosis, and this may lead to the development of early onset autoimmune disease.

REFERENCES

1. Bottazzo, GF, Dean BM, McNally JM, Mackay EH, Swift PGF, Gamble DR. In situ characterization of autoimmune phenomena and expression of HLA molecules in the pancreas in diabetic insulitis. N Engl J Med 1985; 313:353-360
2. Conrad, B, Weidmann E, Trucco G, Rudert WA, Ricordi C, Rodriquez-Rilo H, Behboo R, Finegold D, Trucco M. Evidence for superantigen involvment in insulin-dependent diabetes mellitus etiology. Nature 1994; 371:351-355
3. Bottazzo, GF, Florin-Christensen A, Doniach D. Islet-cell antibodies in diabetes mellitus with autoimmune polyendocrine deficiencies. Lancet 1974; 2:1279-1282
4. Eisenbarth, GS. Type I diabetes mellitus: a chronic autoimmune disease. N Engl J Med 1986; 314:1360-1368
5. Bingley, PJ, Christie MR, Bonifacio E, Bonfanti R, Shattock M, Fonte MT, Bottazzo GF, Gale EAM. Combined analysis of autoantibodies improves prediction of IDDM in islet cell antibody-positive relatives. Diabetes 1994; 43:1304-1310
6. Verge, CF, Gianani R, Kawasaki E, Yu L, Pietropaolo M, Jackson RA, Chase PH, Eisenbarth GS. Prediction of type I diabetes mellitus in first degree relatives using a combination of insulin, glutamic

acid decarboxylase and ICA512bdc/IA-2 autoantibodies. Diabetes 1996; 45:926-933

7. Ziegler, AG, Hummel M, Schenker M, Bonifacio E. Autoantibody appearance and risk for development of childhood diabetes in offspring parents with Type 1 diabetes. The 2-year analysis of the German BABYDIAB study. Diabetes 1999; 48:460-468
8. Pietropaolo, M, Becker DJ, LaPorte RE, Dorman JS, Riboni S, Rudert WA, Mazumdar S, Trucco M. Progression to insulin-requiring diabetes in seronegative prediabetic subjects: the role of two HLA-DQ high risk haplotypes. Diabetologia 2002; 45:66-76
9. Diabetes Prevention Trial-Type 1 Diabetes Study Group. Effects of insulin in relatives of patients with type 1 diabetes mellitus. N Engl J Med 2002; 346:1685-1691
10. Herold, KC, Hagopian W, Auger JA, Poumian-Ruiz E, Taylor L, Donaldson D, Gitelman SE, Harlan DM, Xu D, Zivin RA, Bluestone JA. Anti-CD3 monoclonal antibody in new-onset type 1 diabetes mellitus. N Engl J Med 2002; 346:1692-1698
11. Pietropaolo M, Trucco M. "Major histocompatibility locus and other genes that determine the risk of development of Type 1 diabetes mellitus." In *Major histocompatibility locus and other genes that determine the risk of development of Type 1 diabetes mellitus*, D. LeRoith, S. I. Taylor, and J. M. Olefsky ed. Philadelphia: Lippincott Williams & Wilkins, 2000.
12. Todd, JA, Bell JI, McDevitt HO. HLA-DQβ gene contributes to susceptibility and resistance to insulin-dependent diabetes mellitus. Nature 1987; 329:599-604
13. Morel, PA, Dorman JS, Todd JA, McDevitt HO, Trucco M. Aspartic acid at position 57 of the HLA-DQ beta chain protects against Type I diabetes: a family study. Proc Natl Acad Sci (USA) 1988; 85:8111-8115
14. Concannon, P, Gogolin-Ewens KJ, Hinds DA, Wapelhorst B, Morrison VA, Stirling B, Mitra M, Farmer J, Williams SR, Cox NJ, Bell GI, Risch N, Spielman RS. A second-generation screen of the human genome for susceptibility to insulin-dependent diabetes mellitus. Nature Genet 1998; 19:292-296
15. Lander, ES, Kruglyak L. Genetic dissection of complex traits: guidelines for interpreting and reporting linkage results. Nature Genet 1995; 11:241-247

16. Kruglyak, L, Daly M, Reeve-Daly MP, Lander ES. Parametric and nonparametric linkage analysis: a unified multipoint approach. Am J Hum Genet 1996; 58:1347-1363
17. Thomson, G. Strategies involved in mapping diabetes genes: an overview. Diabetes Rev 1997; 5:106-115
18. Kruglyak, L, Lander ES. Complete multpoint sib-pair analysis of qualitative and quantitative traits. Am J Hum Genet 1995; 57:439-454
19. Lernmark, Å, Ott J. Sometimes it's hot, sometimes it's not. Nature Genet 1998; 19:213-214
20. Wen, L, Wong FS, Tang J, Chen NY, Altieri M, David C, Flavell R, Sherwin R. In vivo evidence for the contribution of human histocompatibility leukocyte antigen (HLA)-DQ molecules to the development of diabetes. J Exp Med 2000; 191:97-104
21. Miyazaki, T, Uno M, Uehira M, Kikutani H, Kishimoto T, Kmoto M, Nishimoto H, Miyazaki JI. Direct evidence for the contribution of unique I-A^{NOD} to the development of insulitis in non-obese diabetic mice. Nature 1990; 345:722-724
22. Slattery, RM, Kjer-Nielsen L, Allison J, Charlton B, Mandel TE, Miller JFAP. Prevention of diabetes in non-obese diabetic I-Ak transgenic mice. Nature 1990; 345:724-726
23. Lund, T, O'Reilly L, Hutchings P, Kanagawa O, Simpson E, Gravely R, Chandler P, Dyson J, Picard JK, Edwards A, Kioussis D, Cook A. Prevention of insulin-dependent diabetes mellitus in non-obese diabetic mice by transgenes encoding modified I-A beta chain or normal I-E alpha chain. Nature 1990; 345:727-729
24. Boitard, C, Bendelac A, Richard MF, Carnaud C, Bach JF. Prevention of diabetes in nonobese diabetic mice by anti-I-A monoclonal antibodies: transfer of protection by splenic T cells. Proc Natl Acad Sci (USA) 1988; 85:9719-9723
25. Brown, JH, Jardetzky TS, Gorga JC, et al. Three-dimensional structure of the human class II histocompatibility antigen HLA-DR1. Nature 1993; 364:33-39
26. Lee, KH, Wucherpfennig KW, Wiley DC. Structure of a human insulin peptide-HLA-DQ8 complex and susceptibility to type 1 diabetes. Nat Immunol 2001; 2:501-507
27. Cornell, C. N., Stankiewicz, W., Asher, D., Babu, S., Yu, L., Bao, F., Yu, J., Nelson, J., Bugawan, T., Korman, E., Eisenbarth, G. S., and Rewers, M. J. Absence of islet autoantibodies at diabetes onset

does not rule out Type 1A diabetes. Diabetes 49 (Suppl. 1), A68. 2000.
Ref Type: Abstract

28. She, J-X, Marron MP. Genetic susceptibility factors in type 1 diabetes: linkage, disequilibrium and functional analyses. Curr Opin Immunol 1998; 114:370-376
29. Oldstone, MBA. Viral persistence. Cell 1989; 56:517-520
30. Oldstone, MBA, Nerenbergh M, Southern P, Price J, Lewicki H. Virus infection triggers insulin-dependent diabetes mellitus in a transgenic model: role of anti-self (virus) immune response. Cell 1991; 65:319-331
31. von Herrath, MG, Dockter J, Oldstone MBA. How virus induces a rapid or slow onset insulin-dependent diabetes mellitus in a transgenic model. Immunity 1994; 1:231-242
32. Luppi, P, Zanone MM, Rudert WA, et al. Restricted TCR V beta gene expression and enterovirus infection in type I diabetes: a pilot study. Diabetologia 1999; 43:1484-1497
33. Kaufman, DL, Erlander MG, Clare-Salzler M, Atkinson MA, Maclaren NK, Tobin AJ. Autoimmunity to two forms of glutamate decarboxylase in insulin- dependent diabetes mellitus. J Clin Invest 1992; 89:283-292
34. Horwitz, MS, Bradley LM, Harbertson J, et al. Coxsackie virus-induced diabetes: initiation by bystander damage and not molecular mimicry. Nature Medicine 1998; 4:781-
35. Tough, DF, Borrow P, Sprent J. Induction of bystander T cell proliferation by viruses and type 1 interferon in vivo. Science 1996;1947-1950
36. Nahill, S, Welsh R. High frequency of cross-reactive cytotoxic T lymphocytes elicited during the virus-induced polyclonal cytotoxic T lymphocyte response. J Exp Med 1993; 177:317-327
37. Tripp, RA, Hou S, McMickle A, Houston J, Doherty PC. Recruitment and proliferation of CD8+ T cells in respiratory virus infections. J Immunol 2003; 154:6013-6021
38. Bach, J-F, Chatenaud L. Tolerance to islet autoantigens in type 1 diabetes. Annu Rev Immunol 2001; 19:131-161
39. Pietropaolo, M, Eisenbarth GS. Autoantibodies in human diabetes. Curr Dir Autoimmun 2001; 4:252-282
40. The Expert Committee on the Diagnosis and Classification of Diabetes Mellitus. Report of the Expert Committee on the Diagnosis

and Classification of Diabetes Mellitus. Diabetes Care 1997; 20:1183-1197

41. Pietropaolo, M, Peakman M, Pietropaolo SL, Zanone MM, Foley TP, Becker DJ, Trucco M. Combined analysis of GAD65 and ICA512(IA-2) autoantibodies in organ and non-organ specific autoimmune diseases confers high specificity for insulin-dependent diabetes mellitus. J Autoimmun 1998; 11:1-10
42. Greenbaum, CJ, Palmer JP, Kuglin B, Kolb H, and Participating Laboratories. Insulin autoantibodies measured by radioimmunoassay methodology are more related to insulin-dependent diabetes mellitus than those measured by enzyme-linked immunosorbent assay: Results of the fourth international workshop on the standardization of insulin autoantibody measurement. J Clin Endocrinol Metab 1992; 74:1040-1044
43. Baekkeskov, S, Aanstoot H, Christgau S, Reetz A, Solimena MS, Cascalho M, Folli F, Richter-Olsen H, DeCamilli P. Identification of the 64K autoantigen in insulin dependent diabetes as the GABA-synthesizing enzyme glutamic acid decarboxylase. Nature 1990; 347:151-156
44. Rabin, DU, Pleasic S, Palmer-Crocker R, Shapiro JA. Cloning and Expression of IDDM-Specific Human Autoantigens. Diabetes 1992; 41:183-186
45. Lan, MS, Lu J, Goto Y, Notkins AL. Molecular cloning and identification of a receptor-type protein tyrosine phosphatase, IA-2, from human insulinoma. DNA Cell Biol 1994; 13:505-514
46. Wasmeier, C, Hutton JC. Molecular cloning of phogrin, a protein tyrosyne phosphatase homologue localized to insulin secretory granule membranes. J Biol Chem 1996; 271:18161-18170
47. Roep, BO, Kallan AA, Hazenbos WLW, Bruining GJ, Bailyes EM, Arden S, Hutton JC, DeVries RRP. T-cell reactivity to a 38kD insulin-secretory-granule protein in patients with recent-onset type 1 diabetes. Lancet 1991; 337:1439-1441
48. Christie, MR, Hollands JA, Browm TJ, Michelsen BK, Delovitch TL. Detection of pancreatic islet 64,000 Mr autoantibodies in insulin-dependent diabetes distinct from glutamate decarboxylase. J Clin Invest 1993; 92:240-248
49. Karjalainen, J, Martin JM, Knip M, Ilonen J, Robinson BH, Savilahti E, Akerblom HK, Dosch HM. A bovine albumin peptide as a possible trigger of insulin-dependent diabetes mellitus. N Engl J Med 1992; 327:302-307

50. Pietropaolo, M, Castano L, Babu S, Buelow R, Kuo Y-LS, Martin S, Martin A, Powers AC, Prochazka M, Naggert J, Leiter EH, Eisenbarth GS. Islet cell autoantigen 69 kDa (ICA69): Molecular cloning and characterization of a novel diabetes associated autoantigen. J Clin Invest 1993; 92:359-371
51. Miyazaki, I, Gaedigk R, Hui MF, Cheung RK, Morkowski J, Rajotte RV, Dosch HM. Cloning of human and rat p69, a candidate autoimmune target in type I diabetes. Biochem Biophys Acta 1994; 1227:101-104
52. Elias, D, Cohen IR, SHECHTER Y, Spirer Z, Golander A. Antibodies to insulin receptor followed by anti-idiotype. Diabetes 1987; 36:348-354
53. Birk, OS, Douek DC, Elias D, Dewchand H, Gur SL, Walker MD, Van der Zee R, Cohen IR, Altmann DM. A role of Hsp60 in autoimmune diabetes: analysis in a transgenic model. Proc Natl Acad Sci USA 1996; 93:1032-1037
54. Atkinson, MA, Maclaren NK, Scharp DW. No evidence for HSP65 in insulin dependent diabetes. Lancet 1990; 337:263-264
55. Georgopoulos, C, McFarland H. Heat shock proteins in multiple sclerosis and other autoimmune diseases. Immunol Today 1993; 14:373-375
56. Honeyman, MC, Cram DS, Harrison LC. Transcription factor jun-B is target of autoreactive T-cells in IDDM. Diabetes 1993; 42:626-630
57. Mallone, R, Ortolan E, Baj G, Funaro A, Giunti S, Lillaz E, Saccucci F, Cassader M, Cavallo-Perin P, Malavasi F. Autoantibody response to CD38 in Caucasian patients with type 1 and type 2 diabetes: immunological and genetic characterization. Diabetes 2001; 50:752-762
58. Winer, S, Tsui H, Lau A, Song A, Li X, Cheung RK, Sampson A, Afifiyan F, Elford A, Jackowski G, Becker DJ, Santamaria P, Ohashi P, Dosch HM. Autoimmune islet destruction in spontaneous type 1 diabetes is not beta-cell exclusive. Nature Medicine 2003; 9:198-205
59. Atkinson, MA, Maclaren NK. Islet cell autoantigens in insulin-dependent diabetes. J Clin Invest 1993; 92:1608-1616
60. Pietropaolo M, Eisenbarth GS. "Molecular targets of the autoimmunity of type I diabetes." In *Molecular targets of the autoimmunity of type I diabetes*, B. Draznin and D. LeRoith ed. Totowa, NJ: Humana Press Inc., 1994.

61. Bell, GI, Karam JH, Rutter WJ. Polymorphic DNA region adjacent to the 5' end of the human insulin gene. Proc Natl Acad Sci USA 1981; 78:5759-5763
62. Rotwein, P, Chyn R, Chirgwin J, Cordell B, Goodman HM, Permutt MA. Polymorphism in the 5'-flanking region of the human insulin gene and its possible relation to Type II diabetes. Science 1981; 213:1117-1120
63. Yu, L, Robles DT, Abiru N, Rewers M, Kelemen K, Eisenbarth GS. Early expression of antiinsulin autoantibodies of humans and the NOD mouse: evidence for early determination of subsequent diabetes. Proc Natl Acad Sci USA 2000; 97:1701-1706
64. Owerbach, D, Nerup J. Restriction fragment length polymorphism of the insulin gene in diabetes mellitus. Diabetes 1982; 31:275-277
65. Ziegler, AG, Ziegler R, Vardi P, Jackson RA, Soeldner JS, Eisenbarth GS. Life table analysis of progression to diabetes of anti-insulin autoantibody-positive relatives of individuals with type I diabetes. Diabetes 1989; 38:1320-1325
66. Pugliese, A, Bugawan T, Moromisato R, Awdeh ZL, Alper CA, Jackson RA, Erlich HA, Eisenbarth GS. Two subsets of HLA-DQA1 alleles mark phenotypic variation in levels of insulin autoantibodies in first degree relatives at risk for insulin-dependent diabetes. J Clin Invest 1993; 93:2447-2452
67. Davies, JL, Kawaguchi Y, Bennett ST, Copeman JB, Cordell HJ, Pritchard LE, Reed PW, Gough SCL, Jenkins SC, Palmer SM, Balfour KM, Rowe BR, Farrall M, Barnett AH, Bain SC, Todd JA. A genome-wide search for human type I diabetes susceptibility genes. Nature 1994; 371:130-136
68. Bennett, ST, Lucassen AM, Gough SCL, Powell EE, Undlien DE, Pritchard LE, Merriman ME, Kawaguchi Y, Dronsfield MJ, Pociot F, Nerup J, Bouzekri N, Cambon-Thomsen A, Ronningen KS, Barnett AH, Bain SC, Todd JA. Susceptibility to human type I diabetes at IDDM2 is determined by tandem repeat variation at the insulin gene minisatellite locus. Nature Genet 1995; 9:284-292
69. Bennett, ST, Wilson AJ, Cucca F, Nerup J, Pociot F, McKinney PA, Barnett AH, Bain SC, Todd JA. *IDDM2-VNTR*-encoded susceptibility to type 1 diabetes: dominant protection and parental transmission of alleles of the insulin gene-linked minisatellite locus. J Autoimmun 1996; 9:415-421
70. Bennett, ST, Wilson AJ, Esposito L, Bouzekri N, Undlien DE, Cucca F, Nisticò L, Buzzetti R, the IMDIAB Group, Bosi E, Pociot

F, Nerup J, Cambon-Thomsen A, Pugliese A, Shield JPH, McKinney PA, Bain SC, Polychronakros C, Todd JA. Insulin VNTR allele-specific in type 1 diabetes depende on identity of untransmitted paternal allele. Nature Genet 1997; 17:350-352
71. Lucassen, AM, Screaton GR, Julier C, Elliot TJ, Lathrop M, Bell JI. Regulation of insulin gene expression by the IDDM associated, insulin locus haplotype. Hum Mol Genet 1994; 4:501-506
72. Kennedy, GC, German MS, Rutter WJ. The minisatellite in the diabetes susceptibility locus IDDM2 regulates insulin transcription. Nature Genet 1995; 9:293-298
73. Owerbach, D, Gabbay KH. The search for IDDM susceptibility genes: the next generation. Diabetes 1996; 45:544-551
74. Krontiris, TG. Minisatellites and human disease. Science 1995; 269:1682-1683
75. Krontiris, TG, Delvin B, Karp DD, Robert NJ, Risch N. An association between the risk of cancer and mutation in the HRAS1 minisatellite locus. N Engl J Med 1993; 329:517-523
76. Kiaris, H, Spandidos DA, Jones AS, Vaughan ED, Field JK. Mutations, expression and genomic instability of the H-ras proto-oncogene in squamous cell carcinomas of the head and neck. Br J Cancer 1995; 72:123-128
77. Wang, YH, Griffith J. Expanded CTG triplet block from the myotonic dystrophy gene create the strongest known nucleosome positioning elements. Nature Genet 1995; 25:570-573
78. Pugliese, A, Zeller M, Fernandez JrA, Zalcberg LJ, Barlett RJ, Ricordi C, Pietropaolo M, Eisenbarth GS, Bennett ST, Patel DD. The insulin gene is transcribed in the human thymus and transcription levels correlate with allelic variation at the *INS* VNTR-*IDDM2* susceptibility locus for type 1 diabetes. Nature Genet 1997; 15:293-297
79. Vafiadis, P, Bennett ST, Todd JA, Nadeau J, Grabs R, Goodyear CG, Wickramasinghe S, Colle E, Polychronakros C. Insulin expression in the thymus is modulated by *INS* VNTR alleles at the *IDDM2* locus. Nat Genet 1997; 15:289-292
80. Sospedra, M, Ferrer-Francesch X, Pujol-Borrell R, Juan M, Foz-Sala M. Transcription of a broad range of self-antigen in human thymus suggests a role for central mechanisms in tolerance toward peripheral antigens. J Immunol 1998; 161:5918-5929
81. Pugliese, A, Brown D, Garza D, Murchison D, Zeller M, Redondo M, Diez J, Eisenbarth GS, Patel DD, Ricordi C. Self-antigen-

presenting cells expressing diabetes-associated autoantigens exist in both thymus and peripheral lymphoid organs. J Clin Invest 2001; 107:555-564
82. Werdelin, O, Cordes U, Jenson T. Aberrant expression of tissue-specific proteins in the thymus: a hypothesis for the development of central tolerance. Scand J Immunol 1998; 47:95-100
83. Pietropaolo, M, Giannoukakis N, Trucco M. Cellular environment and freedom of gene expression. Nat Immunol 2002; 3:335-
84. Chentoufi, AA, Polychronakros C. Insulin expression levels in the thymus modulate insulin-specific autoreactive T-cell tolerance: the mechanism by which the IDDM2 locus may predispose to diabetes. Diabetes 2002; 51:1383-1390
85. Henderson, L. O., Atkinson, M., Bingley, P. J., Bonifacio, E., Bosi, E., Ellis, T. E., Eisenbarth, G. S., Hagopian, W. A., Hannon, W. H., Jackson, R., Lernmark, A., Lou, D., Mei, J., Orban, T., Smith, S. J., Vogt, R. J., Wasserfall, C., Williams, A. J. K., Yu, L., and Study Group-DBSTAR Group. Dried blood-spots as a matrix for Type 1-diabetes autoantibody detection. Diabetes 49 (Suppl. 1), A36. 2000. Ref Type: Abstract
86. Gerling, IC, Serreze DV, Christianson SW, Leiter EH. Intrathymic islet cell transplantation reduces β-Cell autoimmunity and prevents diabetes in NOD/Lt Mice. Diabetes 1992; 41:1672-1676
87. Posselt, AM, Barker CF, Friedman AL, Naji A. Prevention of autoimmune diabetes in the BB rat by intrathymic islet transplantation at birth. Science 1992; 256:1321-1324
88. Smith, KM, Olson DC, Hirose R, Hanahan D. Pancreatic gene expression in rare cells of thymic medulla: evidence for functional contribution to T cell tolerance. International Immunol 1997; 9:1355-1365
89. Clare-Salzler, M, Brooks J, Chai A, Van Herle K, Anderson C. Prevention of diabetes in nonobese diabetic mice by dendritic cell transfer. J Clin Invest 1992;741-748
90. Feili-Hariri, M, Dong X, Alber SM, Watkins SC, Salter RD, Morel PA. Immunotherapy of NOD mice with bone marrow-derived dendritic cells. Diabetes 1999; 48:2300-2308
91. Papaccio, G, Nicoletti F, Pisanti FA, Bendtzen K, Galdieri M. Prevention of spontaneous autoimmune diabetes in NOD mice by transferring *in vitro* antigen-pulsed syngeneic dendritic cells. Endocrinology 2000; 141:1500-1505

92. Nepom, GT, Kwok WT. Molecular basis for HLA-DQ association in IDDM. Diabetes 1998; 47:1177-1184
93. Pearson, T, Markees TG, Wicker LS, Serreze DV, Peterson LB, Mordes JP, Rossini AA, Greiner DL. NOD Congenic Mice Genetically Protected From Autoimmune Diabetes Remain Resistant to Transplantation Tolerance Induction. Diabetes 2003; 52:321-326
94. Bach, J-F. Immunotherapy of insulin-dependent diabetes mellitus. Curr Opin Immunol 2001; 13:601-605
95. Kukreja, A, Cost G, Marker J, Zhang C, Sun Z, Lin-Su K, Ten S, Sanz M, Exley M, Wilson B, Porcelli S, Maclaren N. Multiple immuno-regulatory defects in type-1 diabetes. J Clin Invest 2002; 109:131-140
96. Masteller, EL, Bluestone JA. Immunotherapy of insulin-dependent diabetes mellitus. Curr Opin Immunol 2002; 14:652-659
97. Chatenaud, L, Primo J, Bach J-F. CD3 antibody-induced dominant self tolerance on overtly diabetic NOD mice. J Immunol 1997; 158:2947-2954
98. Long-term survival of skin allografts induced by donor splenocytes and anti-CD154 antibody in thymectomized mice requires CD4(+) T cells, interferon-gamma, and CTLA4. J Clin Invest 1998; 101:2446-2455
99. Iwakoshi, NN, Markees TG, Thornley T, Cuthbert A, Leif J, Phillips NE, Mordes JP, Greiner DL, Rossini AA. Skin allograft maintenance in a new synchimeric model system of tolerance. J Immunol 2001; 167:6623-6630
100. Taylor, PA, Noelle RJ, Blazar BR. CD4 $^{+}$CD25^{+} immune regulatory cells are required for induction of tolerance to alloantigen via costimulatory blockade. J Exp Med 2001; 193:1311-1317
101. van Maurik, A, Herber M, Wood KJ, Jones ND. Cutting edge: CD4^{+}CD25^{+} alloantigen-specific immunoregulatory cells that can prevent CD8+ T cell-mediated graft rejection: implications for anti-CD154 immunotherapy. J Immunol 2002; 169:5401-5404
102. Homann, D, Jahreis A, Wolfe T, Hughes A, Coon B, van Stipdonk MJ, Prilliman KR, Schoenberger SP, von Herrath MG. CD40L blockade prevents autoimmune diabetes by induction of bitypic NK/DC regulatory cells. Immunity 2002; 16:403-415
103. Wilson, SB, Kent SC, Horton HF, Hill AA, Bollyky PL, Hafler DA, Strominger JL, Byrne MC. Multiple differences in gene expression

in regulatory Vα24JαQ T cells from identical twins discordant for type I diabetes. Proc Natl Acad Sci USA 2000; 97:7411-7416

104. Sharif, S, Arreaza GA, Zucker P, Mi QS, Delovitch TL. Regulation of autoimmune disease by natural killer T cells. J Mol Med 2002; 80:290-300

105. Wilson, SB, Kent SC, Patton KT, Orban T, Jackson RA, Exley M, Porcelli S, Schatz DA, Atkinson MA, Balk SP, Strominger JL, Hafler DA. Extreme Th1 bias of invariant Vα24JαQ T cells in type 1 diabetes. Nature 1998; 391:177-181

106. Lee, PT, Putnam A, Benlaga K, Teyton L, Gottlieb PA, Bendelac A. Testing the NKT cell hypothesis of human IDDM pathogenesis. J Clin Invest 2002; 110:793-800

107. Shi, FD, Flodström M, Balasa B, Kim SH, Van Gunst K, Strominger JL, Wilson SB, Sarvetnick N. Germ line deletion of the CD1 locus exacerbates diabetes in the NOD mouse. Proc Natl Acad Sci USA 2001; 98:6777-6782

108. Naumov, YN, Bahjat KS, Gausling R, Abraham R, Exley MA, Koezuka Y, Balk SB, Strominger JL, Clare-Salzler M, Wilson SB. Activation of CD1d-restricted T cells protects NOD mice from developing diabetes by regulating dendritic cell subsets. Proc Natl Acad Sci USA 2001; 98:13838-13843

109. Sonoda, KH, Faunce DE, Taniguchi M, Exley M, Balk S, Stein-Streilein J. NK T cell-derived IL-10 is essential for the differentiation of antigen-specific T regulatory cells in systemic tolerance. J Immunol 2001; 166:42-50

110. Seini, KI, Fukao K, Muramoto K, Yanagisawa K, Takada Y, Kakuta S, Iwakura Y, Iwakura Y, Takeda K, Nakayama T, Taniguchi M, Bashuda H, Yagita H, Okumura K. Requirement for natural killer T (NKT) cells in the induction of allograft tolerance. Proc Natl Acad Sci USA 2001; 98:2581-

111. Björses, P, Aaltonen J, Vikman A, Perheentupa J, Ben-Zion G, Chiumello G, Dahl N, Heideman P, Hoorweg-Nijman JJG, Mathivon L, Mullis PE, Pohl M, Ritzen M, Romeo G, Shapiro MS, Smith CS, Solyom J, Zlotogora J, Peltonen L. Genetic homogeneity of autoimmune polyglandular disease type I. Am J Hum Genet 1996; 59:879-886

112. Aaltonen, J, Horelli-Kuitunen N, Fan J-B, Perheentupa J, Myers R, Palotie A, Peltonen L. High-resolution physical and transcriptional mapping of the autoimmune polyendocrinopathy-candidiasis-

ectodermal dystrophy locus on chromosome 21q22.3. Genome Res 1997; 7:820-829

113. Bennett, CL, Yoshioka R, Kiyosawa H, Barker DF, Fain PR, Shigeoka AO, Chance PF. X-Linked syndrome of polyendocrinopathy, immune dysfunction, and diarrhea maps to Xp11.23-Xq13.3. Am J Hum Genet 2000; 66:461-468
114. The Finnish-German APECED Consortium. An autoimmune disease, APECED, caused by mutations in a novel gene featuring two PHD-type zinc-finger domains. Nature Genet 1997; 17:399-403
115. Nagamine, K, Peterson P, Scott HS, Kudoh J, Minoshima S, Heino M, Krohn KJE, Lalioti MD, Mullis PE, Antonarkis SE, Kawasaki K, Asakawa S, Ito F, Shimizu N. Positional cloning of the APECED gene. Nature Genet 1997; 17:393-398
116. Redondo, MJ, Eisenbarth GS. Genetic control of autoimmunity in Type I diabetes and associated disorders. Diabetologia 2002; 45:605-622
117. Pitkänen, J, Doucas V, Sternsdorf T, Nakajima T, Aratani S, Jensen K, Will H, Vähämurto P, Ollia J, Vihinen M, Scott HS, Antonarakis SE, Kudoh J, Shimizu N, Krohn K, Peterson P. The autoimmune regulator protein has transcriptional transactivating properties and interacts with the common coactivator CREB-binding protein. J Biol Chem 2000; 275:16802-16809
118. Zuklys, S, Balciunaite G, Agarwal A, Fasler-Kan E, Palmer E, Hollander GA. Normal thymic architecture and negative selection are associated with AIRE expression, the gene defective in the autoimmune-polyendocrine-candidiasis-ectodermal dystrophy (APECED). J Immunol 2000; 165:1976-1983
119. Anderson, MS, Venanzi ES, Klein L, Chen Z, Berzins SP, Turley SJ, von Boehmer H, Bronson R, Dierich A, Benoist C, Mathis D. Projection of an immunological self shadow within the thymus by the Aire protein. Science 2002; 298:1395-1401
120. Bennett, CL, Christie J, Ramsdell F, Brunkow ME, Ferguson PJ, Whitesell L, Kelly TE, Saulsbury FT, Chance PF, Ochs HD. The immune dysregulation, polyendocrinopathy, enteropathy, X-linked syndrome (IPEX) is caused by mutations of *FOXP3*. Nat Genet 2001; 27:21-22

Chapter 3
TYPE 2 DIABETES IN CHILDREN AND ADOLESCENTS

Lawrence M. Dolan, MD
Children's Hospital Medical Center, Cincinnati, OH

INTRODUCTION

Within the past decade there has been a sharp increase in the frequency of type 2 diabetes in adolescents and children[1-12]. Although this increase has been associated with a rise in the frequency of obesity in the pediatric population, the etiology of type 2 diabetes in the pediatric subjects remains unclear. To better understand the similarities and the differences between pediatric and adult type 2 diabetes and the potential risks type 2 diabetes poses to our youth and future generations, this chapter will compare and contrast the pathophysiology and treatment of both adult and pediatric type 2 diabetes.

TYPE 2 DIABETES IN ADULTS

Type 2 diabetes mellitus is a metabolic disorder resulting from the development of insulin resistance and the progressive deterioration of pancreatic beta cell function[13]. The National Health and Nutrition Survey III (NHANES III), collecting data from 1988-1994 in the adult population in the United States, documented that 5.1% had diagnosed diabetes, 2.7% had undiagnosed diabetes, and 6.9% had carbohydrate intolerance[14]. A recent report projected an increase in the frequency of the diabetic population worldwide from 135 million in 1995 to 300 million by 2025[15]. Type 2 diabetes is a major cause of ophthalmologic, renal, neurologic, and cardiovascular morbidity and mortality[13]. The cost of medical care for diabetes in the United States in 1998 exceeded $60 billion[15, 16].

Type 2 diabetes is seen most frequently in obese, sedentary, middle aged adults with a higher frequency in minority than non-Hispanic white populations[17]. Sixty to eighty percent of adults with type 2 diabetes are obese[18].The frequency of diabetes increases with advancing age affecting 1.6% of 20 to 39 year olds, 6.5% of 40 to 49 year olds, 12.6% of 50 to 59 year olds, and 19% of those greater than 59 years of age having diabetes.

The gender distribution is equal until 60 years of age. Thereafter, the male to female ratio is 1.1/1. Native Americans and other minority populations have a higher prevalence of type 2 diabetes than non-Hispanic Whites. After controlling for standard risk factors, the relative risk for type 2 diabetes in Pima Indians is 5 fold, in Hispanics 1.9 to 2.3 fold, and in African-Americans 1.6 to 2 fold greater risk than non-Hispanic whites[14, 19, 20]

Type 2 diabetes is a silent, progressive disease with devastating consequences. Studies estimate that most patients have unrecognized elevation of plasma glucose for 7-12 years prior to diagnosis[21, 22]. This chronic, occult elevation of the plasma glucose frequently results in the presence of microvascular and macrovascular complications at diagnosis. These findings include 77% with hyperlipidemia, 57% with hypertension, 20% with retinopathy, 10% with nephropathy, and 10% with coronary or peripheral vascular disease[21, 22].

Pathophysiology of Type 2 Diabetes

Despite extensive study over many years, the pathophysiology of type 2 diabetes is not understood. Investigators have identified a number of key factors required for the development of type 2 diabetes. The components of diabetes include: 1) a strong genetic contribution; 2) environmental factors, 3) end organ resistance to the action of insulin, and 4) beta cell failure[13].

Studies of monozygotic (MZ) and dizygotic (DZ) twins, families, and different ethnic groups support the role of a genetic contribution to the development of type 2 diabetes[23]. Two studies of twins, the Veterans Twin Study and the Finish Registry Study, that do not contain referral bias reported 58% and 34% concordance for MZ and 17% and 16% concordance for DZ twins, respectively[24, 25]. The Veterans Study also reported higher plasma glucose values in discordant MZ twins suggesting that the frequency of carbohydrate abnormalities in MZ twins is underestimated. Studies of offspring and siblings reveal a 50% and 35% risk of developing diabetes, respectively[23]. Other evidence for a genetic contribution includes a difference in the frequency of diabetes by ethnic group (Native American 5 fold, Hispanic 1.9 to 2.3 fold, and African-American 1.6 to 2 fold compared to non-Hispanic whites) that remains after controlling for common risk factors[20]. Despite significant clinical evidence of a major genetic component to the development of type 2 diabetes, studies of candidate genes have yet to define the genetic etiology of type 2 diabetes.

Studies of ethnic groups with the same genetic background but living in different environments provide information concerning the role of environmental factors in the development of type 2 diabetes[26]. Examples include: 1) a frequency of diabetes of 37% and 54% in female and male adult Arizona Pima Indians versus 11% and 6% in northwest Mexican Pima Indians; 2) a frequency of diabetes in Asian Indians of 1% in rural and 2% in urban India versus 5% in South Africa, 9% in Singapore, and 13% in Fiji; and 3) a frequency of diabetes in the Japanese in Hiroshima, Japan of 7% and in Hawaii of 12%[26-28]. Environmental factors implicated include sedentary versus active life style, obesity, socio-economic status, and differences in dietary intake including increased total caloric intake, saturated fats, unrefined sugar and decreased fiber[29-33].

Insulin resistance is a key factor in the development of type 2 diabetes[34]. Extensive investigations have demonstrated decreased insulin sensitivity in liver, adipose tissue, and skeletal muscle in patients with type 2 diabetes. Cellular abnormalities include decreased recruitment of glut-4 glucose transporters, decreased activity of insulin receptor tyrosine kinase, and decreased storage of glucose as glycogen in skeletal muscle[17, 35-42].

While obesity is a major contributor to insulin resistance, obesity is not the sole cause of insulin resistance[34]. Investigators have suggested a number of potential abnormalities in target organs of insulin action that may contribute to insulin resistance. These studies have identified a number of genes that may contribute to insulin resistance. The candidate genes include potential mutations in the insulin signaling chain that include but are limited to the insulin receptor, insulin receptor substrates, liver glucokinase promoter, GLUT-4, and glycogen synthetase[43].

Beta cell failure is also a key factor in the development of type 2 diabetes[26]. Initially, beta cells respond to insulin resistance by increasing insulin production in order to maintain glucose homeostasis[44]. This results in increased fasting and 2-hour post glucose load plasma insulin concentrations. With time the ability of the beta cells to secrete insulin is exhausted. The first sign of beta cell failure is a decline in 2-hour post glucose load plasma insulin concentrations[44]. The exact etiology of beta cell failure remains unclear. Suggested mechanisms of beta cell failure include decreased beta cell mass, an abnormality in the glucose sensing mechanism or aberrant intracellular glucose metabolism[45, 46]. Primary (genetic) and acquired (glucose or other metabolic toxicity) beta cell defects have been postulated[13].

Model for the Development of Type 2 Diabetes

Both insulin resistance and beta cell dysfunction are required for the development of type 2 diabetes[47]. Although the sequence of events in each ethnic population has not been defined, longitudinal and cross-sectional data from many populations suggest that all ethnic groups share the same basic pathway to diabetes.

Pima Indian Model for the Development of Type 2 Diabetes

Based on longitudinal data collected in adult Pima Indians, investigators have proposed the following model for the development of type 2 diabetes[13, 44]. Individuals proceed from normal glucose metabolism to insulin resistance to impaired glucose tolerance to diabetes.

This model was developed from the study of 1,459 Pima Indians (544 males, 915 females: all >15 years of age with mean age of 35 years) who were followed every 2 years with fasting and 2-hour post glucose load plasma glucose and insulin concentrations for a median of 6.3 years (maximum of 16.3 years)[44]. During the study 306 subjects developed impaired glucose tolerance and 54 developed diabetes. At the beginning of the study subjects whose glucose metabolism deteriorated were older, more obese, and had higher fasting and 2-hour post glucose load plasma glucose and insulin concentrations. Predictors of progression from normal to impaired glucose tolerance were age, higher body mass index, and increased 2-hour post glucose load plasma glucose and insulin concentrations. Predictors of progression from impaired glucose tolerance to diabetes were increased 2-hour post glucose load plasma glucose but declining 2-hour post load plasma insulin concentrations. Importantly, higher body mass index was not a predictor of progression from carbohydrate intolerance to diabetes. However, duration of obesity, when adjusted for current body mass index, was highly correlated with the development of diabetes[48]. Although insulin resistance was not identified as a separate stage in this study, the pattern of higher fasting insulin and body mass index (BMI) prior to progression from normal to carbohydrate intolerance supports the presence of insulin resistance as a stage preceding carbohydrate intolerance. Biochemical (silent, pre-clinical) diabetes preceded overt diabetes[44]. These longitudinal data document the progression through specific stages in the development of type 2 diabetes with predictors of progression at each stage of developing diabetes.

Pima Model: Rate of Progression to Diabetes

Three studies in adult Pima Indians provide data to estimate the rate of progression through each of the stages prior to the development of overt diabetes[44, 49, 50]. These studies in middle aged Pima Indians suggest progression rates over 5 years of 11% to 20% for normal glucose tolerance to carbohydrate intolerance and 17.6% to 43% for carbohydrate intolerance to diabetes.

Pattern of Progression through the Stages of Diabetes in Other Populations

Prospective studies in other populations of adults indicate that the sequence of events in the Pima model is present in all ethnic groups. Elevated fasting plasma insulin concentration is a major risk factor for the development of type 2 diabetes in normal or impaired glucose tolerant non-Hispanic whites, Hispanics, Swedes, and Frenchmen[32, 51-53]. Studies of insulin secretion also established that declining insulin secretion predicted progression to diabetes. In normal glucose tolerant non-Hispanic whites and Nauruans, an increased 2-hour post-glucose load plasma insulin concentration predicted progression to type 2 diabetes. In glucose intolerant French-men, Nauruans, and Japanese, a decline in 2-hour post-glucose load plasma insulin concentration predicted progression to diabetes[34, 51, 53, 54]. In addition, Israeli investigators have reported that increased body mass index leads to glucose intolerance but prolonged duration of obesity is required to progress from carbohydrate intolerance to diabetes[55]. Finally, investigators compared predictive factors for the development of type 2 diabetes in two populations, one at lower risk of developing diabetes (non-Hispanic whites) and one at higher risk (Hispanics) [56]. As seen in the Pima Indians, increased fasting plasma insulin concentration and decreased insulin secretion were the strongest independent risk factors for developing diabetes[56]. The authors suggest that despite the ethnic variation in frequency of disease, the pathway to diabetes is the same as in the Pima model[56].

There is limited cross-sectional and no longitudinal data concerning the development of type 2 diabetes in African-Americans. However, the following data support that African-American adults also follow the Pima model. Specifically, non-diabetic African-Americans have a greater frequency of insulin resistance than non-Hispanic whites[57]. In addition, virtually all obese and 60% of non-obese type 2 African-American diabetics are insulin resistant[58]. Although there are no studies examining insulin secretion in developing type 2 diabetes in African-Americans, African-Americans with type 2 diabetes are at greater risk than non-Hispanic whites to present at diagnosis in diabetic ketoacidosis documenting relative insulin deficiency (beta cell failure)[59, 60]. Thus, although longitudinal data are not available, the limited cross-sectional data are consistent with the Pima model of early insulin resistance and late beta cell failure.

ADOLESCENT AND CHILDHOOD TYPE 2 DIABETES

Historical Perspective

In 1979 investigators published the first report of an increase in the frequency of type 2 diabetes in the pediatric population[12]. This paper described a prevalence of 0.4% (females 0.72%, males 0%) in 10-14 year olds and 2.3% (females 2.73%, males 2.43%) in 15-19 year olds in adolescent Pima Indians. Because of the known increased prevalence of type 2 diabetes in adult Pima Indians, this report drew little attention.

The next report of an increase in the frequency of type 2 diabetes in pediatric patients was in 1988[61]. Canadian investigators published case reports of type 2 diabetes in the First Nation Children in Manitoba.

In 1990 Japanese investigators described an increased incidence of type 2 diabetes. They documented an increase from 1.8/100,000 in 1975 to 3.8/100,000 in 1986. In addition to documenting a rise in the frequency of type 2 diabetes, the authors also documented the first evidence of the onset of diabetic complications early in the course of the disease. Abnormal flourescein angiography was present in 35% (16/45) at diagnosis and 39% two years after diagnosis[62].

In 1996 investigators in Cincinnati using a population-based study design documented an increase in the frequency of type 2 diabetes in African-Americans and non-Hispanic whites. The incidence of type 2 diabetes increased from 0.7/100,000 in 1982 to 7.2/100,000 in 1994. The frequency of type 2 diabetes in all newly diagnosed patients 0-19 years of age increased from 4% prior to 1992 to 16% in 1994. In the 10-19 year old group, 33% of all newly diagnosed patients in 1994 had type 2 diabetes. African-Americans composed 68% of the cases with 32% non-Hispanic whites. The female/male ratio was 1.7/1.0. The average BMI at diagnosis was 37.7 ± 9.6 kg/m2. The average age at diagnosis was 13.8 ± 1.9 years [1]. In 1998 investigators from Arkansas reported similar findings in an African-American and non-Hispanic white populations[3].

In 1998 investigators reported an additional rise in the frequency of type 2 diabetes in the Pima Indians. The frequency in 10-14 year olds increased from 0.4% in 1976 to 2.3% in 1996 and in 15-19 year olds from 2.3% in 1976 to 4.0% in 1996. Gender specific data in the 10-14 year olds demonstrated that the frequency rose in female Pima Indians from 0.72% (1976) to 2.88% (1996) and in males from 0% (1976) to 1.4% (1996). Gender specific data in 15-19 year olds revealed a frequency increase in females from 2.73% (1976) to 5.31% (1996) and in males from 2.43% (1976) to 3.78% (1996). This report also documented a high frequency of obesity (85% of the patients had body weight > 140% of ideal body weight for age), hypertension (18% of the patients had blood pressure > 140/90 mmHg), and microalbuminuria (22%)[5-7].

In 1998 investigators in San Diego also reported an increase in type 2 diabetes in individuals of Central or South American descent[2]. Fifty percent of the patients were obese with an age range of 5 to 17 years. The investigators provided documentation of elevated fasting and stimulated plasma c-peptide concentrations. The mean fasting plasma c-peptide was 3.6 ng/ml and peak stimulated plasma c-peptide after Sustacal challenge was 8.9 ng/ml. These values are significantly greater than c-peptide values reported for type 1 patients in the Diabetes Complications and Control Trial of 0.6 ng/ml and 1.5 ng/ml with duration of disease less than 5 years[63]. The data from San Diego provide biochemical evidence of insulin resistance.

Recent reports also confirm an increase in the frequency of type 2 diabetes in the Asian population in the San Francisco Bay Area, Seattle, and Hawaii where Filipino, Japanese, Chinese, and Hawaiian type 2 adolescents are being identified[64-66]. These patients share the clinical characteristics described in the other ethnic populations.

Diagnosis of Type 2 Diabetes in Adolescents and Children

The diagnosis of type 2 diabetes is made using a combination of clinical, historical and biochemical information. The major criteria include: 1) demonstrating the lack of the need for exogenous insulin to prevent the metabolic cascade of diabetic ketoacidosis (DKA) in the basal state: 2) documenting the absence of autoimmune (type 1A) and "Other Specific Types" of diabetes; and 3) defining insulin resistance by plasma insulin or c-peptide concentration.

The lack of a requirement of exogenous insulin to prevent DKA in the basal state is a key clinical characteristic of type 2 diabetes. The lack of need for insulin for greater than 6 months without ketosis or DKA strongly supports a diagnosis of type 2 diabetes in pediatric subjects. Prior to making the diagnosis of type 2 diabetes, autoimmune diabetes with a prolonged honeymoon and "Other Specific Types" of diabetes must be excluded as described below.

Autoimmune or type1A diabetes is diagnosed by the presence of autoimmune markers in plasma[67]. Typically pediatric subjects also require daily insulin administration in the basal state to prevent DKA. However, some patients, especially older subjects, may experience less rapid beta cell destruction and a more variable insulin requirement.

Autoimmune markers for type 1A diabetes include cytoplasmic islet cell antibodies documented by immunoflouresence or the measurement of antibodies to glutamic acid decarboxylase, islet cell antibody 512, or insulin autoantibodies[67, 68]. Although there are reports of positive antibodies in adults with type 2 diabetes, analysis of these patients' clinical course and phenotype suggest that these patients have more characteristics of type 1 diabetes than type 2 diabetes[69]. These adults appear to have a slower onset variant of autoimmune diabetes and the term late autoimmune diabetes in adults (LADA) has been applied to some of these patients.

Investigators anticipate that as more tools become available to better define autoimmune diabetes new subtypes of autoimmune diabetes will be identified. For example, only 85% of type 1 diabetes have positive autoimmune markers[67]. The remaining patients, type 1B diabetes, have insulinopenia due to either an unidentified autoimmune process (marker) or a non-autoimmune (idiopathic) etiology of their diabetes. Variants of idiopathic insulinopenic diabetes are seen in African-American and Asian patients who experience episodic DKA with varying degrees of insulin deficiency between episodes[67].

If autoimmune markers are measured after insulin administration or a period of time after diagnosis, the antibody titers must be interpreted carefully. Insulin autoantibodies must be measured in insulin naïve patients or within 10 days of initiating insulin therapy to prevent false positive titers[70]. If insulin has been administered for more than 10 days, a positive titer for insulin autoantibodies may be due to insulin administration rather than an underlying autoimmune process. As duration of disease increases the frequency of positive antibody titers declines. By ten years' duration only 65% of patients test positive for at least one of the autoimmune markers[71, 72].

A detailed description of "Other Specific Types" of diabetes as defined by the American Diabetes Association (ADA) Expert Committee was published recently[67]. In brief, the category "Other Specific Types" (also referred to in some texts as secondary diabetes) identifies types of diabetes resulting from diseases of the exocrine pancreas, endocrinopathies, drugs, chemicals, infections, genetic syndromes, genetic defects in insulin action and genetic defects in beta cell function. These types of diabetes are easily distinguished from type 2 diabetes by the clinical history and physical examination.

Two categories of "Other Specific Types" of diabetes that are sometimes difficult to distinguish from type 2 diabetes are maturity onset diabetes of the young (MODY) and atypical diabetes in African-Americans (ADAA). These entities are discussed in detail in a separate chapter. In brief, MODY is the result of a genetic mutation in either the glucose sensing or the insulin production systems[73, 74]. The patients are identified clinically by an autosomal dominant pattern (direct transmission in 3 successive generations) of a MODY type of diabetes. Characteristics of MODY diabetes include onset under 25 years of age, typically a thin phenotype, no gender predominance, and mild diabetes identified by intermittent or low exogenous insulin requirement. Five specific types of MODY types have been identified. MODY types 1 through 4 have been found in non-Hispanic white families with MODY 5 identified in a Japanese family. To date, MODY has not been identified in the Hispanic or African-American population. These clinical criteria can be used to identify suspected cases of MODY with genetic tests performed to confirm the diagnosis where indicated.

Distinguishing ADAA from type 2 diabetes can be a more difficult task[73, 75]. Patients with ADAA have an autosomal dominant inheritance pattern of ADAA. At diagnosis they present with an acute onset of diabetes with DKA but subsequently lack the need for exogenous insulin to prevent DKA. Fifty percent of these individuals are thin and fifty percent are obese. There is a female predominance (female/male 3:1). With increased duration of disease type 1 and type 2 patients lose beta cell function. ADAA patients, however, do not lose beta cell function over time. Genetic mutations in two families have been identified. One family had a glucokinase mutation and the other a mitochondrial DNA mutation[73].

Documenting plasma c-peptide can be helpful to identify insulin resistance if the measurement is performed in a controlled setting and the results interpreted carefully. C-peptide reflects endogenous insulin production. C-peptide is typically measured in the fasting state or after administration of a mixed meal challenge[63, 76-78]. Difficulties in interpreting c-peptide concentrations include the limitation of c-peptide production by the beta cells due to glucose toxicity, progressive beta cell dysfunction with increased duration of disease, and a paucity of data concerning the plasma c-peptide concentration in diabetic and non-diabetic subjects. Specifically, glucose toxicity results in lower plasma c-peptide concentrations due to beta cell dysfunction that can be reversed, at least in part, with an improvement in plasma glucose concentration[13]. In addition, as the duration of disease increases, beta cell failure rises resulting in lower plasma c-peptide concentrations[79, 80].

Data from the Diabetes Control and Complications Trial (DCCT) define "cut-points" for c-peptide to identify type 1A patients[63]. In subjects with diabetes less than 5 years duration, a fasting c-peptide < 0.6 ng/ml and peak mixed meal stimulated value < 1.5 ng/ml were found in type 1 patients. The exception to this rule is a type 1 patient early in the disease process or a patient with a prolonged honeymoon[81]. Such patients are identified by the presence of autoimmune markers in their plasma. In addition, investigators found that DCCT type 1 patients with duration of diabetes > 5 years had both fasting and peak stimulated plasma c-peptide values < 0.6 ng/ml.

There are no data that define insulin resistance in diabetic patients. However, there are data in non-diabetic children and adolescents in the Bogalusa Heart studies that help address this question[82]. The investigators report fasting c-peptides and percentiles for these values in healthy African-American and non-Hispanic white male and female teenagers. The 95th percentile for non-Hispanic white males was 3.35 ng/ml, African American males was 2.93 ng/ml, non-Hispanic white females was 3.38 ng/ml, and African-American females was 3.66 ng/ml. These data provide a reference point for the upper limit of normal in this age group. One limitation of the Bogalusa data is that obese subjects were not excluded from the analysis. As a result the c-peptide values are higher than would be expected in a non-obese population. Use of the 95th percentile from the Bogalusa data will probably underestimate subjects with insulin resistance. Data from non-obese children and adolescents taking into account ethnic background, gender, and pubertal development are required to identify the upper range of normal c-peptide in non-diabetic pediatric subjects in order to better define insulin resistance by plasma c-peptide concentration.

Clinical Characteristics

Despite the fact that there has been a marked increase in the frequency of type 2 diabetes in a number of different ethnic groups throughout the world, the total number diagnosed patients at any one center remains relatively low. As a result extensive clinical information on each ethnic population is not available. However, common clinical themes are present in the literature concerning type 2 diabetes in adolescents. These themes include: a higher frequency in minority populations, a female predominance, obesity, clinical evidence of insulin resistance, and preliminary data suggesting that a higher frequency of early complications of diabetes may develop.

The following paragraphs provide a description of the clinical data available in the Cincinnati population, one of the largest populations characterized. The data is presented as an example of the findings of type 2 diabetes in two ethnic populations, African-Americans and non-Hispanic Whites. The data described here are similar to that reported in African-Americans and non-Hispanic whites in Arkansas, Hispanics in San Diego, Asians in the San Francisco Bay Area, and the Pima Indians[2, 3, 5-7, 64].

Chart reviews to assess various clinical characteristics at presentation have been performed in the past three years. The following is a summary of the clinical information collected during those reviews. The difference in the denominators reflects differences in the total number of patients diagnosed at the time of the chart review.

Demographics and Prevalence Estimate

As of February 2001 the Cincinnati population consists of 173 patients. There are 112 females and 61 males (Female/male = 1.83) with 105 (61%) African-American, 64 (37%) non-Hispanic white, and 3 (2%) Other. The average age at diagnosis is 14.5 ±2.3 years. The age range is 8 to 21 years. The prevalence of type 2 diabetes using epidemiology techniques previously described [1] are shown in table 1.

Table 1: Prevalence February 2001: 0-19 years of age (per 1,000)

All Groups	Non-Hispanic White	African-American	Female	Male
0.17	0.08	0.80	0.23	0.11

Table 2: Prevalence February 2001 (per 1,000)

10-14 years old	0.15
15-19 year olds	0.51

Although these data provide an estimate of the true prevalence, the data under estimate the true frequency of the disease because of the limitations of the epidemiologic techniques employed and the high likelihood that there is a clinically silent period of hyperglycemia of unknown duration prior to diagnosis (see below).

Obesity

Obesity is a major characteristic but not a diagnostic criterion. The body mass index (BMI) at diagnosis for the Cincinnati population is 36±7.7 kg/m2. Ninety three percent of the group had BMI > the 95th percentile for chronologic age, gender and race. The remaining seven percent had BMI > the 75th percentile for chronologic age. No type 2 patient had a BMI < the 75th percentile for age, gender, and race.

Clinically Silent Disease

Type 2 diabetes in adults has a long clinically silent period prior to presentation. Data document that adults have type 2 diabetes 7-12 years prior to clinical diagnosis[21, 22]. To address this issue 113 patient charts were reviewed and the chief complaint was recorded. Twelve charts had no chief complaint recorded. Thus, records from 101 subjects were analyzed.

Fifty seven percent (58/101) of the patients presented with a chief complaint of polyuria and polydipsia. Forty three percent (43/101) presented with non-classical symptoms of diabetes. One third of this group

(14/43) were identified by positive urinalysis for glucose during a routine physical examination. Eighty percent of the group who were identified by routine urinalysis were female with 73% of the females non-Hispanic whites.

These data document: 1) non-classical presentation of type 2 diabetes in adolescents is frequent; 2) silent diabetes is present in adolescents; and 3) non-Hispanic white females are at greatest risk to present with only a positive urinalysis. The reason(s) for the difference in presentation by ethnicity is not clear.

Diabetic Ketoacidosis

DKA is considered to be the classic presentation of type 1 diabetes. Both adult and pediatric African-American type 2 patients can present in DKA[59, 60]. To assess the frequency of DKA at diagnosis we reviewed 113 patient records. DKA was defined as serum bicarbonate level < 15 meq/l.

Fourteen percent (16/113) of the patients had DKA at diagnosis. Nine were female and 7 were male. Fourteen (7 female, 7 male) were African-American accounting for 19% of all African-American patients. The two remaining patients were non-Hispanic white females.

These data document: 1) the presence of DKA does not rule out a diagnosis of type 2 diabetes; 2) African-Americans present more frequently in DKA than non-Hispanic whites; and 3) there is an equal gender frequency of DKA in African-Americans despite a female predominance in the overall frequency of the disease. The reason(s) for the equal gender distribution in a disease that has a female predominance is not clear.

Complications of Diabetes at Diagnosis

Adults frequently present at diagnosis with the complications of diabetes: 77% with hyperlipidemia, 50% with hypertension, 20% with retinopathy, 10% with microalbuminuria and 10% with cardiovascular disease[21, 22, 83]. To examine whether there was evidence of some of these complications of diabetes in adolescents at diagnosis, the frequency of hyperlipidemia and elevated blood pressure was examined.

Hyperlipidemia

The frequency of an abnormal fasting lipid profile was examined in 128 patient records. Lipid profile data was only included in the analysis if a fasting lipid profile was obtained within 3 months of diagnosis when the patient was metabolically stable. Nineteen patients met these criteria. Fifty seven percent had both elevated triglycerides and low HDL-cholesterol[84]. These data document: 1) abnormal lipid values are seen frequently in adolescents; 2) as seen in adults with type 2 diabetes, low HDL-C and elevated TG are commonly observed; and 3) since elevated TG is one of the strongest risk factors for premature heart disease in adults with type 2 diabetes, adolescents also appear to be at increased risk for premature heart disease.

Elevated Blood Pressure

The presence of increased blood pressure was examined in 113 patient records. The records were included in the analysis if the following criteria were met. Sixty-six patient records had a casual resting blood pressure performed within 3 months of diagnosis when the patient was metabolically stable. Blood pressure > 90th percentile after correction for age and height was considered elevated. The data documented that 56% of non-Hispanic whites and 42% of African-Americans had an elevated systolic or diastolic blood pressure while elevations in both measurements were found in 17% and 11% of these populations, respectively[85]. These data suggest that elevated blood pressure is found in adolescents with a frequency similar to adults with type 2 diabetes. A systematic, detailed approach is needed to document the frequency of hypertension in this population.

Summary

The Cincinnati data document an increased frequency of type 2 diabetes in adolescents that began in 1992. The disease has a higher frequency in obese, African-American females and has rarely been recognized before the onset of puberty. Due to the frequency of diagnosis of the disease by a positive urinalysis on routine physical examination, a clinically silent period of unknown duration is likely. In addition, the presence of DKA does not exclude a diagnosis of type 2 diabetes. Hyperlipidemia and elevated blood pressure are frequent findings at diagnosis suggesting that adolescents are at risk for developing cardiovascular disease at an early age. These data suggest that type 2 diabetes in adolescents follow a pattern of presentation similar to type 2 diabetes in adults. However, the marked female predominance in adolescents suggests that important differences maybe present between adolescent and adult type 2 diabetes.

TREATMENT OF TYPE 2 DIABETES IN ADULTS

Step-wise Addition Therapy

The cornerstones of the treatment of type 2 diabetes are diet and exercise followed by pharmacologic intervention. The recommendation of the American Diabetes Association is to maintain a hemoglobin A1c less than 8%. If this level of blood sugar control cannot be achieved, additional therapeutic interventions should be considered. The United Kingdom PDS and other studies have demonstrated that non-pharmacologic therapy is effective in only 25% of patients after a time of three years from diagnosis[79]. With advancing duration of disease, there is progressive deterioration of beta cell function such that only ten percent of patients can be treated with non-pharmacologic intervention at nine years duration of disease[80]. As a result clinicians employ the concept of step-wise addition of pharmacologic agents rather than substitution or subtraction of pharmacologic agents in order to maximize glycemic control.

Pharmacologic Agents

There are four classifications of pharmacologic agents employed to achieve glycemic control: inhibitors of carbohydrate absorption, stimulators of insulin release, agents that reduce insulin resistance, and the use of exogenous insulin to overcome insulin resistance[43, 86, 87].

Inhibitors of Carbohydrate Absorption

Alpha-glucosidase, approved for use in September 1995, inhibits the digestion of complex carbohydrates thus limiting the availability of simple sugars for absorption. This action decreases post-prandial glycemic excursion thus improving plasma glucose control. Specific contraindications include the presence of chronic gastrointestinal disease. Alpha-glucosidase administration is most effective in patients where post-prandial hyperglycemia is the major issue[43, 86, 87].

Stimulators of Insulin Release

Sulfonlyureas

Sulfonlyureas have been used to treat type 2 diabetes since 1942. Sulfonlyureas require the presence of a functioning beta cell. Sulfonylureas bind to a specific surface cell receptor on the beta cell resulting in the closure of ATP-potassium dependent channels. Closure of the potassium channels depolarizes the cell membrane activating calcium channels and increasing cytoplasmic calcium. Increased cytoplasmic calcium stimulates insulin release. Second and third generation sulfonylureas have identical cellular mechanisms of action but differ in potency and duration of action.

Sulfonylureas are degraded by the liver and excreted in the urine. Thus, their use with significant renal or kidney disease may result in hypoglycemia. These agents are teratogenic in animals and are therefore not recommended for use during pregnancy[86, 88]. Side effects include hypoglycemia, weight gain, gastrointestinal intolerance, and cholestatic jaundice. The possibility of increased cardiovascular mortality was reported in the University Group Diabetes Program (UGDP). Subjects who received 1.5 grams of tolbutamide per day had a 2.5 fold increase in cardiovascular mortality compared to diet alone, resulting in a discontinuation of the study. Since then no study has observed an increased risk of cardiovascular mortality and the UGDP study design has been criticized. It is prudent, however, to know that controversy surrounds early forms of these drugs. Sufonylureas are considered a first line therapeutic intervention in non-obese subjects whose main problem is impaired insulin secretion and who have a duration of diabetes less than 5 years. Sulfonylureas are used as a second line drug when insulin sensitizing agents have failed. Due to progression of beta cell failure, the secondary failure rate of sulfonylureas is 3-5% per year[43, 86, 87].

Repaglinide

Repaglinide was approved by the FDA in December 1997. Repaglinide binds to non-sulfonylurea receptors that also close ATP-potassium dependent channels and utilize the same cascade as sulfonlyureas to stimulate insulin release. Repaglinide has a short duration of action therefore it must be taken before each meal. Repaglinide is degraded by the liver and excreted in the urine. With significant liver or kidney disease a prolonged metabolic effect is possible. No data are available concerning its use in pregnancy[86, 88]. Due to the recent approval of repaglinide the frequency of hypoglycemia and other potential side effects are not known. The indications for use are the same as the sulfonylureas[43, 86, 87].

Insulin Sensitizing Agents

Biguanides

Biguanides have been used to treat diabetes since 1957. Phenformin was removed form the US market in 1975 due to the risk of developing lactic acidosis. At that time metformin was introduced in Europe, Canada, and Mexico. In December 1994 metformin was approved for use in the United States.

The precise cellular mechanism of action of metformin is not known. Metformin's biological effects include decreasing absorption of glucose from the gastrointestinal tract, inhibiting endogenous glucose production by reducing gluconeogenesis and glycogen breakdown, and increasing glucose stimulated glucose disposal by muscle by increasing non-oxidative pathways (storage of glucose as glycogen, conversion of glucose to lactate, incorporation of glucose into triglycerides). The increase in peripheral glucose disposal is accompanied by lower plasma insulin concentrations.

Metformin is excreted by the kidney. Therefore, renal disease or any process that reduces glomerular filtration rate necessitates a reduction or discontinuation of metformin. Metformin also increases lactic acid production by the intestine. Normally, the lactic acid is efficiently cleared by the liver. If impaired hepatic function is present, this limitation can result in lactic acidosis that is potentially fatal. Thus, with impaired liver function, metformin treatment is contraindicated. As with tolbutamide, the possibility of increased cardiovascular mortality was reported in the University Group Diabetes Program (UGDP). Subjects who received 100 mg of phenformin per day had a 2.5 fold increase in cardiovascular mortality compared to diet alone resulting in a discontinuation of the study. Since then no study has observed an increase risk of cardiovascular mortality and the UGDP study design has been criticized. It is prudent, however, to know that controversy surrounds early forms of this type of drug. Safety in pregnancy has not been established[86, 88].

The known side effects of metformin are gastrointestinal symptoms – nausea, anorexia, vomiting and diarrhea. Five to twenty percent of patients experience these symptoms. The symptoms appear to be dose related and are responsive to a reduction in the amount of metformin administered. There is no risk of hypoglycemia.

UKPDS demonstrated that metformin was most effective in overweight patients. Metformin promoted weight loss in addition to improving glycemic control. Metformin also resulted in improved macrovascular outcomes. Although the exact mechanism for improved macrovascular outcomes is not known, metformin has been shown to reduce plasminogen activator inhibitor-1 and reduce platelet aggregation. Other potential benefits from metformin therapy include a reduction in plasma triglycerides and a lowering of total cholesterol and LDL-cholesterol[43, 86, 87].

Thiazolidinediones (TZDs)

Research on TZDs began in 1983 and trogitozone was approved for use in January 1997. Thereafter, two additional TZDs, rosiglitozone and pioglitozone, were approved for clinical use.

TZDs are known to bind to a PPAR gamma subtype receptor. PPAR gamma receptor has been shown to induce fat cell differentiation. Whether this is the cellular mechanism by which TZDs affect insulin sensitivity is unclear.

One suggested systemic mechanism for TZDs to improve carbohydrate metabolism is the ability of TZDS to increase fatty acid uptake by the adipose tissue thus reducing plasma fatty acid concentrations. Fatty acids are known to inhibit peripheral glucose uptake and increase hepatic glucose production. A reduction in plasma fatty acid concentration would increase peripheral glucose disposal and reduce hepatic glucose output.

The major side effect of TZDs is weight gain. Hypoglycemia is not seen with monotherapy.

Due to elevated liver enzyme and potential hepatic toxicity, troglitozone was withdrawn from the US in March 2000. Rosiglitozone and pioglitozone have not been associated with hepatic toxicity but it is recommended to follow liver function tests prior to and periodically during therapy. The TZDS have also been associated with expanded intravascular volume. As a result TZDs are contraindicated with renal or cardiac disease. The safety of TZDs in pregnancy has not been established[86, 88].

TZDs have been used as primary therapy in type 2 diabetes. The promotion of weight gain has limited their use in obese diabetics. TZDs have also been used as secondary therapy when metformin or insulin stimulating agent therapy has failed. TZDs provide an added benefit of increasing HDL-Cholesterol[43, 86, 87].

Exogenous insulin

Exogenous insulin is used to treat type 2 diabetes for a number of reasons. First, short-term insulin administration is used to eliminate glucose toxicity in order to make oral therapy more effective. Second, nocturnal administration of insulin is used to inhibit nighttime gluconeogenesis and improve fasting plasma glucose. Third, when other therapies fail, multiple daily injections of insulin are employed to maximize glucose control. The major side effects of insulin therapy are weight gain and hypoglycemia.

TREATMENT OF TYPE 2 DIABETES IN ADOLESCENTS AND CHILDREN

Glycemic Control

A majority of the patients diagnosed with type 2 diabetes in the pediatric population are obese. Considering the treatment options and lessons learned from adults, there appear to be two logical, initial pharmacologic therapies to enhance the effects of proper diet and exercise. First, the use of metformin as a primary monotherapy. Second, with a significant elevation of plasma glucose, the use of short-term exogenous insulin to eliminate glucose toxicity accompanied or followed by metfomin administration as exogenous insulin is gradually discontinued. Due to the anticipated progression of beta cell failure with increased duration of disease, additive rather than substitution or subtraction therapy appears to be the best choice for the long-term management of glycemic control. Additional therapies should be chosen with the goal of exploiting different mechanisms of pharmacologic action in order to attack both insulin resistance or beta cell failure.

A second issue is the high frequency of females in the pediatric population. Since these individuals are entering child bearing years and a majority of the pharmacologic agents have not been shown to be safe in pregnancy, this issue needs to be discussed in detail and options considered to prevent an untoward effect on a developing fetus[86, 88].

Primary Metformin Therapy

Primary metformin therapy is the only treatment that has undergone systematic, scientific evaluation[89]. In a randomized, double blind, placebo controlled study 82 subjects with type 2 diabetes (age range 14-16 years, 70% female, 37 non-Hispanic white, 24 African-American, 18 Hispanic, all having Sustacal stimulated plasma c-peptide concentrations greater than 1.5 ng/ml) received either placebo or 500 mg of metformin twice a day with an increase to 1000 mg twice a day over two weeks for 16 weeks. At the end of the study, the metformin treated group had a lower mean fasting plasma glucose (63 mg/dl lower) and a lower mean hemoglobin A 1c (7.5% vs 8.6%) @ $p < 0.001$ than control subjects. The percentage of subjects who reported gastrointestinal complaints were not significantly different (43% in metformin and 30% in controls). Lipid profile did not change over the 16 weeks of therapy. Blood pressure was not reported. This study demonstrates the efficacy of short-term metformin therapy in adolescents with type 2 diabetes.

Short-Term Exogenous Insulin

Short-term exogenous insulin has been reported anecdotally to be successful to reduce glucose toxicity in subjects with significantly elevated blood sugars associated with concomitant oral therapy (usually metformin) or subsequent administration of metformin with tapering and elimination of insulin therapy. However, no clinical trial has tested the effectiveness of this approach compared to other potential modes of therapy.

Other Glycemic Interventions

Although there are no studies published to demonstrate the safety and efficacy in the pediatric population of other therapeutic interventions used in adults to treat type 2 diabetes, clinicians have used the insulin stimulating and sensitizing agents and alpha glucosidase inhibitors in adolescents. If, due to failure of primary treatment with metformin, a clinician chooses to use these agents prior to the publication of clinical trials demonstrating the safety and efficacy of these agents, the step-wise additive approach used in adults is an excellent model to employ. Each additional agent should be chosen to attack a different point in the disease process (insulin secretion, insulin resistance, glucose absorption) with the additive therapy enhancing blood glucose control.

Non-Glycemic Therapy

Obesity is a consistent but not necessary finding in adults and pediatric patients with type 2 diabetes. The rise in obesity in both populations associated with the increase in type 2 diabetes suggests that obesity is a major contributing factor to the process.

In adults the National Health and Nutrition Education Survey II (NHANES II) (1976-1980) documented a frequency of obesity of 25.5% using BMI > 85th percentile for NHANES II. NAHANES III (1988-1994) using the same criteria for obesity documented a frequency of obesity of 33.3%. This is a rate of increase of obesity of 0.72% per year[90, 91].

In adolescents there has been a similar increase in the frequency of obesity. NHANES studies, using a different definition of obesity (the 95th percentile for BMI in NHANES II) documented an increase in the frequency of obesity from 5.7% (NHANES II, 1976-1980) to 10.8% (NHANES III, 1988-1994)[92]. Population based studies in an urban-suburban school district in Cincinnati using the 85th percentile for BMI for NHANES II demonstrated a frequency of obesity in 3rd to 5th graders of 12.4% in 1975 and 25.3% in 1990,[93] an increase of 0.86% per year. In addition to an increase in the overall frequency of diabetes, specific patterns of obesity are being identified with heavier students becoming more obese than thinner students. In the 3rd to 5th graders in the Cincinnati study, students whose BMI was greater than the 40th percentile were getting more obese than students whose BMI was less than the 40th percentile. In addition, students with BMI greater than the 75th percentile were experiencing the greatest increase in BMI[93]. Recent publications support a continued increase in the frequency of obesity in the pediatric population at all ages[94, 95].

Recent work has suggested a number of physiologic mechanisms for the development of insulin resistance in obese subjects. One very attractive mechanism is the effect of an increase in the amount of visceral adipose tissue. Visceral adipose tissue has been shown to be metabolically different from other types of adipose tissue. Visceral fat releases greater amounts of free fatty acids[96, 97]. Free fatty acids have been shown to induce insulin resistance at both the liver and peripheral tissues[43]. This results in an increase in hepatic glucose output by the liver and reduces insulin stimulated glucose uptake by muscle. This model provides an plausible mechanism for the development of type 2 diabetes in populations experiencing an increase in the frequency of obesity. If this mechanism is a major or sole contributor to the development of type 2 diabetes, then primary and secondary efforts to prevent an increase in visceral adiposity should be an equal or greater focus than the treatment of a complication of obesity – type 2 diabetes.

Recent publications suggest that clinicians need to reconsider their approach and attitude towards obesity[98, 99]. The authors suggest that considering obesity as a disease similar to hypertension may result in more creative, aggressive, and effective methods of treatment. Physical activity and good dietary habits remain the cornerstones of treatment. However, if these therapies fail, secondary intervention with pharmacologic agents in both the short-term and the long-term needs to be considered. Potential types of intervention include agents that block absorption of food or alter central regulation of food intake or thermogenesis[100]. In very selected populations, the risks and potential benefits of surgical intervention also need to be considered. Unfortunately, there are no studies that have demonstrated safety and efficacy of current anti-obesity agents in pediatric patients. However, there are a number of studies in progress and many advances are being made toward understanding the mechanisms involved in the development of obesity. As new knowledge and agents become available, investigators need to apply the information in clinical trials in order to develop safe and effective methods of preventing and treating obesity and reducing the frequency of type 2 diabetes.

SUMMARY

Although the exact prevalence and incidence of type 2 diabetes in the pediatric population has not yet been defined, a number of studies have demonstrated a marked increase in the frequency of the disease in the past decade. Pediatric type 2 diabetes shares many of the characteristics seen in adult type 2 diabetes. Both processes are primarily seen in obese subjects and there is a higher frequency in non-Hispanic white populations. Preliminary data in adolescents suggest that as in type 2 adults, adolescents may have a period of clinically silent hyperglycemia with evidence of cardiovascular, ophthalmologic and renal compromise at or shortly after clinical diagnosis. One major difference between adult and pediatric type 2 diabetes is the marked female gender predominance in pediatrics versus an equal gender distribution in adults. If a female predominance remains or other differences are found as larger pediatric populations are characterized, pediatric type 2 diabetes may result from a different physiologic process than type 2 in adults.

The increased frequency of type 2 diabetes in the pediatric population raises major issues for the individual with the disease, our population as a whole, and future generations. First, the increased personal burden of the disease includes the performance of daily cares for the management of diabetes and the possibility of end organ damage at a younger age. The latter concept is supported by a report of earlier complications in diabetic patients in Japan who were diagnosed with type 2 diabetes in the third decade of life. Of the 135 patients in the report 60% had clinical nephropathy by age 31 years, 23% renal failure requiring dialysis by age 35 years, 24% were blind by age 32 years, and 10% had atherosclerosis by age 36 years[101]. Although these data are not directly applicable to adolescents, the data suggest that development of diabetes at an earlier age will result in more rapid progression to end organ damage. Second, due to the increased frequency of the disease and earlier onset of complications, the financial burden to the population as a whole will rise and limit resources that could be used for other purposes. Finally, data from the Pima Indians document that the presence of maternal diabetes increases the frequency of diabetes in the offspring. Specifically, when maternal diabetes, maternal impaired glucose tolerance, or normal glycemia was present during the pregnancy, 45%, 8.6%, and 1.4% of offspring developed diabetes as young adults, respectively[102]. These data and the increased frequency of type 2 diabetes in a predominantly female population as they enter their child bearing years suggest that the increased frequency of type 2 diabetes in the pediatric population will also place future generations at increased risk for this devastating disease.

REFERENCES

1. Pinhas-Hamiel, O., et al., Increased incidence of non-insulin-dependent diabetes mellitus among adolescents [see comments]. J Pediatr, 1996. 128(5 Pt 1): p. 608-15.
2. Glaser, N.S. and K.L. Jones, Non-insulin dependent diabetes mellitus in Mexican-American children. West J Med, 1998. 168(1): p. 11-6.
3. Scott, C.R., et al., Characteristics of youth-onset noninsulin-dependent diabetes mellitus and insulin-dependent diabetes mellitus at diagnosis. Pediatrics, 1997. 100(1): p. 84-91.
4. Harris, S.B., B.A. Perkins, and E. Whalen-Brough, Non-insulin-dependent diabetes mellitus among First Nations children. New

entity among First Nations people of north western Ontario. Can Fam Physician, 1996. 42: p. 869-76.

5. Fagot-Campagna, A., Knowler, W.C., Pettitt, D.J., Type 2 Diabetes in Pima Indian children: Cardiovascular risk factors at diagnosis and 10 years later. Diabetes, 1998. 47: p. A155.
6. Fagot-Campagna, A., N.R. Burrows, and D.F. Williamson, The public health epidemiology of type 2 diabetes in children and adolescents: a case study of American Indian adolescents in the Southwestern United States. Clin Chim Acta, 1999. 286(1-2): p. 81-95.
7. Dabelea, D., et al., Increasing prevalence of Type II diabetes in American Indian children. Diabetologia, 1998. 41(8): p. 904-10.
8. Hale, D.E., Danney, M.M., Non-insulin dependent diabetes in Hispanic youth (Type 2Y). Diabetes, 1998. 47(Suppl 1): p. A82.
9. Libman, I.M., et al., Was there an epidemic of diabetes in nonwhite adolescents in Allegheny County, Pennsylvania? Diabetes Care, 1998. 21(8): p. 1278-81.
10. Pihoker, C., et al., Non-insulin dependent diabetes mellitus in African-American youths of Arkansas. Clin Pediatr (Phila), 1998. 37(2): p. 97-102.
11. Fagot-Campagna, A., et al., Type 2 diabetes among North American children and adolescents: an epidemiologic review and a public health perspective. J Pediatr, 2000. 136(5): p. 664-72.
12. Savage, P.J., et al., High prevalence of diabetes in young Pima Indians: evidence of phenotypic variation in a genetically isolated population. Diabetes, 1979. 28(10): p. 937-42.
13. Olefsky, J.M., Diabetes mellitus (type II): etiology and pathogenesis, in Endocrinology, L.J. DeGroot, Editor. 1995, W. B. Saunders Company: Philadelphia. p. 1436-63.
14. Harris, M.I., et al., Prevalence of diabetes, impaired fasting glucose, and impaired glucose tolerance in U.S. adults. The Third National Health and Nutrition Examination Survey, 1988-1994 [see comments]. Diabetes Care, 1998. 21(4): p. 518-24.
15. Narayan, K.M.V., et al., Diabetes - a common, growing, serious, costly, and potentially preventable public health problem. Diabetes Research and clinical Practice, 2000. 50(Suppl. 2): p. S77-S84.
16. Javitt, J.C. and Y.-P. Chiang, Economic impact of diabetes, in Diabetes in America, N.I.o. Health, Editor. 1995, National Institutes of Health: Washington D.C. p. 601-11.
17. Thorburn, A.W., et al., Multiple defects in muscle glycogen synthase activity contribute to reduced glycogen synthesis in non-

insulin dependent diabetes mellitus. J Clin Invest, 1991. 87(2): p. 489-95.
18. Cowie, C.C. and M.I. Harris, Physical and metabolic characteristics of persons with diabetes, in Diabetes in America, N.I.o. Health, Editor. 1995, National Institutes of Health: Washington D.C. p. 117-64.
19. Harris, M.I., et al., Prevalence of diabetes and impaired glucose tolerance and plasma glucose levels in U.S. population aged 20-74 yr. Diabetes, 1987. 36(4): p. 523-34.
20. Haffner, S.M., Epidemiology of type 2 diabetes: risk factors. Diabetes Care, 1998. 21 Suppl 3: p. C3-6.
21. Harris, M.I., Undiagnosed NIDDM: clinical and public health issues. Diabetes Care, 1993. 16(4): p. 642-52.
22. Harris, M.I., et al., Onset of NIDDM occurs at least 4-7 yr before clinical diagnosis. Diabetes Care, 1992. 15(7): p. 815-9.
23. Rewers, M. and R.F. Hamman, Risk factors for non-insulin-dependent diabetes, in Diabetes in America, N.I.o. Health, Editor. 1995, National Institutes of Health: Washington D.C. p. 179-220.
24. Newman, B., et al., Concordance for type 2 (non-insulin-dependent) diabetes mellitus in male twins. Diabetologia, 1987. 30(10): p. 763-8.
25. Kaprio, J., et al., Concordance for type 1 (insulin-dependent) and type 2 (non-insulin- dependent) diabetes mellitus in a population-based cohort of twins in Finland [see comments]. Diabetologia, 1992. 35(11): p. 1060-7.
26. Bennett, P.H., Epidemiology of non-insulin-dependent diabetes, in Diabetes mellitus: A fundamental and clinical text, D. LeRoith, S.I. Taylor, and J.M. Olefsky, Editors. 1996, Lippincott-Raven: Philadelphia. p. 455-459.
27. Ravussin, E., et al., Effects of a traditional lifestyle on obesity in Pima Indians. Diabetes Care, 1994. 17(9): p. 1067-74.
28. Kawate, R., et al., Diabetes mellitus and its vascular complications in Japanese migrants on the Island of Hawaii. Diabetes Care, 1979. 2(2): p. 161-70.
29. Helmrich, S.P., et al., Physical activity and reduced occurrence of non-insulin-dependent diabetes mellitus [see comments]. N Engl J Med, 1991. 325(3): p. 147-52.
30. Manson, J.E., et al., A prospective study of exercise and incidence of diabetes among US male physicians. Jama, 1992. 268(1): p. 63-7.
31. Manson, J.E., et al., Physical activity and incidence of non-insulin-dependent diabetes mellitus in women. Lancet, 1991. 338(8770): p. 774-8.

32. Lundgren, H., et al., Fasting serum insulin concentration and early insulin response as risk determinants for developing diabetes. Diabet Med, 1990. 7(5): p. 407-13.
33. Bennett, P.H., W.C. Knowler, and H.R. Baird, Diet and development of non-insulin-dependent diabetes mellitus: An epidemiological perspective, in Diet, diabetes, and atherosclerosis, P.G. Micossi, A.L. Catapano, and R. Paoletti, Editors. 1984, Raven Press: New York. p. 109.
34. Bogardus, C., Metabolic abnormalities in the development of non-insulin-dependent diabetes mellitus, in Diabetes mellitus: A fundamental and clinical text, D. LeRoith, S.I. Taylor, and J.M. Olefsky, Editors. 1996, Lippincott-Raven: Philadelphia. p. 459-467.
35. Caro, J.F., et al., Cellular alterations in liver, skeletal muscle, and adipose tissue responsible for insulin resistance in obesity and type II diabetes. Diabetes Metab Rev, 1989. 5(8): p. 665-89.
36. Olefsky, J.M., et al., Cellular mechanisms of insulin resistance in non-insulin-dependent (type II) diabetes. Am J Med, 1988. 85(5A): p. 86-105.
37. Arner, P., et al., Defective insulin receptor tyrosine kinase in human skeletal muscle in obesity and type 2 (non-insulin-dependent) diabetes mellitus. Diabetologia, 1987. 30(6): p. 437-40.
38. Obermaier-Kusser, B., et al., A defective intramolecular autoactivation cascade may cause the reduced kinase activity of the skeletal muscle insulin receptor from patients with non-insulin-dependent diabetes mellitus. J Biol Chem, 1989. 264(16): p. 9497-504.
39. Damsbo, P., et al., Reduced glycogen synthase activity in skeletal muscle from obese patients with and without type 2 (non-insulin-dependent) diabetes mellitus. Diabetologia, 1991. 34(4): p. 239-45.
40. Nyomba, B.L., et al., Insulin-sensitive tyrosine kinase: relationship with in vivo insulin action in humans. Am J Physiol, 1990. 258(6 Pt 1): p. E964-74.
41. Shulman, G.I., et al., Quantitation of muscle glycogen synthesis in normal subjects and subjects with non-insulin-dependent diabetes by 13C nuclear magnetic resonance spectroscopy [see comments]. N Engl J Med, 1990. 322(4): p. 223-8.
42. Kelley, D.E., M. Mokan, and L.J. Mandarino, Intracellular defects in glucose metabolism in obese patients with NIDDM. Diabetes, 1992. 41(6): p. 698-706.
43. Matthaei, S., et al., Pathophysiology and pharmacological treatment of insulin resistance. Endocr Rev, 2000. 21(6): p. 585-618.

44. Saad, M.F., et al., A two-step model for development of non-insulin-dependent diabetes. Am J Med, 1991. 90(2): p. 229-35.
45. Gepts, W. and P.M. Lecompte, The pancreatic islets in diabetes. Am J Med, 1981. 70(1): p. 105-15.
46. Saito, K., N. Yaginuma, and T. Takahashi, Differential volumetry of A, B and D cells in the pancreatic islets of diabetic and nondiabetic subjects. Tohoku J Exp Med, 1979. 129(3): p. 273-83.
47. Ward, W.K., et al., Pathophysiology of insulin secretion in non-insulin-dependent diabetes mellitus. Diabetes Care, 1984. 7(5): p. 491-502.
48. Everhart, J.E., et al., Duration of obesity increases the incidence of NIDDM. Diabetes, 1992. 41(2): p. 235-40.
49. Lillioja, S., et al., Insulin resistance and insulin secretory dysfunction as precursors of non-insulin-dependent diabetes mellitus. Prospective studies of Pima Indians. N Engl J Med, 1993. 329(27): p. 1988-92.
50. Saad, M.F., et al., The natural history of impaired glucose tolerance in the Pima Indians. N Engl J Med, 1988. 319(23): p. 1500-6.
51. Charles, M.A., et al., Risk factors for NIDDM in white population. Paris prospective study. Diabetes, 1991. 40(7): p. 796-9.
52. Haffner, S.M., et al., Incidence of type II diabetes in Mexican Americans predicted by fasting insulin and glucose levels, obesity, and body-fat distribution. Diabetes, 1990. 39(3): p. 283-8.
53. Sicree, R.A., et al., Plasma insulin response among Nauruans. Prediction of deterioration in glucose tolerance over 6 yr. Diabetes, 1987. 36(2): p. 179-86.
54. Kadowaki, T., et al., Risk factors for worsening to diabetes in subjects with impaired glucose tolerance. Diabetologia, 1984. 26(1): p. 44-9.
55. Modan, M., et al., Effect of past and concurrent body mass index on prevalence of glucose intolerance and type 2 (non-insulin-dependent) diabetes and on insulin response. The Israel study of glucose intolerance, obesity and hypertension. Diabetologia, 1986. 29(2): p. 82-9.
56. Haffner, S.M., H. Miettinen, and M.P. Stern, Are risk factors for conversion to NIDDM similar in high and low risk populations? Diabetologia, 1997. 40(1): p. 62-6.
57. Haffner, S.M., et al., Increased insulin resistance and insulin secretion in nondiabetic African-Americans and Hispanics compared with non-Hispanic whites. The Insulin Resistance Atherosclerosis Study. Diabetes, 1996. 45(6): p. 742-8.

58. Banerji, M.A., et al., Does intra-abdominal adipose tissue in black men determine whether NIDDM is insulin-resistant or insulin-sensitive? Diabetes, 1995. 44(2): p. 141-6.
59. Umpierrez, G.E., et al., Diabetic ketoacidosis in obese African-Americans. Diabetes, 1995. 44(7): p. 790-5.
60. Pinhas-Hamiel, O., L.M. Dolan, and P.S. Zeitler, Diabetic ketoacidosis among obese African-American adolescents with NIDDM. Diabetes Care, 1997. 20(4): p. 484-6.
61. Dean, H. and M.E. Moffatt, Prevalence of diabetes mellitus among Indian children in Manitoba. Arctic Med Res, 1988. 47(Suppl 1): p. 532-4.
62. Owada, M., et al., Descriptive epidemiology of non-insulin dependent diabetes mellitus detected by urine glucose screening in school children in Japan. Acta Paediatr Jpn, 1990. 32(6): p. 716-24.
63. Diabetes Control and Complications Trial (DCCT): results of feasibility study. The DCCT Research Group. Diabetes Care, 1987. 10(1): p. 1-19.
64. Egli, C.A., Increase of early-onset Type 2 Diabetes observed in Asian-Americans as well as other minority youth. Diabetes, 1999. 48(Suppl.): p. A390.
65. Rodriguez, B.L., Personal communication. 2001.
66. Pihoker, C., Personal communication. 2001.
67. Report of the Expert Committee on the Diagnosis and Classification of Diabetes Mellitus. Diabetes Care, 2001. 24(Suppl. 1): p. S5-S20.
68. Verge, C.F., et al., Combined use of autoantibodies (IA-2 autoantibody, GAD autoantibody, insulin autoantibody, cytoplasmic islet cell antibodies) in type 1 diabetes: Combinatorial Islet Autoantibody Workshop. Diabetes, 1998. 47(12): p. 1857-66.
69. Turner, R., et al., UKPDS 25: autoantibodies to islet-cell cytoplasm and glutamic acid decarboxylase for prediction of insulin requirement in type 2 diabetes. UK Prospective Diabetes Study Group. Lancet, 1997. 350(9087): p. 1288-93.
70. Mueller, P., Personal communication. 2001.
71. Savola, K., et al., Autoantibodies associated with Type I diabetes mellitus persist after diagnosis in children. Diabetologia, 1998. 41(11): p. 1293-7.
72. Kolb, H., et al., Prospective analysis of islet cell antibodies in children with type 1 (insulin-dependent) diabetes. Diabetologia, 1988. 31(4): p. 189-94.
73. Winter, W.E., M. Nakamura, and D.V. House, Monogenic diabetes mellitus in youth. The MODY syndromes. Endocrinol Metab Clin North Am, 1999. 28(4): p. 765-85.

74. Winter, W.E. and J.H. Silverstein, Molecular and genetic bases for maturity onset diabetes of youth. Curr Opin Pediatr, 2000. 12(4): p. 388-93.
75. Winter, W.E., et al., Maturity-onset diabetes of youth in black Americans. N Engl J Med, 1987. 316(6): p. 285-91.
76. Savage, P.J., et al., C-Peptide and insulin secretion in Pima Indians and Caucasians: constant fractional hepatic extraction over a wide range of insulin concentrations and in obesity. J Clin Endocrinol Metab, 1979. 48(4): p. 594-8.
77. Lev-Ran, A. and D.L. Hwang, C-peptide in NIDDM. Follow-up for 4-6 yr. Diabetes Care, 1993. 16(1): p. 76-81.
78. Heding, L.G. and S.M. Rasmussen, Human C-peptide in normal and diabetic subjects. Diabetologia, 1975. 11(3): p. 201-6.
79. Levy, J., et al., Beta-cell deterioration determines the onset and rate of progression of secondary dietary failure in type 2 diabetes mellitus: the 10-year follow-up of the Belfast Diet Study. Diabet Med, 1998. 15(4): p. 290-6.
80. Turner, R.C., et al., Glycemic control with diet, sulfonylurea, metformin, or insulin in patients with type 2 diabetes mellitus: progressive requirement for multiple therapies (UKPDS 49). UK Prospective Diabetes Study (UKPDS) Group. Jama, 1999. 281(21): p. 2005-12.
81. Jenson, H.B., et al., Treatment of multiple brain abscesses caused by Bacillus cereus. Pediatr Infect Dis J, 1989. 8(11): p. 795-8.
82. Jiang, X., et al., Racial (black-white) differences in insulin secretion and clearance in adolescents: the Bogalusa heart study. Pediatrics, 1996. 97(3): p. 357-60.
83. Cowie, C.C., M.I. Harris, and M.S. Eberhardt, Frequency and determinants of screening for diabetes in the U.S. Diabetes Care, 1994. 17(10): p. 1158-63.
84. Young, L.A., et al., Lipid abnormalities in adolescents with type 2 diabetes (DM). Diabetes, 2000. 49(Suppl.): p. A352.
85. Young, L.A., et al., Prevalence of blood pressure (BP) elevation at diagnosis in adolescents with type 2 diabetes (DM). Diabetes, 1999. 48(Suppl.): p. A368.
86. Kastrup, E.K., ed. Drug Facts and Comparisons. 2001, Wolters Kluwer Company: St. Louis. 291-312.
87. Mahler, R.J. and M.L. Adler, Clinical review 102: Type 2 diabetes mellitus: update on diagnosis, pathophysiology, and treatment. J Clin Endocrinol Metab, 1999. 84(4): p. 1165-71.
88. Preconception care of women with diabetes. Diabetes Care, 2001. 24(Suppl. 1): p. S66-S68.

89. Jones, K., et al., Metformin improves glycemic control in children with Type 2 Diabetes. Diabetes, 2000. 49(Suppl.): p. A75.
90. Update: prevalence of overweight among children, adolescents, and adults--United States, 1988-1994. MMWR Morb Mortal Wkly Rep, 1997. 46(9): p. 198-202.
91. Must, A., et al., The disease burden associated with overweight and obesity. Jama, 1999. 282(16): p. 1523-9.
92. Prevalence of overweight among adolescents--United States, 1988-91. MMWR Morb Mortal Wkly Rep, 1994. 43(44): p. 818-21.
93. Morrison, J.A., et al., Sex and race differences in cardiovascular disease risk factor changes in schoolchildren, 1975-1990: the Princeton School Study. Am J Public Health, 1999. 89(11): p. 1708-14.
94. Bundred, P., Evidence that young children have joined the race towards obesity. British Medical Journal, 2001. 322: p. 326.
95. Rosner, B., et al., Percentiles for body mass index in U.S. children 5 to 17 years of age. J Pediatr, 1998. 132(2): p. 211-22.
96. Matsuzawa, Y., et al., Pathophysiology and pathogenesis of visceral fat obesity. Ann N Y Acad Sci, 1995. 748: p. 399-406.
97. Goran, M.I. and B.A. Gower, Relation between visceral fat and disease risk in children and adolescents. Am J Clin Nutr, 1999. 70(1): p. 149S-56S.
98. Kopelman, P.G., Obesity as a medical problem. Nature, 2000. 404(6778): p. 635-43.
99. Friedman, J.M., Obesity in the new millennium. Nature, 2000. 404(6778): p. 632-4.
100. Bray, G.A. and L.A. Tartaglia, Medicinal strategies in the treatment of obesity. Nature, 2000. 404(6778): p. 672-7.
101. Yokoyama, H., et al., Existence of early-onset NIDDM Japanese demonstrating severe diabetic complications. Diabetes Care, 1997. 20(5): p. 844-7.
102. Pettitt, D.J., et al., Congenital susceptibility to NIDDM. Role of intrauterine environment. Diabetes, 1988. 37(5): p. 622-8.

Chapter 4
MATURITY-ONSET DIABETES OF THE YOUNG:
Autosomal Dominant Forms of Youth-Onset Diabetes

William E. Winter, M.D.
University of Florida
Department of Pathology, Immunology, & Laboratory Medicine and Pediatrics

INTRODUCTION

In order to gain an understanding of maturity-onset diabetes of youth (MODY), we need to understand the general classification of diabetes mellitus [1,2,3]. Diabetes mellitus is classified as Type 1 diabetes (T1DM), Type 2 diabetes (T2DM), other specific types of diabetes (2^0 diabetes) and gestational diabetes (GDM)[4]. Type 1 diabetes is primary insulinopenic diabetes and is sub-classified as type 1a: autoimmune (e.g., islet autoantibody positive; T1ADM) and type 1b: idiopathic (e.g., islet autoantibody negative; T1BDM)[5]. Autoantibodies against the islets are the best evidence for autoimmunity in individual T1DM subjects[6]. The most helpful autoantibodies in this regard are islet cell cytoplasmic autoantibodies (ICA)[7,8], insulin autoantibodies (IAA)[9], glutamic acid decarboxylase autoantibodies (GADA)[10], and insulinoma-associated-2 autoantibodies (IA-2A)[11]. Type1B diabetes has been hypothesized to result from viral infection and destruction of the beta cells but evidence for this is limited [12].

Six genetic loci have been confirmed that influence the development of type 1 diabetes: IDDM1; 6p21: the human leukocyte antigen complex (HLA; susceptibility alleles:DR3, DR4, DQB1*0302, *0201; protective alleles: DR2, DBQ1*0602); IDDM2; 11p15: the insulin gene VNTR (variable number of tandem repeats)[13]; IDDM4; 11q13; IDDM5; 6q25; IDDM8; 6q27; and IDDM12; 2q33 (possibly CTLA4)[14].

Type 2 diabetes (T2DM) results from insulin resistance plus relative insulinopenia, and is non-autoimmune [15, 16]. T2DM can be subdivided by age at onset into adult/maturity-onset T2DM [non insulin-dependent diabetes mellitus (NIDDM), adult-onset diabetes (AOD) or maturity-onset diabetes (MOD)] and pediatric-onset T2DM [e.g., early-onset diabetes or non-insulin-dependent diabetes of youth (NIDDY)][17]. Pediatric T2DM is becoming increasingly common[18,19]. T2DM usually involves defects in the beta cell secretion of insulin (e.g., progressive relative and later possible absolute insulinopenia) and liver (e.g., excess hepatic glucose output) and muscle/adipose tissue responses to insulin (e.g., decreased glucose clearance) [20]. The liver can be either a net glucose consumer (e.g, the postprandial state) or a net glucose producer (e.g., durin fasting). Adipose and muscle tissue are major sites of insulin action and serve t clear glucose from the circulation. Insulin resistance in insulin sensitive tissue is a common finding in T2DM[21].

Other specific types of diabetes that *may* cause non-insulin depender forms of diabetes in children include genetic defects of ß-cell function. Geneti defects of ß-cell function include maturity-onset diabetes of youth (MODY)[22, 2 mitochondrial diabetes syndromes[24], insulinopathies and hyperproinsulinemias [2 MODY gene defects may account for 2 to 3% of adult EuropeanT2DM[26].

Mitochondrial diabetes syndromes are recognized by their maternal mod of inheritance (e.g., disease is passed only from mothers to their offspring; sperr do not pass on mitochondria)[27]. The severity of mitochondrial diseases depend upon the specific mutation and the mutations "prevalence" among the subject' mitochondria and distribution among their tissues. Variable numbers and kind of mitochondria (e.g., normal and abnormal) is termed "heteroplasmy." As th percentage of abnormal mitochondria increases, the likelihood of more sever disease increases. The proportion of normal and abnormal mitochondria als varies among tissues at random and thus tissues with a higher percentage o abnormal mitochondria will be more severely affected. Heteroplasmy and variabl tissue distribution can account for the wide clinical variability observed for an single mitochondrial DNA mutation. Mitochondrial diabetes has been reporte as an isolated finding or as part of a multi-component syndrome such as MELAS (mitochondrial encephalopthy, lactic acidosis and stroke-like syndrome) o MERRF(myoclonic epilepsy and ragged red fiber disease). In Japan 1 to 3% o cases of T2DM are ascribed to mitochondrial mutations. Mechanisitically it i hypothesized that the mitochondrial mutations interfere with beta-cell energy production and this leads to hypoinsulinism[28]. The most common mitochondria mutation associated with diabetes is A3243G involving the $tRNA^{Leu(UUR}$ anc deafness[29]. Several other diabetogenic mutations can occur concurrently with the A3243G such as C946A (12SrRNA) and A1041G (12SrRNA), T3394C (NADH dehydrogenase 1) and G4491A (NADH dehydrogenase 2). Some of these mutations are associated with cardiomyopathy or Leiber hereditary optic neuropathy (LHON). Other diabetogenic mitochondrial mutations occur independently of A3243G: A3252G ($tRNA^{Leu(UUR)}$), C3256T ($tRNA^{Leu(UUR)}$), A3260G ($tRNA^{Leu(UUR)}$), T3271C ($tRNA^{Leu(UUR)}$), G3316A (NADH dehydrogenase 1) and T14709C ($tRNA^{Glu}$). These later mutations may be variously associated with myopathy, cardiomyopathy, LHON or MELAS. Mitochondrial diabetes syndromes are uncommonly insulin-dependent. Insulinopathies and hyperproinsulinemias are very rare.

CLINICAL DIAGNOSIS OF DIABETES

Because therapy is predicated on pathophysiology, identification of the specific type of diabetes affecting an individual is critical to proper diabetes management[30,31]. A clinical approach to diabetes classification is to divide diabetes into acute-onset diabetes versus insidious-onset diabetes because mode-of-presentation is the first clinical expression of disease that the treating physician observes.

Insulin treated, ketotic, lean children with diabetes most likely have T1DM. In African American youth with acute onset-diabetes who have a strong family history of early-onset T2DM, atypical diabetes mellitus (ADM) must be considered (see below)[32]. Uncommonly, severely obese minority (African, Hispanic or Native American) adolescents may present with ketosis or DKA and later be diagnosed with T2DM [33].

In insidious-onset diabetes, obese minority children are likely to have T2DM[34]. If the Caucasian child with insidious-onset diabetes is lean and has a strong family history of autosomal dominant diabetes, MODY is diagnosed[22]. If the mode of inheritance is maternal, mitochondrial diabetes is a likely diagnostic consideration.

MODY: CLINICAL DIAGNOSIS

Fajans and coworkers[35] originally described the clinical characteristics of MODY ~30 years ago. By definition according to Fajans [36], 1) the onset of MODY occurs prior to age 25 years; 2) MODY is non-insulin requiring and non-ketotic; and 3) MODY is inherited as an autosomal dominant trait. Fajans' definition was based primarily upon his experience with the large RW pedigree[37]. MODY in this family was ultimately shown to result from a mutation in hepatocyte nuclear factor-4α ("MODY1"). MODY is now identified worldwide affecting almost every major ethnic group[38].

First described in 1987, ADM is a subtype of MODY that occurs in ~10% of African American children with youth-onset diabetes[32]. The age of onset of ADM is generally <40 years old. ADM presents acutely (often with ketosis or even diabetic ketoacidosis, e.g., DKA) distinguishing ADM from classic Caucasian MODY. ADM is non-insulin requiring after months to years following initial diagnosis. This transition from a "type 1" to a "type 2" phenotype distinguishes ADM from most cases of insidious-onset pediatric T2DM. Only ~40 to 50% of ADM children are obese which likely represents the high frequency of obesity in the background African American population. On the other hand, children with T2DM are essentially always massively obese. ADM subjects are insulinopenic[32] and lack a first phase insulin response to intravenous glucose administration. In one member of an ADM family, a glucokinase mutation was discovered[39] while in another family a mitochondrial variation or mutation was identified[40].

In Caucasians and Japanese with MODY, 5 molecular causes of MODY have been identified[41,22,23]:(1) MODY1: Hepatocyte nuclear factor-4 alpha (HNF-4α) mutations; (2) MODY2: Glucokinase (GCK) mutations; (3) MODY3: Hepatocyte nuclear factor-1 alpha (HNF-1α) mutations; (4) MODY4: Insulin promoter factor-1 (IPF-1) mutations; and (5) MODY5: Hepatocyte nuclear factor-1 beta (HNF-1ß) mutations (Table 1).

Table 1: Classification of the MODY syndromes

MODY Type	Defective gene	Abbreviation
MODY1	Hepatocyte nuclear factor-4α	HNF-4α
MODY2	Glucokinase	GCK
MODY3	Hepatocyte nuclear factor-1α	HNF-1α
MODY4	Insulin promoter factor-1	IPF-1
MODY5	Hepatocyte nuclear factor-1ß	HNF-1ß

Clinical Classification	Major population group affected
Classic MODY	Caucasians
Atypical Diabetes Mellitus	African Americans

Four of these 5 causes of MODY involve transcription factor mutations (e.g. the HNF and IPF-1 forms of MODY). The penetrance of diabetes in carriers of the transcription factor forms of MODY is usually >80% by age 40 but not absolute[42]. On the other hand because of its mild nature, as few as 50% of GCK mutation carriers may present with clinical diabetes unless routine oral glucose tolerance testing is carried out. Prior to the discovery of the individual MODY mutations, a wide spectrum of beta-cell abnormalities were described and thus no consistent metabolic phenotype for MODY emerged from the early studies[43].

MODY2

MODY2: Glucokinase Mutations

MODY2 results from mutations in the glucokinase (GCK) gene [44]. GCK mutations were the first molecular etiology for MODY identified although the MODY1 genetic locus had previously been mapped to chromosome 20. MODY2 is discussed first among the various MODY syndromes because GCK mutations were indeed the first molecular causes of MODY identified. Furthermore, GCK mutations produce the diabetic state in a manner fundamentally different from the transcription factor mutations (MODY1, MODY3, MODY4 and MODY5).

Froguel's initial 1992 report of the linkage of MODY to GCK involved studies of 16 French MODY families[45]. Between 45% and 95% of these families demonstrated coinheritance of the MODY phenotype and GCK alleles. One month later Vionnet et al.[46] described the first GCK mutation in MODY: in exon 7 in the F8 MODY kindred, glutamic acid at residue 279 was shown to be replaced by an amber stop codon (E279X). Whereas the normal codon at position 279 was GAG, the mutated GCK gene displayed GAT introducing the termination codon into the GCK sequence. The truncated GCK product would be only ~60% of the full length GCK gene (normally 465 amino acids).

Presently more than 80 GCK mutations have been described (for example,[48] Guazzini[47]. MODY2 is the most common cause of MODY in France and the second most common cause of MODY in the U.K. (note: the most common cause of MODY in the U.K. is HNF-1α mutations). The difference in the distribution of causes of MODY between France and the U.K. may be due to different criteria used to search for MODY families in these countries where the French investigate families with more modest degrees of hyperglycemia than the British investigators.

MODY2: Metabolism

Clinically, MODY2 patients display essentially non-progressive or only mildly progressive insulinopenia with relatively mild diabetes and fasting hyperglycemia. There is an apparent low rate of complications. MODY2 patients may be asymptomatic or female carriers may present with GDM. Usually 50% of carriers of GCK mutations eventually develop diabetes.

On average, plasma glucose levels in GCK deficiency are ~40 mg/dL higher than in controls but ~100 mg/dL below those levels observed in patients with classic T2DM. Typical of most diabetic states, MODY2 patients exhibit hyperglucagonemia. Counterregulatory responses to hypoglycemia are also activated at a higher than normal glucose level in individuals with GCK mutations[49].

Nonglucose secretagogues induce insulin secretion in MODY2 subjects to a degree similar to controls. This is should not be surprising as nutrient amino acid stimulation of beta-cell energy production would occur independent of GCK and at a metabolic step distal to GCK's actions.

Glucose in newborns is mildly increased above normal and birth weight is decreased by ~500 gms presumably because of intrauterine insulin deficiency. However if the mother is affected with a GCK mutation, mild maternal hyperglycemia (inducing fetal hyperglycemia) may balance intrinsic fetal hypoinsulinemia and produce an infant of normal birth weight for gestational age. Mild neonatal diabetes has been reported to result from a novel hemizygous GCK mutation. Two cases of severe, permanent neonatal diabetes due to complet (homozygous) GCK deficiency have also been reported[50]. One infant wa Norwegian and one infant was Italian. Homozygous transcription factor mutation have not been described.

MODY2: Pathobiology

Over 10 years ago, Matschinsky [51] proposed that GCK functions as th beta-cell glucose sensor. His hypothesis was proven when French MODY familie were first found to harbor GCK mutations[52]. Localized to chromosome 7p15-p13 the GCK gene has 12 exons. The first three exons are termed 1B (1a), 1H (1b and 2a (1c) where 1B is the first exon transcribed in beta cells and 1H is the firs exon transcribed in hepatocytes (Figure 1). The remaining 9 exons are numbere 2 through 10. In the beta cell, alternative splicing of GCK mRNA aligns exon 1I with exons 2 through 10. In the liver, GCK transcription begins with exon 1H an then continues with exon 2 having spliced out exon 2A. The less abundant form of hepatocyte GCK mRNA includes exon 2.

Once GCK was discovered to be a cause of MODY, investigators sough the mechanism of action whereby GCK mutations might cause diabetes[53]. Early on, mutations in GCK were hypothesized to alter glucose and/or ATP binding[5 to the enzyme. GCK, also known as hexokinase D or type IV, is expressed in bet cells and hepatocytes. GCK functions as the glucose sensor of the beta cell. In th hepatocyte, GCK plays a role in glucose clearance. Normally when glucose enter the beta cell via the facilitative glucose transporter-2 (GLUT2), GCK i responsible for the phosphorylation of glucose to glucose-6-phosphate.

Because of the kinetics of GCK activity (low affinity for glucose, high K_m and high V_{max}), the rate of formation of glucose-6-phosphate normally reflect the extracellular glucose concentration. GCK is not inhibited by its product glucose-6-phosphate. In contrast other hexokinases exhibit low K_m , low V_{ma} kinetics and are inhibited by glucose-6-phosphate. The rate of formation o glucose-6-phosphate then controls the rate of energy production within the bet cell with the production of ATP from ADP and inorganic phosphate (Figure 2) The mitochondria play a major role in energy production as pyruvate derived fron glycolysis enters the Krebs citric acid cycle. During the Krebs cycle for each acetyl-CoA entering the cycle (2 per glucose molecule burned), hydrogen i liberated in the form of 3 NADH and 1 $FADH_2$ molecules. Mitochondria oxidative phosphorylation of NADH and $FADH_2$ subsequently produces large amounts of ATP during electron transport.

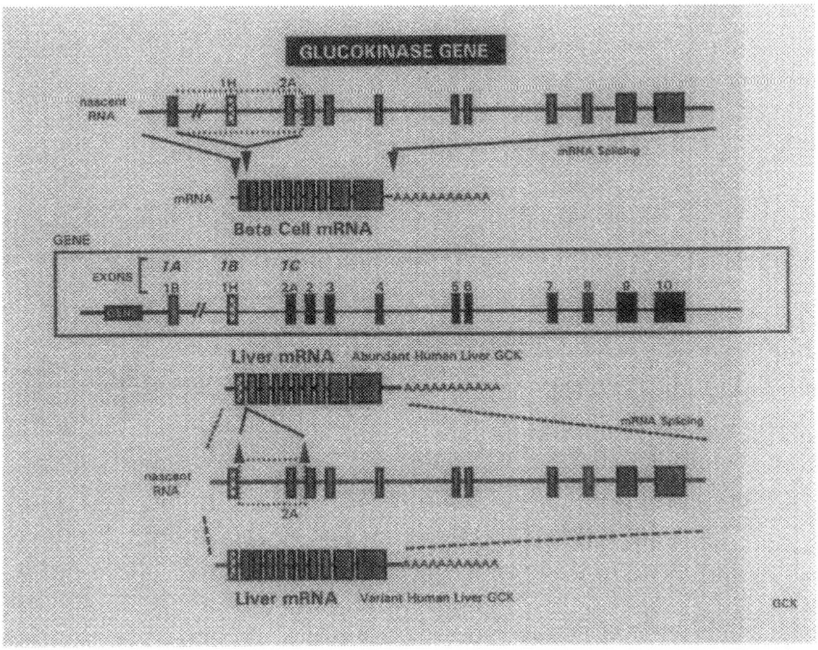

Figure 1: The germline glucokinase (GCK) gene is depicted in the rectangle. The GCK gene is transcribed differentially in the beta cell (top) and hepatocyte (bottom). In the hepatocyte, variable splicing of the nascent mRNA transcript leads to the production of two hepatocyte mRNAs.

As the ratio of ATP to ADP plus inorganic phosphate rises and ADP and inorganic phosphate concentrations fall, a beta-cell ATP-sensitive potassium channel is inhibited. This potassium channel normally allows K+ to leave the beta cell. The channel is composed of two types of subunits: the inwardly rectifying potassium channel $K_{ir}6.2$ and the sulfonylurea receptor (SUR). Kir6.2 is encoded on chromosome 11p14.1 whereas the SUR gene is located close by on chromosome 11p15.1. With a rise in intracellular potassium, the beta cell depolarizes. Subsequent to depolarization, the voltage-dependent calcium channel opens. As intracytoplasmic concentrations of ionized calcium rise, fusion of insulin-containing granules with the beta-cell plasma membrane occurs triggering insulin exocytosis.

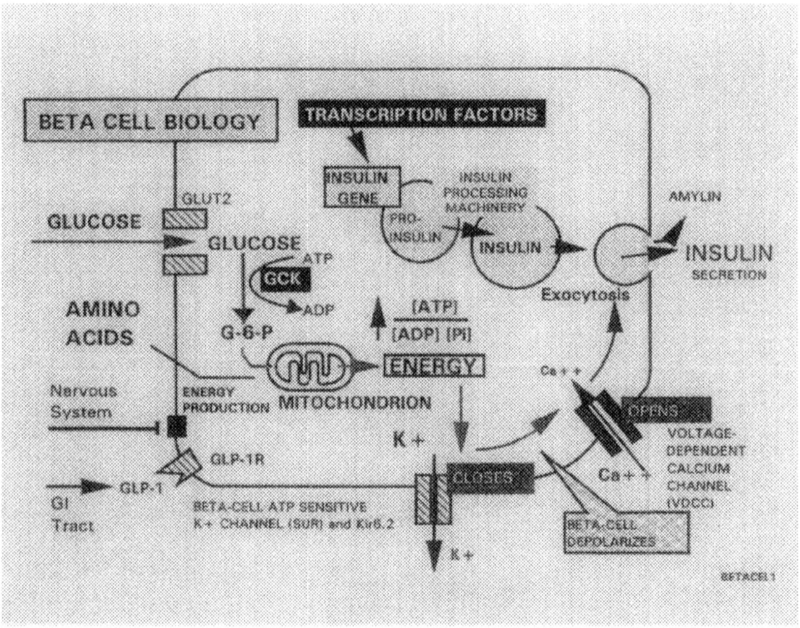

Figure 2: Beta cell insulin release responds to many stimuli: glucose, amino acids, nervous system innervation, and gastrointestinal tract hormones such as glucagon-like peptide-1 (GLP-1). Glucose enters the beta-cell via the facilitative glucose transporter GLUT2. Within the beta cell, glucose is phosphorylated to glucose-6-phosphate (G-6-P) via the catalytic action of glucokinase (GCK). Via glycolysis, the mitochondrial Krebs citric acid cycle and oxidative phosphorylation, energy is produced as beta-cell ATP concentrations rise and ADP and inorganic phosphate (Pi) concentrations decline. Subsequently, the potassium channel closes. This channel is constituted by the sulfonylurea receptor (SUR) and the inwardly-rectified Kir6.2 K+ subunit. With a rise in intracellular K+ concentrations, the beta cell depolarizes. Next, the voltage-dependent calcium channel opens. Increased cytoplasmic free calcium induces insulin exocytosis as insulin granules fuse with the plasma membrane to release insulin as well as other beta-cell products such as amylin (islet-associated polypeptide). Because amino acids can provide cellular energy, amino acids can release insulin. Amino acids acid distal to the action of glucose and GCK.

In subjects with MODY2, if the beta cell is less responsive to plasma glucose than normal because of a GCK loss-of-function mutation, e.g., the beta-cell is glucose "resistant" or insensitive, and beta-cell insulin release is decreased[55]. Such is the case for GCK mutations. Consequently the positive relationship between change in insulin secretion rate versus plasma glucose is shifted to the right. Whereas the insulin secretion rate is lower than normal at baseline, the insulin secretion rate does, nevertheless, rise with increasing glucose concentrations in the plasma. Very different from bothT1DM, T2DM and other forms of MODY, MODY2 subjects display a first phase insulin release to acute intravenous glucose injection although this is less profound than in controls[56].

As early as 1993, defects in the hepatic GCK gene were shown to contribute to hyperglycemia in MODY2[57]. Hepatic GCK is necessary for plasma glucose clearance and a defect in hepatic GCK would lead to decreased hepatic glucose clearance and hyperglycemia following meals. As well, decreased hepatic GCK activity could impair the normal suppression in hepatic glucose output that should occur with plasma hyperglycemia. Because insulin regulates hepatic GCK synthesis, via hypoinsulinism defects limited to the beta-cell portion of the GCK gene can produce hepatic GCK deficiency. The interrelationship between beta-cell GCK function and hepatocyte GCK function is illustrated in Figure 3.

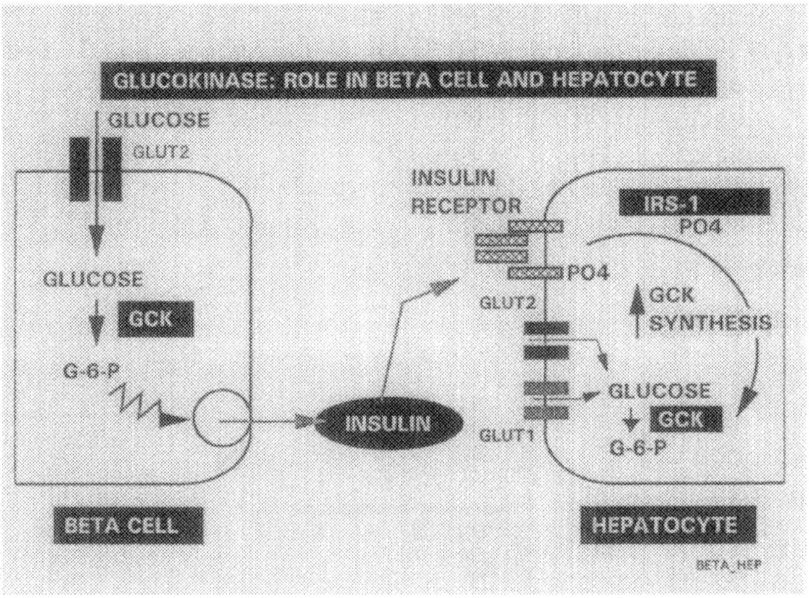

Figure 3: Appropriate beta-cell release of insulin is dependent on normal beta-cell glucokinase (GCK) function. In the hepatocyte, GCK synthesis is insulin regulated. Thus indirectly, the beta-cell GCK controls hepatocyte GCK expression. When insulin binds to the insulin receptor, the insulin receptor acquires tyrosine kinase activity that leads to autophosphorylation and phosphorylation of insulin receptor substrate-1 (ISR-1). GLUT1: facilitative glucose transporter-1; GLUT2: facilitative glucose transporter-2; GLUT4: facilitative glucose transporter-4; glucose-6-phosphate: G-6-P; PO4: phosphate.

MODY2: Prevalence

As noted above, MODY2 mutations are common in MODY pedigrees. However, GCK , 1997 mutations are an uncommon cause (<0.2%) of adult T2DM in the U.S.[58] and Japan[59]. In contrast to the above studies that found little relationship between GCK and "classic" T2DM, a compound-imperfect dinucleotide $(CA)_n$ repeat ~10 kb 3' of GCK was identified as a genetic marker of T2DM in African Americans[60].

MODY1

MODY1: Hepatocyte Nuclear Factor-4α Mutations

MODY1 results from mutations in the transcription factor HNF-4α (chr. 20q12-q13.1) (Figure 4). This was the second MODY transcription factor mutation discovered in 1996[61]. Previously in the early 1990's using linkage studies, MODY in the large RW pedigree had been mapped to chromosome 20q near the adenosine deaminase (ADA) gene[62]. Thus the chromosome 20q-linked form of MODY was termed "MODY1." While MODY1 was the first MODY locus mapped, GCK was the first MODY gene discovered (MODY2). After HNF-1α mutations were discovered as the cause of MODY3[63], HNF-4α in the RW pedigree was studied because HNF-4α was on chromosome 20q between D20S169 and D20S176. The discovery that MODY1 was caused by HNF-4α mutations is a seminal example of positional cloning that directly followed from the discovery of HNF-1α as the MODY3 gene.

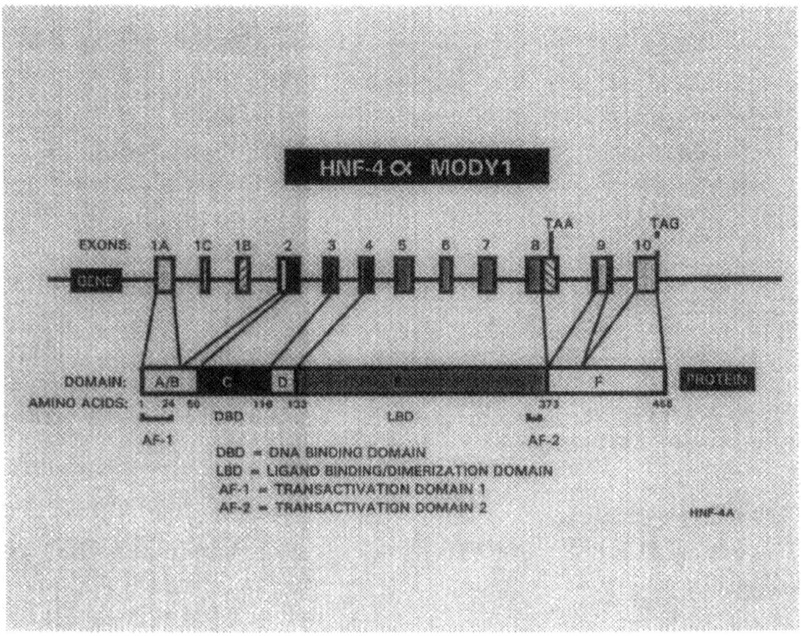

Figure 4: The cause of MODY1 is mutations in the hepatocyte nuclear factor-4α gene (HNF-4α). The gene and protein product are depicted. TAA and TAG are stop codons.

MODY1: Metabolism

Beta-cell dysfunction in MODY1 was recognized years before HNF-4α was discovered to be the cause of MODY1[37]. Clinically, MODY1 patients display progressive insulinopenia with increasing age. MODY1 is more severe than MODY2 as MODY1 subjects exhibit substantial micro and macrovascular complications.

Using a stepped (graded) glucose infusion protocol, non-diabetic carriers of MODY1 mutations demonstrated a decreased insulin secretion rate (ISR) once plasma glucose exceeded ~126 mg/dL[64] (Figure 5). In this protocol, the glucose is initially brought to ~90 mg/dL using a small bolus of insulin followed by continuous insulin infusion. After 20 minutes without insulin infusion (insulin "washout"), 3 samples separated by 10 minutes each are obtained to determine the basal insulin, glucose, and C-peptide concentrations. Subsequently 40 minute infusions rising in a step-wise manner are accomplished (1, 2, 3, 4, 6, and 8 mg • kg^{-1} • min^{-1}). At 10 minute intervals into each 40 minute step, insulin, glucose, and C-peptide are measured. Thus at each step, ISR is determined and is graphed versus the glucose concentration. To determine if glucose priming of the beta cells improves a subsequent exposure to stepped glucose infusions, the subject is infused with glucose at 4-6 mg • kg^{-1} • min^{-1} for 42 hours. The glucose infusion is then weaned to zero over 60 minutes and 30 minutes later the stepped glucose infusions are repeated. In MODY1 non-diabetic carriers, the ISR up to plasma glucose levels of ~120 to ~130 mg/dL is not significantly less than controls (Figure 6 large rectangle). However above this range, whereas the control subjects' ISR continues to rise as plasma glucose rises, the rate of rise in the ISR in MODY1 carriers is marginal and post-challenge hyperglycemia ensues. Non-diabetic MODY1 carriers display no increase in ISRs after priming (Figure 6 lower middle panel) (Table 2). Using these same protocols, the ISR curve in MODY2 carriers was right-shifted (as described above, Figure 6, large rectangle) and glucose-priming did increase the subsequent ISR measurement (Figure 6: lower left panel).

Table 2: Metabolic Characteristics of MODY1, MODY2, and MODY3

	MODY1 (HNF-4α)	MODY2 (GCK)	MODY3 (HNF-1α)
Insulin secretory rate (ISR) up to ~110-126 mg/dL	~Normal	Deficient	~Normal
Rate of rise in ISR above ~110-126mg/dL	Deficient to flat	Greater than MODY1 and MODY3, but less than controls	Deficient to flat
ISR potentiation following glucose infusion	None	Yes	Yes
Response to non-glucose secret-agogues	Deficient	Normal	Not reported

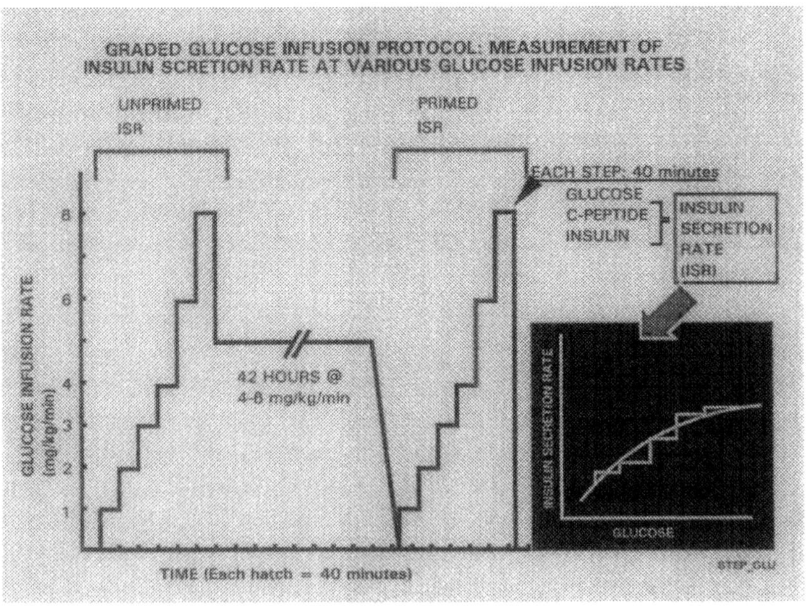

Figure 5: The stepped-glucose infusion protocol allows measurement of the insulin secretion rate (ISR) (see text for a detailed description of the protocol). For subsequent illustrative purposes in

Figure 6, the stepped ISR data has been smoothed (right side of figure).

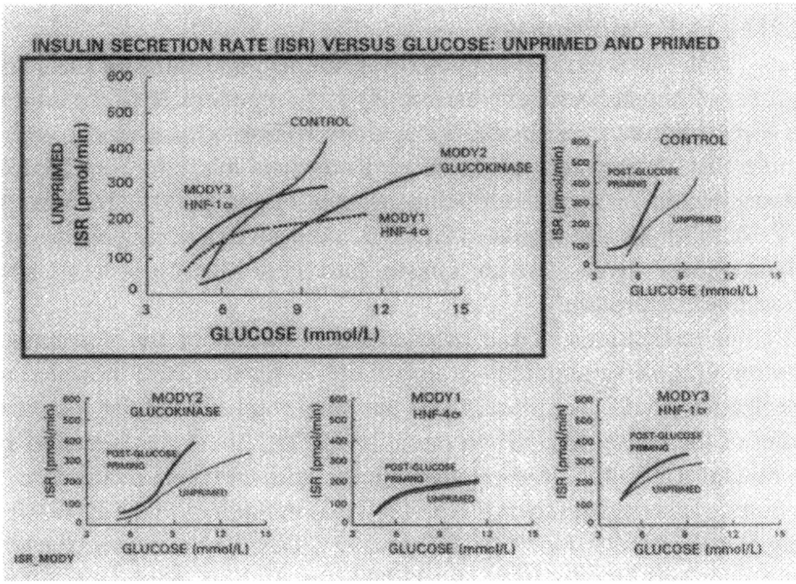

Figure 6: Rectangle: Unprimed, non-diabetic MODY2 carriers display a right-ward shift in the ISR to glucose response curve. Because of relative beta-cell insensitivity, higher than normal glucose levels must be reached before insulin is released. For MODY1 and MODY3 carriers, at near-normal levels of plasma glucose (~6 mmol/L, 108 mg/dL), ISR rates are not significantly lower than in controls. However above this range, while controls exhibit a steady rise in ISR with increasing glucose, MODY1 and MODY3 carriers display an attenuated ISR response. Outside the rectangle: The top right graph demonstrates that following priming, normal controls show an Increased ISR response to glucose. MODY2 and MODY3 carriers display a modest increase in ISR with priming (lower left graph and lower right graph) whereas MODY1 carriers do not experience an increase in ISR with priming (lower middle graph). (conversion for glucose: 1 mmol/L = 18 mg/dL)

Low C-peptide and low proinsulin responses to glucose have been demonstrated in MODY1[65]. Diminished glucagon secretion in response to arginine may be a unique metabolic feature of MODY1[66]. Reduced pancreatic polypeptide responses to hypoglycemia and reduced amylin secretion in response to arginine have also been noted[67]. This suggests a pan-islet lesion in MODY1. Somatostatin secretion has not been reported in MODY1. Loss of first phase insulin response to intravenous glucose injection is observed in MODY1 subjects[68]. Recall that MODY2 subjects do exhibit a first phase response to intravenous glucose challenge. Lipid abnormalities have been reported in

MODY1 subjects: ~3 fold elevated Lp(a) concentrations[65] and low concentrations of triglycerides and apo CIII[68].

MODY1: Pathobiology

HNF-4α is expressed in the liver, kidney, intestine and islets and is a ke regulator of hepatic gene expression. HNF-4α regulates HNF-1α which, in tur is a direct regulator of insulin gene transcription. Coactivators with HNF-4 include SRC-1 (protooncogene SRC, Rous sarcoma, chr. 20q12-q13), GRIP (glucocorticoid receptor interacting protein 1) and p300[69]. Besides regulatin HNF-1α, HNF-4α also regulates GLUT2, aldolase B, glyceraldehyde-3-phospha dehydrogenase, liver pyruvate kinase, fatty acid binding proteins and cellul retinol binding protein[70].

Investigations of the mechanism of action of the nonsense HNF-4 mutation Q268X (glutamine --> stop codon at residue 268) indicated that whi dimerization could take place, there was abnormal subcellular localization[71]. I studies of the missense HNF-4α mutation E276Q, there was impaired synergy c the mutant HNF-4α transcription factor with chicken ovalbumin upstrea promoter transcription factor II (COUP TFII) in binding to the HNF-1α promote using electrophoretic mobility shift assays[72]. Despite the expression of HNF-4 in the liver and kidney, liver and kidney function in individuals affected wit HNF-4α mutations is normal[65].

MODY1: Prevalence

HNF-4α mutations are not common causes (<0.0001%) of adult-onse T2DM [73]. Sakurai et al.[74] described 2 of 100 T2DM subjects (2%) with onset afte age 25 with a cytosine to thymidine nucleotide substitution at the -5 nucleotid position in the HNF-4α intron 1b. Otherwise all populations studied to date do no exhibit high frequencies of HNF-4α mutations in subjects with T2DM. Studie in the Caucasian U.S. T2DM population[75] and in Pima Indians with early-onse T2DM[76] have been negative.

MODY3

MODY3: Hepatocyte Nuclear Factor-1α Mutations

MODY3 results from mutations in the transcription factor HNF-1α (ch 12q24.2) (Figure 7)[63]. Similar to MODY1, MODY3 subjects display progressive insulinopenia with increasing age and present with clinical symptoms of diabete during adolescence or young adulthood. There is a favorable therapeutic respons to oral sulfonylureas although insulin may be required at a later date a insulinopenia advances with age. Some MODY3 subjects may be very well controlled on sulfonylureas or even exhibit hypoglycemia in response tc sulfonylurea therapy.

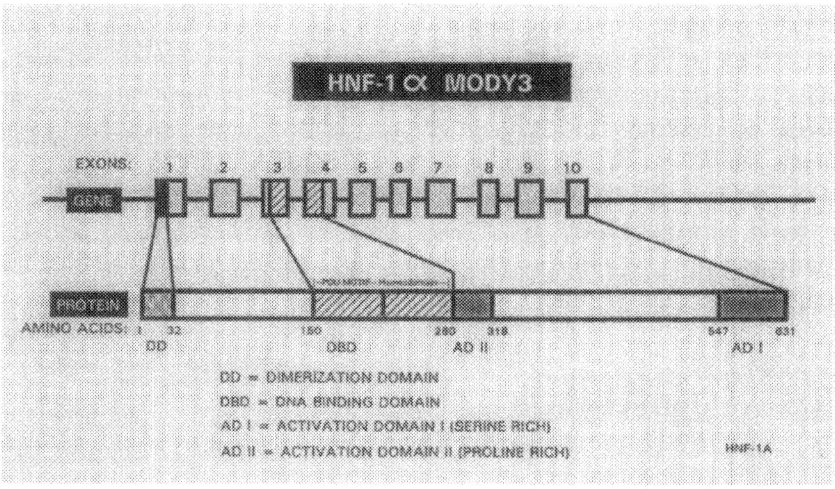

Figure 7: The cause of MODY3 is mutations in the hepatocyte nuclear factor-1α gene (HNF-1α). The gene and protein product are depicted.

Diabetic complications are not uncommon in MODY3 subjects. Isomaa et al.[77] found that microvascular complications were as common in MODY3 subjects as in T1DM or T2DM subjects. Similar to MODY2, MODY3 displays perinatal effects. Birth weight is decreased by ~120 gms. Also similar to MODY2, reduced birth weight likely reflects intrauterine insulin deficiency. While most individuals with HNF-1α mutations exhibit a MODY phenotype, some individuals may display a clinical phenotype otherwise identified as T1DM. Yamada et al.[78] detected HNF-1α mutations in 5.4% (3 of 55) of their T1DM subjects.

MODY3: Metabolism

Post-glucose challenge, in MODY3 subjects the elevation in glucose is greater than the elevation in fasting glucose level above normal. Hypoinsulinism was documented in Finnish MODY3 subjects and in non-diabetic MODY3-carriers[79].

Using the stepped glucose infusion protocol[80], in the fasting state the insulin secretion rate (ISR) below 120 to 130 mg/dL in non-diabetic MODY3-carriers was similar to non-diabetic MODY1-carriers and controls. However above 120 to 130 mg/dL, the ISR did not rise as rapidly in MODY3-carriers (or MODY1-carriers) as in controls (Figure 6: large rectangle). This likely accounts for the accentuated post-glucose challenge hyperglycemia observed in MODY3 subjects. In contrast to non-diabetic MODY1-carriers where 42 hours of glucose priming did not increase ISR, priming did increase ISR in non-diabetic MODY3-carriers (Figure 6: lower right panel). However, *diabetic* MODY3 subjects showed no increment in ISR with glucose priming and ISRs were lower in the diabetic MODY3 subjects than in the non-diabetic MODY3-carriers. In addition to their adverse effect on beta-cell function, HNF-1α mutations appear to affect the renal threshold for glycosuria. Whereas the mean renal threshold for glycosuria in T1DM subjects was 193 mg/dL, in subjects with the R272H HNF-1α mutation the mean renal threshold for glycosuria was 117 mg/dL[81].

MODY3: Pathobiology

The HNF-1α transcription factor is expressed in liver and beta cells. The *TCF1* gene (interferon production regulator factor (HNF1), albumin proximal factor) encodes HNF-1α. HNF-4α regulates HNF-1α providing a conceputal and physical link between MODY1 and MODY3. Insulin is regulated by both HNF-1α and HNF-1ß[82]. HNF-1α mutations may exert their deleterious effects as loss-of-function mutations (e.g., mutations in the promoter or dimerization domains) or as dominant negatives[83]. There is an apparent mutational hotspot in exon 4 of HNF-1α for the Pro291fsinsC mutation[84]. Because this mutation is found in many diverse MODY3 families, the commonality of the mutation must result from recurrence of the mutation and not a founder effect.

MODY3: Prevalence

MODY3 is a very common cause of MODY with more than 60 mutations having been described in HNF-1α[84]. If a suspected MODY subject fails to display an HNF mutation, allelic dropout (nonamplification of an allele containing a mutation) should be considered[85]. HNF-1α mutations may cause 1-2% of adult-onset T2DM[73]. Pre-selection of T2DM subjects can increase the likelihood of finding MODY3 mutations. In a group of T2DM subjects selected for diabetes onset before age 35 and a T2DM-affected first degree relative, 36% (9 of 25) of these T2DM subjects displayed an HNF-1α mutation[84]. Particular ethnic groups may also exhibit a higher rate of HNF-1α mutations as Boutin et al.[86] found HNF-1α mutations in 4 of 56 African American T2DM adults (7.1%). There is an extensive data base that in the common form of T2DM, HNF-1α mutations are uncommon. Possibly 1 to 2% of adult T2DM may be due to HNF1α mutations. Baier et al.[76] concluded from their studies of early-onset T2DM in Pimas that HNF-1α was not involved in T2DM pathogenesis.

MODY4

MODY4: Insulin Promoter Factor-1 Mutations

MODY4 is a consequence of IPF-1 gene (chr 13q12.1) mutations[88] (Figure 8, top). IPF-1 stands for insulin promoter factor-1 which is also known as PDX-1 (*p*ancreatic duodenal homeobo*x*-1 protein); - IDX-1 (*i*slet duodenum *homeobox*-1); and STF-1 (Stefin A factor).

The first IPF-1 mutation identified was a cytosine (C) deletion at codon 63 (ΔCmt) (Pro63fsdelC)[88]. A homozygous frameshift mutation was discovered in an infant with pancreatic agenesis (e.g., small-for-gestational age, neonatal diabetes and exocrine pancreatic insufficiency). The heterozygous parents displayed diabetes: father had T2DM and mother had GDM and there was a strong history of diabetes on both sides of the family.

MODY4: Metabolism

In the original MODY4 family, average age at onset of diabetes was 35 years with a range of 17 to 67 years. 75% of the diabetic MODY4 relatives were treated with diet or oral hypoglycemic agents[87].

Using a five-step (1-h intervals) hyperglycemic clamp, MODY4 subjects exhibited impaired insulin secretion and increased insulin sensitivity[89]. The increased insulin sensitivity may represent a consequence of insulinopenia. In response to persistent insulinopenia, insulin sensitive cells can exhibit an increase in insulin receptor number. First phase insulin response is deficient and almost flat in diabetic MODY4 subjects[89]. Typical of diabetic states and in contrast to MODY1, glucagon is persistently elevated during glucose clamp studies in MODY4 subjects compared to family members that do not carry the IPF-1 mutation. During the clamp experiment, although pancreatic polypeptide is initially low in MODY4 subjects, after the first 90 minutes pancreatic polypeptide concentrations are, in general, similar between MODY4 subjects and unaffected relatives. After 90-120 minutes, initially elevated non-esterified fatty acid concentrations in MODY4 subjects return to control levels. In summary, MODY4 mechanistically results from insulinopenia consistent with beta-cell dysfunction.

MODY4: Pathobiology

IPF-1 regulates insulin, GLUT2, GCK and other genes[90]. The infant with the homozygous IPF-1 mutation and pancreatic agenesis highlights the role of various transcription factors in pancreatic development. Furthermore, diabetes could conceptually result from islet or beta cell maldevelopment as well as pancreatic agenesis or hypoplasia in addition to deficient insulin production or secretion. As a pancreatic growth factor, IPF-1 expression increases during pancreatic regeneration in partially pancreatectomized rats[91].

Mechanistically the Pro63fsdelC introduces a frameshift mutation that leads to a truncated protein product less than half the normal size (e.g., 16 kDa versus full-size 42-43 kDa) (Figure 8, middle). Prior to ΔC, the normal open reading frame is utilized for transcription that will include the normal transactivation domain (TA). After ΔC, an abnormal reading frame is used until the premature stop codon is recognized[88]. Alternatively an internal, aberrant AUG start site for transcription can be utilized (Figure 8, bottom). This produces a mutant N-terminus for the HNF-1α protein lacking TA-domain structure that does go into proper reading frame following the mutation[92]. This carboxy-terminal mutant IPF-1 isoform appears to function as a dominant negative. In addition to the original IPF-1 mutation Pro63fsdelC, studies of T2DM subjects have revealed at least 5 additional mutations: C18R, D76N and R197H[93], Q59L and InsCCG243[94].

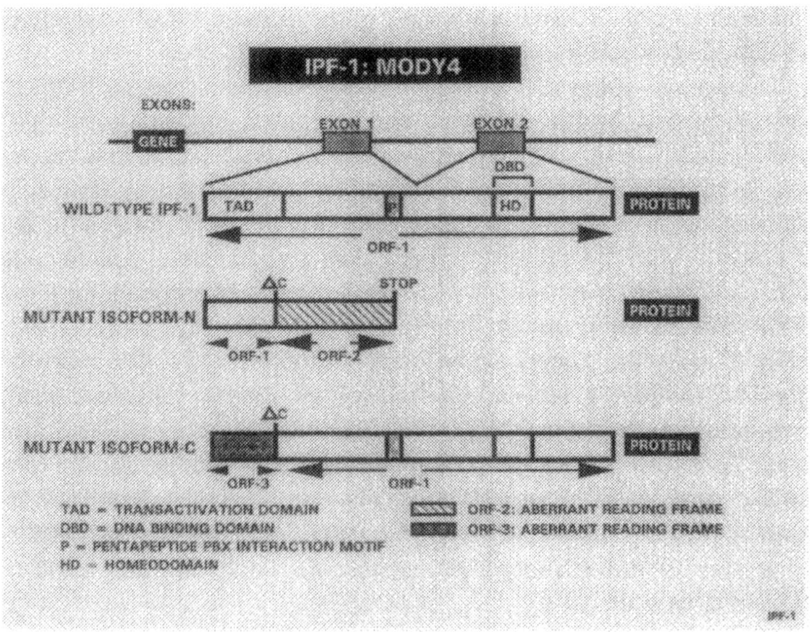

Figure 8: The cause of MODY4 is mutations in the insulin-promoter factor-1 (IPF-1) gene. The

gene and protein products (wild-type, mutant isoform-N and mutant isoform-C) are depicted. ORF = open reading frame.

MODY4: Prevalence

In 12 U.K. families lacking MODY1, MODY2 and MODY3 mutations (e.g., MODY-X families), 2 had IPF-1 mutations (16.7%)[93]. MODY4 mutations have been reported in 5.6% of U.K. T2DM patients with onset before age 40 (2 of 36) and in 2.5% of U.K. T2DM patients with onset between 35 and 70 years (4 of 158) [93]. IPF-1 mutations have also been estimated to occur in 6.2% of French late-onset T2DM subjects[94] and were found in 3.5% of early-onset Scandinavian T2DM and in 2.7% of late-onset Scandinavian T2DM[95]. In a French study[96], IPF-1 was mutated in only 1 of 272 late-onset T2DM subjects (0.37%). Exon 2 mutations were detected in 61 Japanese T2DM subjects[1996]. MODY4 mutations have been detected in families with MODY3 mutations[95].

MODY5

MODY5: Hepatocyte Nuclear Factor-1ß Mutations

MODY5 is a consequence of HNF-1ß mutations (chr.17cen-q21.3). The initial report of an HNF-1ß mutation came from Horikawa et al. [97]. In studying 57 unrelated Japanese MODY subjects, an HNF-1ß mutation (R177X) was discovered in a single individual establishing "MODY5" as a pathological entity. This MODY individual lacked mutations in HNF-4α (MODY1), glucokinase (MODY2) and HNF-1α (MODY3). In screening 40 Japanese individuals with T2DM onset prior to age 35, Nishigori et al.[98] described the second HNF-1ß mutation: A263fsinsGG. Striking clinical findings in MODY5 individuals include renal cysts, proteinuria and a propensity to renal failure. Thus a role for HNF-1ß in renal development was hypothesized. The most recent as well as novel HNF-1ß mutation (R137-K161del) was identified in a Norwegian family with mild diabetes, progressive non-diabetic renal disease and severe genital malformations[99]. Of the 4 female carriers of the HNF-1ß R137-K161del mutation, 2 displayed vaginal aplasia and a rudimentary uterus consistent with Mullerian aplasia.

MODY5: Metabolism

The initial MODY5 subject reported by Horikawa et al. [97] with the HNF-1ß R177X mutation presented with glycosuria at age 10 years when diabetes was diagnosed. After two days of initial treatment with insulin, she was managed with diet for 2 years. Thereafter she was treated with insulin. At age 23, her 24-ho urinary C-peptide was 6% of the normal mean compatible with insulinopenia. Th proband's 31 year old diabetic brother demonstrated no increase in C-peptic after glucagon injection. Metabolic studies in one Norwegian subject with th HNF-1ß R137-K161del mutation showed a reduced 30-minute insuli concentration during an oral glucose tolerance test [99] Future studies wi undoubtedly more clearly define the pathophysiology in MODY5.

MODY5: Pathobiology

The *TCF2* gene (transcription factor-2, hepatic; LF-B3; variant hepati nuclear factor) encodes HNF-1ß. HNF-1ß functions as a homodimer transcriptio factor or as a heterodimer with HNF-1α. HNF-1ß regulates HNF-4α providing link between MODY5 and MODY1. Using a rat albumin promoter-linke reporter gene, the R177X HNF-1ß mutation did not stimulate transcription o obstruct wild-type HNF-1ß activity[97]. Therefore the R177X HNF-1ß mutatio behaves not as a dominant negative but as a loss-of-function mutation. R177X produces a protein of 176 amino acids. The A263fsinsGG mutation reduces HNF 1ß's size to 264 amino acids. In summary, the HNF-1ß mutations described t date include R177X, A263fsinsGG, P328L329fsdelCCTCT and R137-K161del

MODY5: Prevalence

In Horikawa et al.'s initial report [97], HNF-ß mutations were present in 2% of Japanese MODY families (1 of 57). In T2DM Japanese with diabetes onse prior to age 35, 2.5% (1 of 40) had an HNF-1ß mutation [98]. Overall, HNF-1ß mutations are uncommon causes of MODY and are not associated with the common forms of T2DM.

SUMMARY

In the last 10 years, 5 forms of MODY have been mapped and the defective genes identified[22,23]. In 1991, MODY was first mapped to chromosome 20 establishing MODY1. One year later in French MODY1-negative families glucokinase was identified as MODY2. In 1995, in several French MODY families where diabetes was not linked to MODY1 or MODY2, diabetes was mapped to chromosome 12 constituting MODY3. The discoveries of HNF-1α mutations as the cause of MODY3 and HNF-4α mutations as a cause of MODY1 were published in 1996. Mutations in IPF-1 in a case of pancreatic agenesis lead to the recognition of MODY4 in 1997. That same year, a Japanese MODY family was identified with an HNF-1ß mutation originating MODY5. The transcription factor mutations are interrelated pathophysiologically in regard to the regulation of insulin production (Figure 9). Since the discovery of MODY5, in studies of at least 6 candidate transcription factor genes, no new MODY genes have been conclusively demonstrated[100]. In most populations MODY1 through MODY5 account for most cases of MODY[101].

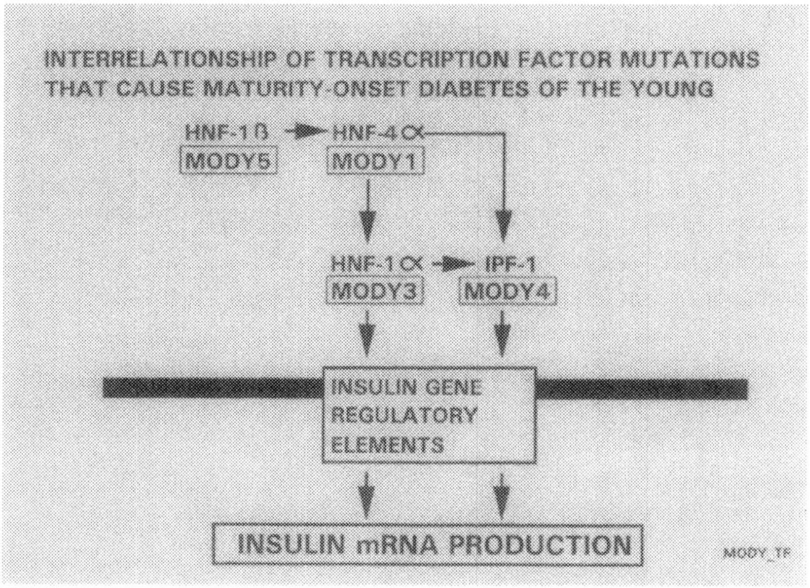

Figure 9: All of the transcription factor mutations that cause MODY are biochemically interrelated.

The MODY syndromes are not common causes of diabetes in either children of adults. At most, 3-5% of youth-onset diabetes results from MODY. In adults, no more than ~5% of cases of T2DM result from MODY mutations. Nevertheless, there is considerable value in diagnosing MODY. Identifying MODY based upon clinical course and family history or through identification of a MODY mutation provides a *specific* diagnosis for the etiology of the subject's diabetes and excludes T1DM and T2DM which are the two most common forms of diabetes. The diagnosis of MODY also supplies specific information concerning the expected response to therapy. For example, while being initially responsive to sulfonylureas, with advancing disease duration MODY1 and MODY3 may require insulin treatment. On the other hand, MODY2 is almost never insulin requiring. MODY4 is intermediate in severity between MODY1/MODY3 and MODY2. In the case of MODY5, there is a high incidence of developmental cystic disease of the kidney and consequent renal failure.

Concerning complications, MODY2, being less severe than other forms of MODY, rarely displays micro or macrovasculopathic complications. However MODY2 may present as a gestational diabetes mellitus when insulin therapy may be required to control hyperglycemia. Excluding MODY2, all forms of MODY present a significant risk for diabetic complications. Finally, the diagnosis of MODY is very important for planning diabetes screening in affected families.

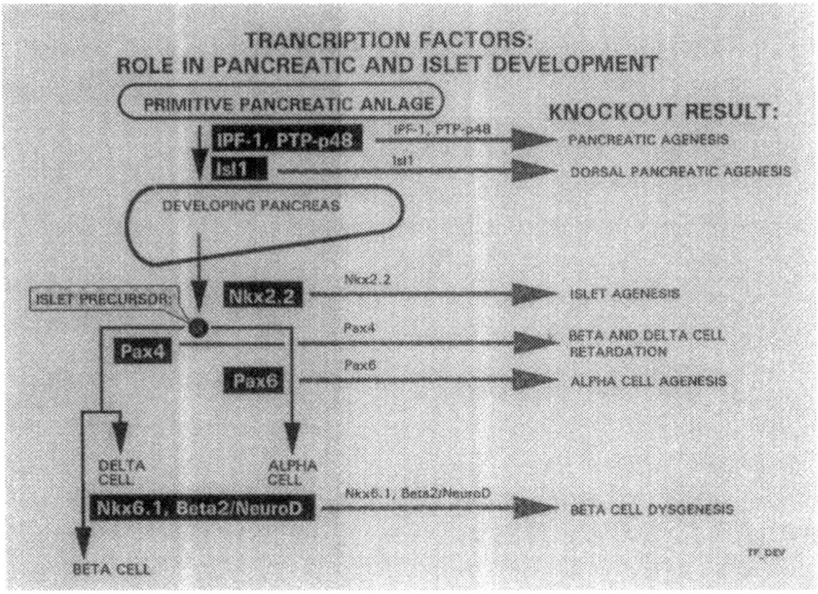

Figure 10: A variety of experimental murine gene knock-out models demonstrate the role of various transcription factors in the development of the pancreas and islets.

Because the MODY syndromes are inherited as autosomal dominants and for the fact that MODY may be sub-clinical or diagnosed only by conducting oral glucose tolerance test, it is clear that all first degree relatives of MODY patients should be screened for diabetes by oral glucose tolerance testing. While an elevated glycohemoglobin is specific for the diagnosis of diabetes (excluding splenectomy where red blood cell life span increases), glycohemoglobin is an insensitive test for the diagnosis of diabetes and should not be used for diabetes screening.

REFERENCES

1. Fajans SS, Conn JW. Prediabetes, subclinical diabetes, and latent clinical diabetes: interpretation, diagnosis and treatment in "On the Nature and Treatment of Diabetes" Leibel DS, Wrenshall GS, Ed. Amsterdam, Excerpta Med., 1965, p. 641 (Int. Congr. Ser., no. 84)

2. Fajans SS, Floyd JC, Tattersall RB, et al: The various faces of diabetes in the young. Arch Intern Med 1976;136:194-202
3. Fajans SS, Cloutier MC, Crowther RL. Clinical and etiologic heterogeneity of idiopathic diabetes mellitus. Diabetes 1978; 27:1112-25
4. Expert Committee: Report of the expert committee on the diagnosis and classification of diabetes mellitus. Diabetes Care 1997, 20:1183-97
5. Winter WE, Maclaren NK. Autoimmune Endocrinopathies. In: Immunologic Disorders in Infants and Children (4th Edition), ER Stiehm (ed): WB Saunders Company, Philadelphia, Pennsylvania, 1996; 824-54
6. House DV, Nakamura M, Winter WE. Autoimmune Markers of Type I Diabetes Mellitus. In: Clinical Diagnostic Immunology: Protocols In Quality Assurance and Standardization. Nakamura RM, Burek CL, Cook L, Folds JD (eds): Blackwell Science, Cambridge, MA 1998; 234-49
7. Bottazzo GF, Florin-Christensen A, Doniach D. Islet-cell autoantibodies in diabetes mellitus with autoimmune polyendocrine deficiencies. Lancet 1974; 2:1279-83
8. Lendrum R, Walker G, Gamble DR. Islet-cell antibodies in juvenile diabetes mellitus of recent onset. Lancet 1975; i:880-3
9. Palmer JP, Asplin CM, Clemons P, Lyen K, Tatpati O, Raghu PK, Paquette TL. Insulin antibodies in insulin-dependent diabetics before insulin treatment. Science 1983; 222(4630): 133-9
10. Baekkeskov S, Aanstoot HJ, Christgau S, Reetz A, Solimena M, Cascalho M, Folli F, Richter-Olesen H, DeCamilli P, Camilli PD. Identification of the 64K autoantigen in insulin-dependent diabetes as the GABA-synthesizing enzyme glutamic acid decarboxylase. Nature 1990; 34:151-6;Rowley MJ, Mackay IR, Chen Y, et al: Antibodies to glutamic acid decarboxylase discriminate major types of diabetes mellitus. Diabetes 1992;41(4):548
11. Rabin DU, Pleasic SM, Shapiro JA, Yoo-Warren H, Oles J, Hicks JM, Goldstein DE, Rae PM. Islet cell antigen 512 is a diabetes-specific islet autoantigen related to protein tyrosine phosphatases. J Immunol 1994 March 15; 152(6):3183-8
12. Yoon J-W, Austin M, Onodera T, et al. Virus-induced diabetes mellitus. N Engl J Med 1979; 300:1173-9
13. Bell GI, Horita S, Karam JH: A polymorphic locus near the human insulin gene is associated with insulin-dependent diabetes mellitus. Diabetes 1984 Feb; 33(2):176-___
14. Winter, W.E.; Chihara, T.; Schatz, D.A.: The genetics of autoimmune diabetes. American Journal of Diseases of Children 1993; 147:1282-90

15. Unger RH, Grundy S. Hyperglycemia as an inducer as well as consequence of impaired islet cell function and insulin resistance: implications for the management of diabetes. Diabetologia 1985; 28:119-21
16. Winter, W.E.: Type 2 diabetes mellitus: the challenge of a metabolic epidemic. Journal of Clinical Ligand Assay 1998: 21 (3) 293-308
17. O'Rahilly S, Spivey RS, Holman RR, et al.: Type II diabetes of early onset: a distinct clinical and genetic syndrome? Brit Med J 1987;294:923-8
18. Pinhas-Hamiel O, Dolan LM, Daniels SR: Increased incidence of non-insulin dependent diabetes mellitus among adolescents. J Pediatr 1996; 128:608-15
19. Jones KL (1998) Non-insulin dependent diabetes in children and adolescents: the therapeutic challenge. Clin Pedatr (2):103-10
20. DeFronzo RA, Bonadonna RC, Ferrannini E: Pathogenesis of NIDDM A balanced overview. Diabetes Care 1992 Mar;15(3):318-68
21. Reaven GM: Syndrome X. Clinical Diabetes. 1994;32-6; Reaven GM Banting lecture 1988. Role of insulin resistance in human disease Diabetes. 1988 Dec;37(12):1595-607
22. Winter WE, Nakamura M, House DV: Monogenic Diabetes Mellitus in Youth: The MODY syndromes. Endocrinology and Metabolism Clinics of North America 1999, 28(4): 765-85
23. Winter WE. Molecular and biochemical analysis of the MODY syndromes. Pediatric Diabetes 2000, 1:88-117
24. van den Ouweland JM, Lemkes HH, Trembath RC, et al: Maternally inherited diabetes and deafness is a distinct subtype of diabetes and associates with a single point mutation in the mitochondrial tRNA(Leu(UUR)) gene. Diabetes 1994 43(6):746-51
25. Haneda M, Polonsky KS, Bergenstal RM, et al.: Familial hyperinsulinia due to secretion of a structurally abnormal insulin. N Engl J Med 1984;310:1288-94
26. Ledermann HM. Is maturity onset diabetes at young age (MODY) more common in Europe than previously assumed? Lancet 1995, 345:648
27. Alcolado JC, Thomas AW: Maternally inherited diabetes mellitus: the role of mitochondrial DNA defects. Diabetes Medicine 1995;12(2):102-8
28. Gerbitz KD, Gempel K, Brdiczka D: Mitochondria and diabetes: Genetic, biochemical, and clinical implications of the cellular energy circuit. Diabetes 1996;45:113-26
29. Kishimoto M, Hashiramoto M, Araki S,et al: Diabetes mellitus carrying a mutation in the mitochondrial tRNA(Leu(UUR)) gene. Diabetologia 1995 Feb; 38(2):193-200
30. American Diabetes Association: Clinical Practice Recommendations

1999: Implications of the Diabetes Control and Complications Trial. Diabetes Care 1999:22(suppl1):S24-S27

31. Shepherd M, Sparkes AC, Hattersley, AT. Genetic testing in maturity onset diabeets of the young (MODY): a new challenge for the diabetic clinic. Pract Diab Int 2001, 18(1):16-21

32. Winter WE, Maclaren NK, Riley WJ, Clarke DW, Kappy MS, Spillar RP: Maturity-onset diabetes of youth in Black Americans. New Engl J Med 1987, 316:285-91

33. Pinhas-Hamiel O, Dolan LM, Zeiter PS: Diabetic ketoacidosis among obese African-American adolescents with NIDDM. Diabetes Care 1997;20:484-6

34. Glaser NS. Non-insulin dependent diabetes mellitus in childhood and adolescence. Pediatr Clin NA 1997, 44(2):307-37

35. Fajans SS, Conn JW: Tolbutamide-induced improvement in carbohydrate tolerance of young people with mild diabetes mellitus. Diabetes 1960;9:83-8

36. Fajans SS: Scope and heterogeneous nature of MODY. Diabetes Care 1990, 13:49-64

37. Herman WH, Fajans SS, Ortiz FJ, et al.: Abnormal insulin secretion, not insulin resistance, is the genetic or primary defect of MODY in the RW pedigree. Diabetes 1994;43:40-6

38. Cameron FJ, Batch JA: Maturity-onset diabetes of the young (MODY): three cases and new prespectives. J Pediatr Endocrinol Metabol 1997;10:63-8

39. Nakamura M, House DV, Winter WE: Novel mutation identified in the glucokinase (GCK) genes of a patient with atypical diabetes mellitus (ADM) of African Americans. Diabetes 1996; 45(Suppl 2):76A

40. Nakamura M , House D V , Winter W E: A novel homoplasmic point mutation at mitochondrial DNA (mtDNA) nucleotide 3308 in a family with atypical diabetes mellitus (ADM) of African Americans (AA). Diabetes 1997, 46, Suppl 1: 175A

41. Stoffers DA. Maturity-onset diabetes of the young (MODY): the past ,present, and future. Growth, Genetics & Hormones. 2000, 16(3):37-41

42. Miedzybrodzka Z, Hattersley AT, Ellard S, Pearson D, de Silva D, Harvey R, Haites N. Non-penetrance in a MODY 3 family with a mutation in the hepatic nuclear factor 1alpha gene: implications for predictive testing. Eur J Hum Genet. 1999 Sep;7(6):729-32

43. Beck-Nielsen H, Nielson OH, Pedersen O, et al: Insulin action and insulin secretion in identical twins with MODY. Diabetes 1988;37:730-5

44. Permutt MA, Chiu KC, Tanizawa Y: Glucokinase and NIDDM: a candidate gene that paid off. Diabetes 1992;41:1367-72
45. Froguel P, Vaxillaire M, Sun F, et al.: Close linkage of glucokinase locus on chromosome 7p to early-onset non-insulin-dependent diabetes mellitus. Nat 1992;356:162-4
46. Vionnet N, Stoffel M, Takeda J, et al.: Nonsense mutations in the glucokinase gene causes early-onset non-insulin-dependent diabetes mellitus. Nat 1992;356:721-2
47. Guazzini B, Gaffi D, Mainieri D, Multari G, Cordera R, Bertolini S, Pozza G, Meschi F, Barbetti F. Three novel missense mutations in the glucokinase gene (G80S; E221K; G227C) in Italian subjects with maturity-onset diabetes of the young (MODY). Mutations in brief no. 162. Online. Hum Mutat. 1998;12(2):136
48. Njolstad PR, Cockburn BN, Bell GI, Sovik O. A missense mutation, Val62Ala, in the glucokinase gene in a Norwegian family with maturity-onset diabetes of the young. Acta Paediatr. 1998 Aug;87(8):853-6
49. Guenat E, Seematter G, Philippe J, Temler E, Jequier E, Tappy L. Counterregulatory responses to hypoglycemia in patients with glucokinase gene mutations. Diabetes Metab. 2000 Nov;26(5):377-84
50. Njolstad PR, Sovik O, Cuesta-Munoz A, Bjorkhaug L, Massa O, Barbetti F, Undlien DE, Shiota C, Magnuson MA, Molven A, Matschinsky FM, Bell GI. Neonatal diabetes mellitus due to complete glucokinase deficiency. N Engl J Med. 2001 May 24;344(21):1588-92
51. Matschinsky FM: Glucokinase as glucose sensor and metabolic signal generator in pancreatic β-cells and hepatocytes. Diabetes 1990;39:647-52
52. Matschinsky FM, Glaser B, Magnuson MA: Pancreatic ß-cell glucokinase, closing the gap between theoretical concepts and experimental realities. Diabetes 1998;47:307-15
53. Weir GC: A defective beta-cell glucose sensor as a cause of diabetes. N Engl J Med 1993;328:729-31
54. Stoffel M, Frogual P, Takeda J, et al.: Human glucokinase gene: isolation, characterization, and identification of two missense mutations linked to early-onset non-insulin-dependent (type 2) diabetes mellitus. Proc Natl Acad Sci USA 1992;89:7698-702
55. Polonsky KS: The ß-cell in diabetes: from molecular genetics to clinical research. Diabetes 1995;44:705-15
56. Velho G, Froguel P, Clement K, et al: Primary pancreatic beta-cell secretory defect caused by mutations in glucokinase gene in kindreds of maturity onset diabetes of the young. Lancet 1992 Aug 22; 340(8817):444-8
57. Sakura H, Kawamori R, Kubota M, Morishima T, Kamada T, Akanuma

Y, Yazaki Y, Kadowaki T. Glucokinase gene mutation and impaired glucose uptake by liver. Lancet. 1993 Jun 12;341(8859):1532-3

58. Chiu KC, Tanizawa Y, Permutt MA: Glucokinase gene variants in the common form of NIDDM. Diabetes 1993;42:579-82

59. Eto K, Sakura H, Shimokawa K, Kadowaki H, Hagura R, Akanuma Y, Yazaki Y, Kadowaki T. Sequence variations of the glucokinase gene in Japanese subjects with NIDDM. Diabetes. 1993 Aug;42(8):1133-7

60. Chiu KC, Province MA, Permutt MA: Glucokinase gene is genetic marker for NIDDM in American Blacks. Diabetes 1992A;41:843-9

61. Yamagata K, Ruruta H, Oda N, et al. Mutations in the hepatocyte nuclear factor-4∝ gene in maturity-onset diabetes of the young (MODY 1). Nature 1996B; 384:458-60

62. Bell GI, Xiang KS, Newman MV,et al: Gene for non-insulin-dependent diabetes mellitus (maturity-onset diabetes of the young subtype) is linked to DNA polymorphism on human chromosome 20q. Proceedings from the Natational Academy of Science USA 1991 Feb 15; 88(4):1484-8

63. Yamagata K, Oda N, Kaisaki PJ, et al.: Mutations in the hepatocyte nuclear factor-1α gene in maturity-onset diabetes of the young (MODY3). Nature 1996A;384:455-8

64. Byrne MM, Sturis J, Fajans SS, et al.: Altered insulin secretory responses to glucose in subjects with a mutation in the MODY1 gene on chromosome 20. Diabetes 1995;44:699-704

65. Lindner T, Gragnoli C, Furuta H, et al.: Hepatic function in a family with a nonsense mutation (R154X) in the hepatocyte nuclear factor-4α/MODY1 gene J Clin Inv 1997;100:1400-5

66. Herman WH, Fajans SS, Smith MJ, et al.: Diminished insulin and glucagon secretory responses to arginine in nondiabetic subjects with a mutation in the hepatocyte nuclear factor-4α/MODY1 gene. Diabetes 1997;46:1749-54

67. Ilag LL, Tabaei BP, Herman WH, Zawacki CM, D'Souza E, Bell GI, Fajans SS. Reduced pancreatic polypeptide response to hypoglycemia and amylin response to arginine in subjects with a mutation in the HNF-4alpha/MODY1 gene. Diabetes. 2000 Jun;49(6):961-8

68. Lehto M, Wipemo C, Ivarsson S-A, Lindgren C, Lipsanen-Nyman M, Weng J, Wibell L, Widén E, Tuomi T, Groop L: High frequency of mutations in MODY and mitochondrial genes in Scandinavian patients with familial early-onset diabetes. Diabetologia 1999, 42:1131-7

69. Wang JC, Stafford JM, Granner DK. SRC-1 and GRIP1 coactivate transcription with hepatocyte nuclear factor 4. J Biol Chem. 1998 Nov

20;273(47):30847-50

70. Stoffel M, Duncan SA. The maturity-onset diabetes of the young (MODY1) transcription factor HNF4alpha regulates expression of genes required for glucose transport and metabolism. Proc Natl Acad Sci U S A. 1997 Nov 25;94(24):13209-14
71. Sladek FM, Dallas-Yang Q, Nepomuceno L. MODY1 mutation Q268X in hepatocyte nuclear factor 4alpha allows for dimerization in solution but causes abnormal subcellular localization. Diabetes. 1998 Jun;47(6):985-90
72. Suaud L, Hemimou Y, Formstecher P, Laine B. Functional study of the E276Q mutant hepatocyte nuclear factor-4alpha found in type 1 maturity-onset diabetes of the young: impaired synergy with chicken ovalbumin upstream promoter transcription factor II on the hepatocyte nuclear factor-1 promoter. Diabetes. 1999 May;48(5):1162-7
73. Yki-Jarvinen H. MODY genes and mutations in hepatocyte nuclear factors. Lancet 1997, 349:516-7
74. Sakura H, Eto K, Kadowaki H, et al.: Structure of the human glucokinase gene and identification of a missense mutation in a Japanese patient with early-onset non-insulin-dependent diabetes mellitus. J Clin Endo Metaob 1992;75(6):1571-3
75. Malecki MT, Antonellis A, Casey P, et al.: Exclusion of the hepatocyte nuclear factor 4α as a candidate gene for late-onset NIDDM linked with chromosome 20q. Diabetes 1998;47:970-2
76. Baier LJ, Permana PA, Traurig M, Dobberfuhl A, Wiedrich C, Sutherland J, Thuillez P, Luczy-Bachman G, Hara M, Horikawa Y, Hinokio Y, Hanson RL, Bogardus C. Mutations in the genes for hepatocyte nuclear factor (HNF)-1alpha, -4alpha, -1beta, and -3beta; the dimerization cofactor of HNF-1; and insulin promoter factor 1 are not common causes of early-onset type 2 diabetes in Pima Indians. Diabetes Care. 2000 Mar;23(3):302-4
77. Isomaa B, Hemricsson M, Lehto M, et al.: Chronic diabetic complications in patients with MODY3 diabetes. DIabetologia 1998;41:467-73
78. Yamada S, Nishigori H, Onda H, Utsugi T, Yanagawa T, Maruyama T, Onigata K, Nagashima K, Nagai R, Morikawa A, Takeuchi T, Takeda J. Identification of mutations in the hepatocyte nuclear factor (HNF)-1 alpha gene in Japanese subjects with IDDM. Diabetes. 1997B Oct;46(10):1643-7
79. Lehto M, Tuomi T, Mahtani MM, et al.: Characterization of the MODY3 phenotype. J Clin Invest 1997;99:582-91
80. Byrne MM, Sturis J, Menzel S, et al: Altered insulin secretory responses to glucose in diabetic and non-diabetic subjects with mutations in the diabetes susceptibility gene MODY3 on chromosome 12. Diabetes 1996;

45:1503-10
81. Menzel R, Kaisaki PJ, Rjasanowski I, Heinke P, Kerner W, Menzel S. A low renal threshold for glucose in diabetic patients with a mutation in the hepatocyte nuclear factor-1alpha (HNF-1alpha) gene. Diabet Med. 1998 Oct;15(10):816-20
82. Okita K, Yang Q, Yamagata K, Hangenfeldt KA, Miyagawa J, Kajimoto Y, Nakajima H, Namba M, Wollheim CB, Hanafusa T, Matsuzawa Y. Human insulin gene is a target gene of hepatocyte nuclear factor-1alpha (HNF-1alpha) and HNF-1beta. Biochem Biophys Res Commun. 1999 Sep 24;263(2):566-9
83. Yamagata K, Yang Q, Yamamoto K, et al.: Mutation P291fsinsC in the transcription factor hepatocute nuclear factor-1α is dominant negative. Diabetes 1998 47;1231-5
84. Kaisaki PJ, Menzel S, Linder T, et al.: Mutations in the hepatocyte nuclear factor-1α gene in MODY and early-onset NIDDM. Diabetes 1997, 46(3):528-35.
85. Ellard S, Bulman MP, Frayling TM, Allen LI, Dronsfield MJ, Tack CJ, Hattersley AT. Allelic drop-out in exon 2 of the hepatocyte nuclear factor-1alpha gene hinders the identification of mutations in three families with maturity-onset diabetes of the young. Diabetes. 1999 Apr;48(4):921-3
86. Boutin P, Chèvre JC, Hami EH, et al.: An automated fluorescent single-strand conformation polymorphism technique for screening mutations in the hepatocyte nuclear factor-1α gene (maturity-onset diabetes of the young). Diabetes 1997;46:2108-9
87. Stoffers DA, Ferrer J, Clarke WL, et al.: Early-onset type-II diabetes mellitus (MODY4) linked to IPF1. Nat Genet 1997A;17:138-9
88. Stoffers DA, Zinkin NT, Stanojevic V, et al.: Pancreatic agenesis attributable to a single nucleotide deletion in the human IPF1 gene coding sequence. Nat Gen 1997B;15:106-10
89. Clocquet AR, Egan JM, Stoffers DA, Muller DC, Wideman L, Chin GA, Clarke WL, Hanks JB, Habener JF, Elahi D. Impaired insulin secretion and increased insulin sensitivity in familial maturity-onset diabetes of the young 4 (insulin promoter factor 1 gene). Diabetes. 2000 Nov;49(11):1856-64
90. Waeber G, Thompson N, Nicod P, Bonny C. Transcriptional activation of the GLUT2 gene by the IPF-1/STF-1/IDX-1 homeobox factor. Mol Endocrinol. 1996 Nov;10(11):1327-34
91. Sharma A, Zangen DH, Reitz P, Taneja M, Lissauer ME, Miller CP,

Weir GC, Habener JF, Bonner-Weir S. The homeodomain protein IDX-1 increases after an early burst of proliferation during pancreatic regeneration. Diabetes. 1999 Mar;48(3):507-13

92. Stoffers DA, Stanojevic V, Habener JF: Insulin promoter factor-1 gene mutation linked to early-onset type 2 diabetes mellitus directs expression of a dominant negative isoprotein. J Clin Invest 1998;102:232-41

93. Macfarlane WM, Frayling TM, Ellard S, Evans JC, Allen LI Bulman MP, Ayres S, Shepherd M, Clark P, Millward A, Demaine A, Wilkin T, Docherty K, Hattersley AT. Missense mutations in the insulin promoter factor-1 gene predispose to type 2 diabetes. J Clin Invest. 1999 Nov;104(9):R33-9

94. Hani EH, Stoffers DA, Chevre JC, Durand E, Stanojevic V, Dina C, Habener JF, Froguel P. Defective mutations in the insulin promoter factor-1 (IPF-1) gene in late-onset type 2 diabetes mellitus. J Clin Invest. 1999 Nov;104(9):R41-8

95. Weng JP, Lehto M, Forsblom C, Huang X, Li H, Groop LC. Hepatocyte nuclear factor-1 beta (MODY5) gene mutations in Scandinavian families with early-onset diabetes or kidney disease or both. Diabetologia. 2000 Jan;43(1):131-2

96. Reis AF, Ye WZ, Dubois-Laforgue D, Bellanne-Chantelot C, Timsit J, Velho G. Mutations in the insulin promoter factor-1 gene in late-onset type 2 diabetes mellitus. Eur J Endocrinol. 2000 Oct;143(4):511-3

97. Horikawa Y, Iwasaki N, Hara M, et al.: Mutation in hepatocyte nuclear factor -1ß gene (TCF2) associated with MODY. Nat Gen 1997;17:384-5

98. Nishigori H, Yamada S, Kohama T, et al.: Frameshift mutation, A263fsinsGG, in the hepatocyte nuclear factor -1ß gene associated with diabetes and renal dysfunction. Diabetes 1998; 47:1354-5

99. Lindner TH, Njolstad PR, Horikawa Y, Bostad L, Bell GI, Sovik O. A novel syndrome of diabetes mellitus, renal dysfunction and genital malformation associated with a partial deletion of the pseudo-POU domain of hepatocyte nuclear factor-1beta. Hum Mol Genet. 1999A Oct;8(11):2001-8

100. Chèvre J-C, Hani EH, Boutin P, Vaxillaire M, Blanche H, Vionnet N, Pardini VC, Timsit J, Larger E, Charpentier G, Beckers D, Maes M, Bellanné-Chantelot C, Velho G, Froguel P: Mutation screening in 18 Caucasian families suggest the existence of other MODY genes. Diabetologia 1998, 41:1017-23

101. Lindner TH, Cockburn BN, Bell GI: Molecular genetics of MODY in Germany. Diabetologia 1999B, 42(1):121-3

Chapter 5

CYSTIC FIBROSIS RELATED DIABETES

James Phillips, M.D and Antoinette Moran, M.D.
University of Minnesota

INTRODUCTION

Cystic Fibrosis (CF) is the most common lethal autosomal recessive disease affecting the Caucasian population. Chronic obstructive pulmonary disease, pancreatic exocrine insufficiency, and abnormally high sweat electrolyte concentrations are characteristic of this disease. In 1989, the defective gene was localized to the long arm of chromosome 7. This region encodes a protein of 1,480 amino acids called the CF transmembrane conductance regulator (CFTR). Defects in CFTR reduce the ability of epithelial cells to transport chloride, altering the fluid and electrolyte composition of cellular secretions. Viscous, dehydrated secretions impair mucociliary clearance in the lungs, and cause progressive obstruction, inflammation, scarring, and destruction of multiple organ systems, particularly in the pulmonary, gastrointestinal, hepatobiliary, and reproductive systems.

CF life expectancy has increased dramatically over the last few decades. With this, CF related diabetes (CFRD) and lesser abnormalities of glucose tolerance have emerged as common complications with a profound impact on the clinical course and survival of CF patients. The primary concern has been the impact of diabetes and insulin deficiency on the nutritional and pulmonary status of CF patients. Abnormal glucose tolerance is associated with progressive clinical deterioration[1-3], and the future rate of decline in pulmonary function is directly proportional to both the magnitude of abnormal glucose tolerance and the degree of insulin deficiency[2]. In a retrospective survival analysis, only 25% of individuals who had CF and diabetes survived to age 30 years, compared to 60% survival at 30 years of age in CF patients without diabetes[3]. It has been postulated that insulin deficiency negatively affects CF clinical status by promoting protein catabolism[4, 5]. Mounting evidence supports the use of insulin to improve pulmonary function and weight parameters[1]. Clearly, the influence of diabetes on morbidity and mortality, and the need to appropriately diagnose and treat this condition, have become crucial issues in CF care.

DEFINITION

Table 1 Differences between CFRD and type 1 and 2 diabetes.

	CFRD	Type 1 Diabetes	Type 2 Diabetes
Most common age of onset	18-21	<20	>40
Usual body habitus	thin	Average	obese
Insulin secretion	↓↓	Absent	*relative ↓
Insulin sensitivity	**↓	↓	↓↓↓
Autoimmune etiology	no	Yes	no
Islet amyloid deposition	yes	No	yes
Ketoacidosis	rare	Yes	rare
Microvascular complications	yes	Yes	yes
Macrovascular complications	no?	Yes	yes

*variably decreased relative to the level needed to correct hyperglycemia, although actual insu may be high, normal or low compared to controls

**mild insulin resistance in baseline state of health can increase dramatically during infection

A classification scheme should identify and differentiate individuals with CF and abnormal glucose tolerance into categories that are useful for clinical management and for epidemiological and research purposes. CFRD shares features of both type 1 and type 2 diabetes, but several important differences necessitate a distinct classification designation (Table 1). The American Diabetes Association (ADA) currently places CFRD in the category of "other specific types (of diabetes), diseases of the exocrine pancreas"[6]. In 1998, a consensus

Table 2. Glucose tolerance categories in CF in response to a standard OGTT.

Status	Fasting Plasma Glucose mg/dl (mM)	2h Plasma Glucose mg/dl (mM)
Normal glucose tolerance (NGT)	< 126 (7.0)	< 140 (7.8)
Impaired glucose tolerance (IGT)	< 126 (7.0)	140-199 (7.8-11.1)
CFRD without fasting hyperglycemia	< 126 (7.0)	≥ 200 (11.1)
CFRD with fasting hyperglycemia	≥126 (7.0)	OGTT not necessary

Classification is based on a standard oral glucose tolerance test (OGTT, 1.75g/kg, maximum 75g), with four diagnostic categories: normal glucose tolerance (NGT), impaired glucose tolerance (IGT), CFRD without fasting hyperglycemia (FH), and CFRD with FH (Table 2).

conference working under the direction of the Cystic Fibrosis Foundation (CFF) established a classification scheme for patients with CF,[7] because prior to that time no unified nomenclature, screening guidelines, diagnostic criteria, or management protocols existed.

This classification system reflects a continuum of glucose tolerance abnormalities. For the most part, it parallels ADA definitions. However, the differentiation of CFRD individuals with and without hyperglycemia in the fasting state is unique to CF and is not included in the ADA scheme[6]. The ADA does not distinguish between these two categories because, in individuals with type 2 diabetes, fasting hyperglycemia and hyperglycemia after a glucose load are equally and independently associated with diabetes microvascular complications[8]. These observations, however, were made in individuals metabolically very dissimilar to CF patients. Patients with CF are thin, have low serum cholesterol levels and normal blood pressure, and who, unless acutely ill, tend to be insulin sensitive. Because no information was available to determine whether individuals with CFRD without FH are at risk for diabetes microvascular complications, the CFRD consensus committee felt it was important to identify and categorize these individuals separately, so that epidemiological data can be gathered to guide future management decisions.

EPIDEMIOLOGY

Prevalence of CFRD is difficult to calculate because of the lack of routine screening at most CF centers. In Denmark, where annual OGTTs are performed, 50% of CF patients aged 30 years or older are reported to have diabetes[9]. At the University of Minnesota, annual OGTT screening revealed a CFRD prevalence of 9% in patients age 5-9 years, 26% in patients age 10-19 years, 35% in patients age 20-30 years, and 43% in patients older than 30 years[10](Figure 1). The only incidence data comes from Denmark, where an annual incidence rate of 3% has been reported[9].

Figure 1. Glucose tolerance categories in CF patients at the University of Minnesota, expressed as percent prevalence within age groups. n=total number of patients within that age group (from reference 10).

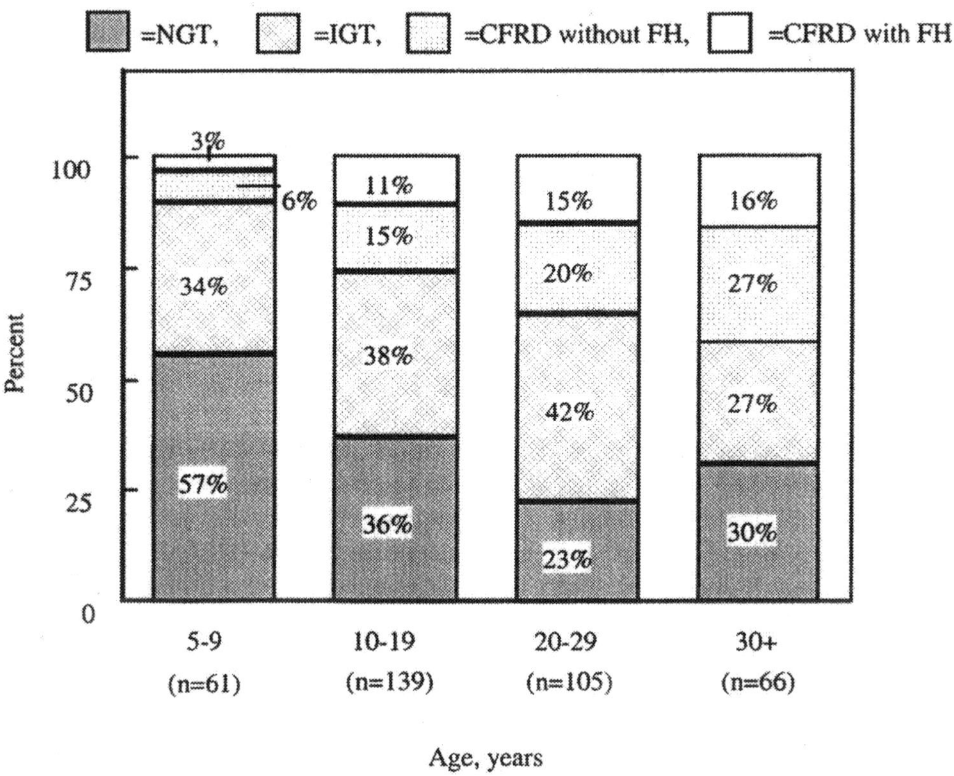

CFRD develops in more female than male patients in the age group younger than 15 years[11]. After the age of 15, male and female patients have equal rates of diagnosis of CFRD[11]. The reason for the earlier onset of diabetes in female patients may be partly due to the insulin resistance of puberty. Although the onset of puberty is often delayed in CF patients, girls with CF still reach puberty at a younger age than boys with CF[12]. CFRD is more likely to affect patients who are delta F508 homozygous, the most common CF mutation[11,13]. This may be because exocrine pancreatic insufficiency, which leads to severe fibrosis of the pancreas, is more common in delta F508 homozygotes.

ETIOLOGY AND PATHOGENESIS

Insulin deficiency is the hallmark of CFRD. The pancreas in CF patients is damaged by progressive obstruction of the pancreatic ducts with thick viscous secretions. Autopsy findings demonstrate fibrosis and fatty infiltration with disruption of the islet architecture and destruction of many, but not all, of the islets[14-16]. This observation supports the hypothesis that mechanical islet destruction results in abnormal glucose homeostasis in the majority of exocrine insufficient CF patients. Islet amyloid deposition may be involved in the progression of abnormal glucose tolerance to overt diabetes. Accumulation of islet amyloid has been noted in type 2 diabetes, but not type 1 diabetes or chronic pancreatitis[17-19]. Islet amyloid is also present in the islets of CF patients with diabetes, but not in those without diabetes[20], suggesting a possible link between CFRD and the genetic predisposition to type 2 diabetes.

CF patients without exocrine disease, who comprise about 5-15% of the CF population, appear to have minimal pancreatic endocrine dysfunction[21]. Abnormal hormone secretion has been noted in the majority of CF patients who are exocrine insufficient. Proinsulin levels are elevated, suggesting beta cell stress or damage[22, 23]. First-phase insulin and C-peptide secretion in response to glucose and other intravenous stimulatory agents is severely impaired[21, 24, 25]. In response to oral stimuli, insulin secretion is delayed and diminished[21]. In addition, glucagon and pancreatic polypeptide secretion are reduced[21], implying destruction of entire islets. Interestingly, levels of somatostatin, an inhibitor of insulin secretion, are increased in CF [26]. Because somatostatin is produced in the pancreas as well as in the central nervous system and throughout the gut, it is unknown if increased levels are of pancreatic origin.

Modest insulin resistance has been found in CF patients with overt diabetes[27-31]. Whether it actually causes diabetes is unclear. Hyperglycemia per se can cause insulin resistance in patients with type 1 diabetes[32], and this is probably also true in CFRD, since insulin resistance is related to glycemic control in this population[30]. Clearly, however, acute infection or severe inflammation may cause insulin resistance and may precipitate diabetes. Insulin sensitivity is more controversial in patients with CF who do not have diabetes, in whom it has been reported to be increased[27, 33], normal[25, 30, 31], or decreased[28, 31]. These differing conclusions are probably due to differing degrees of illness severity in the participants. Insulin resistant patients with CF have been noted to have poorer pulmonary function than patients who are insulin sensitive[28].

Increased fasting hepatic glucose production (HGP) in the presence of normal plasma glucose levels has been reported in patients with CF[27, 31, 34, 35]. In addition, suppression of HGP by physiologic doses of insulin is significantly impaired[27, 34]. Elevated HGP may be a compensatory mechanism to supply substrate for increased energy needs in CF, since HGP normalizes when it is expressed relative to resting energy expenditure[34, 35].

DIAGNOSIS

Cystic fibrosis patients are followed closely by their CF team, with a standard of care that includes quarterly evaluation of pulmonary function and nutrition, and review of the patient's general state of health and medical therapies. Because the onset of diabetes is often insidious, CF caregivers must maintain an elevated index of suspicion for this condition, and annual diabetes screening is necessary.

The 1998 CFRD consensus committee established minimum screening guidelines[7]. It was felt that the most immediate need was to identify individuals with fasting hyperglycemia. Thus, measurement of a fasting plasma glucose level (FPG) is recommended annually on all patients age 14 years or older. Individuals with a FPG $\geq$ 126 mg/dl (7.0 mM) should have a confirmatory FPG obtained the next day or a casual glucose level measured. If the repeat FPG is $\geq$ 126 mg/dl (7.0 mM) or if the casual glucose is $\geq$ 200 mg/dl (11.1 mmol/L), CFRD is diagnosed.

Table 3. Clinical signs of diabetes in CF. While they are not specific for diabetes, CFRD with or without FH should be considered in the differential diagnosis when these signs are present.

- Polyuria
- polydipsia
- delayed progression of puberty
- poor weight gain
- poor growth velocity
- unexplained chronic decline in pulmonary function

Individuals with FPG <126 mg/dl (7.0 mM) who have clinical symptoms of diabetes should have a standard OGTT performed to rule out diabetes without FH

Clinical signs of diabetes in CF include polyuria, polydipsia, delayed progression (but not necessarily onset) of puberty, poor weight gain, poor growth velocity, or an unexplained chronic decline in pulmonary function (Table 3). While these symptoms are not specific for diabetes, diabetes should be considered in the differential diagnosis.

If casual plasma glucose levels are elevated repeatedly or in the presence of symptoms, CFRD can be diagnosed. When used alone, however, casual plasma glucose levels have demonstrated poor sensitivity in the diagnosis of CFRD, since these patients have wide fluctuation in glucose levels throughout the day and a normal value may give false reassurance that the patient does not have diabetes[36]. Hemoglobin A1c measurement is not recommended for the diagnosis of CFRD because it is spuriously low in this population[1, 37]. While an elevated level suggests hyperglycemia has been present, a normal hemoglobin A1c level does not exclude the diagnosis of diabetes.

Pulmonary exacerbations, pregnancy, or glucocorticoid therapy may cause hyperglycemia by inducing insulin resistance. A heightened suspicion of CFRD should be considered in these states and glucose levels should be monitored more closely.

MANAGEMENT OF CFRD WITH FASTING HYPERGLYCEMIA

General Principles

Individuals with CFRD should be seen in a comprehensive setting that allows uncomplicated access to a diabetes team that can provide continuing education and develop an individually tailored management plan. A center accredited by the CF Foundation has the personnel, facilities, and services available for the complex management of CF but may need to develop a new relationship with a diabetes team. In the ideal situation, the diabetes team and CF team can hold a joint clinic in the same location. Patients with diabetes should be seen at least quarterly by the diabetes team.

A management plan that is developed in collaboration with the patient/family and incorporates a flexible, straightforward strategy to achieve blood glucose goals has the greatest likelihood to be successful. The diabetes goals must incorporate the patient's capacity to understand and execute the treatment regimen. Comprehensive self-management training should be provided. Written educational materials for type 1 or type 2 diabetes are not usually appropriate; there is a free CFRD patient manual available from the CF Foundation. Glycemic control targets for individuals with CFRD are similar to those recommended by the ADA for all individuals with diabetes. As for all patients on insulin therapy, frequent SMBG is mandatory to detect asymptomatic hypoglycemia and to adjust the insulin dose to achieve glycemic control targets.

The patient or the healthcare provider may not anticipate a variety of circumstances that impact blood glucose levels. A flexible and responsive therapeutic plan must exist that can accommodate the patient's lifestyle, daily changes in health status, and diabetic management goals. The effectiveness of the overall plan must be continuously evaluated.

Medical therapy

Insulin is the only standard medical treatment recommended at present for patients with CFRD with FH[7, 38]. Usually, unless they are ill, CFRD patients require relatively little basal insulin, and the most effective regimens are those that focus on meal coverage. Conventional therapy with split dose NPH and regular or rapid-acting insulin offers the security and simplicity of a rigid schedule and the convenience of only two or three daily injections. Most CF patients require more flexibility than this, however, since dietary intake can vary tremendously from day to day because of pulmonary and gastrointestinal disease. One frequently successful strategy is to use multiple daily injections (MDI) of rapid acting insulin 3-6 times or more per day, adjusted to match carbohydrate intake. The "carbohydrate counting" method is used, in conjunction with establishment of an insulin to carbohydrate ratio[38]. In otherwise healthy, stable CF patients, 0.5-1.0 units of rapid-acting insulin are usually adequate to cover 1 unit (15 g) of carbohydrate, while sicker patients may need 3 or more units of insulin per carbohydrate unit. With this regimen, basal insulin is seldom needed during the daytime, but modest doses of NPH at night are necessary to normalize fasting glucose levels. Patients may eat whatever they want, whenever they want, as long as they cover it appropriately with insulin. An additional benefit is that many CFRD patients appear to experience less hypoglycemia with this routine than with regimens using longer acting insulin. Anecdotal evidence has suggested that even very low doses of ultralente insulin can lead to hypoglycemia in CFRD patients. Sicker CF patients may have greater insulin resistance, however, and require more background insulin. Insulin pump therapy has been successfully used in CFRD, but very low basal rates are usually needed.

It should be noted that peak insulin levels following subcutaneous insulin lispro administration are somewhat blunted and considerably delayed in CF patients compared to normal control subjects[39]. Some patients may benefit by taking rapid-acting insulin 30 minutes or more before the meal, especially if post-prandial hypoglycemia is a concern.

CF patients who are nauseated or have early satiety sometimes do not know how much food they will be able to tolerate. In this situation, patients are advised to take rapid-acting insulin after eating. This may place the patient at risk for hypoglycemia 3-4 hours later, so these patients should eat or drink additional carbohydrates 2-3 hours after the injection. Every effort should be made to minimize gastrointestinal impediments to good nutrition, including aggressive treatment as needed with acid blockers, proton pump inhibitors or agents that improve gastric motility.

Frequently, because of poor growth or inadequate weight gain, patients with CF receive nighttime continuous drip feedings. A single pre-drip injection of regular insulin to cover the first half of the feeding and NPH to cover the second half is usually effective. The goal is to maintain overnight glucose levels between 80-180 mg/dl (4.4-10.0 mM). For patients who consume oral liquid dietary supplements, those with a relatively high fat concentration cause the least rise in blood glucose levels[40].

The use of oral agents to treat CFRD is controversial, and the CFRD consensus conference recommended that, until further data were available, these drugs should only be considered within the context of controlled research trials[7]. The literature consists primarily of abstracts and uncontrolled studies with small subject numbers[41-44]. There are potential problems with most of the existing FDA approved oral diabetes agents. Because the primary chronic problem in CF is insulin deficiency, drugs that improve insulin sensitivity are not likely to be of major benefit for most patients. Metformin is contraindicated in individuals with hypoxia because of the risk of fatal lactic acidosis, and it has multiple gastrointestinal side-effects which may negatively influence the nutritional status of CF patients. The potential for serious hepatic toxicity with thiazolidinediones may be greater in CF than in the general population because underlying liver damage is common. Drugs which reduce post-prandial glucose excursion by limiting intestinal absorption cannot be recommended to patients who suffer from chronic malabsorption and undernutrition.

Sulfonylureas have been the most commonly used oral agents used in CF. Glyburide, however, is not recommended because 50% of its elimination is in the bile. In the few studies measuring the effect of sulfonylureas on insulin secretion in CF, minimal improvement, if any, was found[42-45]. There are theoretical concerns that these agents may impair the effectiveness of new drugs designed to target the basic CF defect by improving function of the CFTR, because sulfonylureas bind to and inhibit CFTR[46]. The main practical concern with sulfonylureas has been hypoglycemia, which has anecdotally been found to be a common side-effect in CF, limiting the ability to achieve therapeutic doses[47]. Repaglinide-stimulated insulin release is glucose dependent and diminishes at low glucose concentrations (repaglinide product insert, Novo Nordisk Pharmaceuticals). This, combined with its short half-life (one hour), promotes improvement of meal-stimulated insulin secretion while minimizing the chance of between meal or nocturnal hypoglycemia. Theoretically, this profile of action might be ideal for the patient with CFRD without FH, although preliminary studies examining insulin levels after a pre-meal dose of repaglinide in this population suggest that the beta cell response to this drug is limited[39]. Studies are underway to evaluate the safety and efficacy of repaglinide in CFRD.

Nutritional Management

Individuals with CF have many variables that affect energy balance and nutrition. Pancreatic insufficiency with steatorrhea is a common feature. Malabsorption can be exacerbated by the loss of bile salts. Energy requirements may be escalated in CF by infection or pulmonary disease. The resulting malnutrition is associated with stunted growth, pubertal delay, deterioration of lung function, and early death. The need to maintain normoglycemia in CFRD can complicate an already precarious nutritional state.

Because of increased energy requirements and malabsorption, 130-150% of the recommended daily allowance of calories is recommended[48]. The weight goal in CF is 100-110% ideal body weight. Failure to maintain an acceptable weight is associated with poor lung function and decreased survival. Thus, restricting calories in persons with CF is never appropriate.

The dietary strategy in CFRD must provide adequate calories for growth and meet the increased metabolic demands of CF, while achieving a balance of food intake and insulin to maintain as near normal blood glucose levels as possible. Patients with CFRD do not appear to develop diabetes macrovascular complications. Hence, the restrictions in the intake of total fat, saturated fat, and cholesterol are not necessary in this group of patients and, in fact, are an important source of calories. Salt intake is not restricted because CF patients have sodium loss in their sweat. Even in the presence of diabetic nephropathy, protein reduction is probably not appropriate in CF because of the potential for malnutrition. The nutrition therapy features of CFRD, type 1, and type 2 diabetes mellitus are compared in Table 4. The specific goals for medical nutrition developed by the 1998 CFRD Consensus Conference are as follows:[7]

- Sufficient calories, frequently in excess of that required by healthy individuals, must be provided to ensure normal weight gain, growth and development in children and adolescents and normal weight in adults.
- Maintenance of near normal blood glucose levels must be sought to protect the patient from acute and chronic complications of diabetes.
- The dietary plan must include strategies for managing exercise and episodes of illness, and for prevention and treatment of hypoglycemia.
- Flexibility in meal planning is necessary in order to accommodate the patient's lifestyle, variability in energy intake, fluctuations in clinical status and pulmonary treatment regimen.
- Nutritional therapy must take into consideration the patient's psychosocial circumstances, economic issues, education level and cultural or religious beliefs, as well as evaluation of the patient's motivation or ability to learn and potential for making changes.

A meal plan should be developed that accommodates these goals and is within the capabilities of the patient to adhere to. Food intake must be balanced with insulin and metabolic demands to achieve acceptable blood glucose levels. Patients on fixed insulin doses must consume prescribed amounts of carbohydrates at specific times. This strategy sometimes works for individuals with a relatively constant meal and activity schedule. Most CF patients require more flexibility than this and have better metabolic control and better body weight if they count the carbohydrates they consume and adjust their insulin accordingly.

Table 4. Comparison between medical nutrition therapy in CFRD and type 1 and type 2 diabetes.

	CFRD	Type 1 and 2 diabetes
Calories/day	Never restricted---high calorie diet to maintain/achieve normal weight	Often restricted to maintain/achieve weight or glucose goals
Protein	No reduction	May be reduced in nephropathy
Fat	High (40% of daily kcal)	Restricted (<30% of daily kcal)
Carbohydrate	Individualized	Individualized
Sodium	> 4,000 mg/day	< 2,400 mg/day
Vitamins and Minerals	Supplementation required	Supplementation not necessary

Complications

Advances in CF care have extended the life expectancy to greater than 30 years, and many patients live into their fourth, fifth, or even sixth decades. In type 1 and type 2 diabetes mellitus, development of diabetes complications is a function of the duration of diabetes and the degree of glycemic control. It is likely that these same factors are important in CF. The unique pathophysiologic features of CF such as hypoxia and chronic infection and inflammation may also contribute to the development of complications. Health care providers have documented increasing reports of complications of CFRD over the last twenty years, which reflect the increasing life span of individuals with CF as well as better recognition of diabetes complications. Diabetic complications may be acute or chronic.

Acute

Patients with CFRD rarely develop ketoacidosis. The absence of ketoacidosis may be explained by the preservation of sufficient numbers of beta cells to ensure enough insulin secretion to suppress ketogenesis or by the relative deficiency of glucagon.

Despite glucagon deficiency, patients with CF demonstrate normal spontaneous recovery from insulin-induced hypoglycemia due to a brisk catecholamine response[21]. Hypoglycemia has, however, been reported as an acute complication of insulin administration in CF. Patients with CFRD on NPH and regular insulin therapy had serious episodes of hypoglycemia without meticulous attempts to control blood glucose levels[49]. Accidental administration of insulin as well as misadventures in insulin given in conjunction with a continuous-drip feeding have also led to hypoglycemia and, in one case, death[38]. CFRD patients and their families should be taught to recognize hypoglycemia. If hypoglycemia is treated appropriately with dietary management, patients rarely need outside assistance, develop seizures, or experience a loss of consciousness. The use of rapid-acting insulin may minimize the risk of hypoglycemia.

Chronic

In the past, the limited life span of individuals with CF explained the paucity of complications secondary to diabetes in these patients. In recent years, however, retinopathy[9, 50, 51], nephropathy[9, 50-52], and neuropathy[50, 51] have all been reported in CFRD. Complication monitoring can be confounded by damage to these organs from processes other than diabetes. Nephrotoxic antibiotics such as aminoglycosides and penicillins may compromise renal function, although they do not usually cause proteinuria. Because malabsorption is a feature of CF, nerve damage can be caused by essential vitamin or mineral deficiency. It may be difficult to differentiate between diabetic neuropathy and nerve damage induced by malnutrition. Likewise, gastroesophageal reflux, delayed gastric emptying, nausea and abdominal pain are frequent complications of CF which may be difficult to distinguish from diabetes gastrointestinal complications.

In general, cholesterol levels are abnormally low in CF patients, but triglyceride levels may be elevated[53]. Macrovascular complications of diabetes have not been described in CF, and no CF patient has been reported to die from atherosclerotic cardiovascular disease. This assessment may change as patients live longer.

Screening for diabetic complications is recommended in all patients with CFRD[7]. Quarterly measurement of blood pressure and careful examination for the presence of neuropathic foot problems and ischemia should be preformed. Annual dilated eye examination and urine albumin measurement should be done. Screening investigations for diabetic complications should begin at the time of CFRD diagnosis because, due to the insidious onset of CFRD, the true duration of diabetes prior to diagnosis of overt symptoms is often not known.

Psychosocial Aspects of CFRD

CF patients have complex treatment regimens prior to the diagnosis of diabetes. When CFRD is diagnosed, the psychological impact can be devastating. The added weight and responsibility of CFRD may have the greatest psychosocial impact during adolescence. Adolescents may rebel against not only CFRD treatment, but their multifaceted CF regimens as well, with little recognition of the consequences. Families and treatment team members must anticipate this possibility and respond to variable degrees of poor adherence with concern and compassion. A prolonged period of poor adherence, despair, or suggestions of depression should prompt a reassessment of the CFRD management plan and referral to the appropriate services. Routine interaction with a mental health professional from the time of CFRD diagnosis may help prevent more serious problems later. While no patient is eager to start insulin therapy, within a couple months many become convinced that it is worthwhile because they see positive results, particularly in weight gain.

Continuity and consistency of caregivers over time, a flexible management approach, parent and involvement, education and information, and accessible and available care are valuable components of treatment that will foster an environment that lessens the burden of stress to patients and their families[54]. Caregivers must strive to make access to care as uncomplicated, speedy, and economical as possible. Patients and parents must know the expectations of the caregivers as well as the capacity for clinical improvement and the potential for meaningful life.

Inpatient Management

CFRD patients become tremendously insulin resistant when they are acutely ill, and may need considerably larger insulin doses than usual. A dramatic increase in insulin requirements may herald the onset of illness. Blood glucose levels must be monitored closely and insulin dose adjustments made aggressively to minimize hyperglycemia during illness. Insulin requirements tend to decrease over several weeks with resolution of the illness, and thus close blood glucose monitoring and communication with the diabetes team must be continued until the baseline insulin requirements are reached.

Patients who are not known to have diabetes or patients with CFRD without FH may develop fasting hyperglycemia during times of acute illness or corticosteriod treatment. Glucose levels must be monitored during these times. Insulin therapy should be considered in patients who have sustained fasting hyperglycemia for more than 48 hours. Typically, pre-meal insulin requirements range from 0.5-3.0 units insulin per unit (15g) carbohydrate. NPH is usually needed at night to normalize fasting hyperglycemia. Aggressive blood glucose monitoring should be continued throughout the acute illness and for several weeks afterwards, since insulin needs usually decline as the patient's health improves. Approximately half of CF patients who require insulin during acute illness are able to discontinue it several weeks later[10].

Pregnancy

Early fears that pregnancy would shorten survival in women with CF appear, for the most part, to be unfounded[55, 56]. Unfortunately, an unusually rapid deterioration of pulmonary function is noted in the years following pregnancy in women with CF who have diabetes during pregnancy[55]. While this is not an absolute contraindication to pregnancy, it is important that women with CFRD and their partners understand the risks.

Issues of fertility, sexuality and contraception should be introduced early during the adolescent years for all young women with CF and especially for those with diabetes. After transition to the adult CF clinic, all women should again be counseled about the risks of pregnancy, methods of birth control, and the importance of careful metabolic control prior to pregnancy. For women with CFRD wishing to become pregnant, aggressive normalization of blood glucose levels is vital to reduce fetal and perinatal morbidity and mortality. Tight blood glucose control may also help improve overall nutrition in pregnant CF women, since normal weight gain is often difficult in CF pregnancies. As with other diabetic pregnancies, monitoring for microvascular disease should be performed.

Women with CF who are not known to have CFRD may develop gestational diabetes during pregnancy. The optimal timing for performing screening in CF pregnancies is not known. Diabetes may occur earlier than in non-CF pregnancy because CF patients are insulin deficient. Until studies better define this, it is recommended that a baseline OGTT be performed prior to conception if possible, or at the time the pregnancy is confirmed[7]. This should be repeated in the middle of the second and third trimesters, or earlier if maternal weight gain is inadequate. Six weeks or more after the pregnancy ends, an OGTT should be performed and the OGTT category of the mother reclassified.

Management of CFRD without fasting hyperglycemia

Patients with CFRD without FH constitute a group for whom it is not known whether insulin therapy can prevent malnutrition or diabetes complications. No management guidelines are available because there are no data about the risk of diabetes in this group. Studies are underway to determine both the risk of microvascular complications and whether insulin deficiency compromises nutritional status in this population.

If patients with CFRD without FH are clinically stable, current practice is to simply monitor them because they are at risk for progression to fasting hyperglycemia. A home glucose monitoring device is provided and they may be asked to do a glucose profile one day per month and during times of illness[38]. Carbohydrate in the diet is not restricted, but they are taught the method of carbohydrate counting and asked to evenly distribute their carbohydrate intake throughout the day. Insulin therapy is usually not recommended unless symptoms of diabetes are present, such as poor weight gain, poor growth velocity, poor progression of puberty, or unexplained chronic decline in pulmonary function. Under these conditions, a trial of pre-meal insulin therapy should be considered. Chronic complication screening recommendations are the same as for CFRD with FH.

Management of impaired glucose tolerance

Little is known about the prognosis of CF patients with impaired glucose tolerance, other than that they are at greater risk for progression to diabetes than those with a normal glucose tolerance test[37]. Concerns in the general population that IGT may predispose to cardiovascular disease do not appear to be relevant in CF. There are no data to suggest management strategies or risk of complications for this group of patients. CF patients with IGT should be monitored with an annual OGTT and blood glucose levels should be measured during acute illnesses, because of the risk of progression to diabetes[7, 37].

Summary

Advances in care have markedly extended the lifespan of individuals with CF over the last forty years. This has been accompanied by an increased prevalence of CFRD. Only recently has a uniform and suitable approach to nomenclature, diagnosis, and management of CFRD been attempted. The CFRD consensus conference in 1998 established diagnostic categories based on oral glucose tolerance testing and provided recommendations for screening and management[7]. This effort has provided a foundation on which priorities for provider education, research, and patient care can be based.

A current priority is to identify individuals in the CF population who have fasting hyperglycemia because they are at highest risk for progressive clinical deterioration. These patients should be treated with insulin. The diabetes care plan must be flexible and must take into account daily fluctuations in overall health and appetite. Calorie restriction is never appropriate, because attaining and maintaining normal body weight is necessary for survival in CF. Marked insulin resistance is noted during acute illness or corticosteriod therapy, and insulin needs increase dramatically in these circumstances. Although patients with CFRD are at risk for microvascular diabetes complications, they do not appear to suffer macrovascular complications. Few guidelines are available for the management of CFRD individuals without fasting hyperglycemia or those that have impaired glucose tolerance.

Research over the next few years will provide more management guidance and clarification of complications associated with long-standing diabetes. The relationship between glycemic control, nutrition, and pulmonary status needs to be better further delineated. Recent advances have provided the means by which improved strategies to diagnose and manage CFRD today can be implemented and further explored for development of optimal care of CFRD in the future.

REFERENCES

1. Lanng S, Thorsteinsson B, Nerup J, Koch C. Diabetes mellitus in cystic fibrosis: effect of insulin therapy on lung function and infections. Acta Paediatrica 1994; 83:849-53.
2. Milla CE, Warwick WJ, Moran A. Trends in pulmonary function in cystic fibrosis patients correlate with the degree of glucose intolerance at baseline. Am J Resp Crit Care Med 2000; 162:891-5.
3. Finkelstein SM, Wielinski CL, Elliott GR, Warwick WJ, Barbosa J, Wu SC, Klein DJ. Diabetes mellitus associated with cystic fibrosis. J Pediatr 1998; 112:373-7.
4. Moran A, Milla C, DuCret R, Nair KS. Protein metabolism in clinically stable adult CF patients with abnormal glucose tolerance. Diabetes in press:2001.

5. Hardin DS, Leblanc A, Lukenbaugh S, Para L, Seilheimer DK. Proteolysis associated with insulin resistance in cystic fibrosis. Pediatrics 1998; 101:433-7.
6. American Diabetes Association Clinical Practice Recommendations. Diabetes Care Supplement1:1999.
7. Moran A, Hardin D, Rodman D, Allen HF, Beall RJ, Borowitz D, Brunzell C, Campbell PW, Chesrown SE, Duchow C, Fink RJ, FitzSimmons SC, Hamilton N, Hirsch I, Howenstine MS., Klein DJ, Madhun Z, Pencharz PB, Quittner AL, Robbins MK, Schindler T, Schissel K, Schwarzenberg SJ, Stallings VA, Tullis E., Zipf WB. Diagnosis, screening, and management of CFRD: a consensus conference report. J Diabetes Research and Clinical Practice 1999; 45:55-71.
8. Report of the expert committee on the diagnosis and classification of diabetes mellitus. Diabetes Care 1997; 20:1183-97.
9. Lanng S, Thorsteinsson B, Lund-Andersen C, Nerup J, Schiotz PO, Koch C. Diabetes mellitus in Danish CF patients: prevalence and late diabetic complications. Acta Paediatr 1994; 83:72-7.
10. Moran A, Doherty L, Wang X, Thomas W. Abnormal glucose metabolism in cystic fibrosis. J. Pediatr 1998; 133:10-16.
11. Rosenecker J, Eichler I, Kuhn L, Harms HK, von der Hardt **J.** Genetic determination of diabetes mellitus in patients with cystic fibrosis. J Pediatr 1995; 127:441-3.
12. Reiter E, Stern R, Root A. The reproductive endocrine system in CF: basal gonadotropin and sex steroid levels. Am J Dis Child 1981; 135:422-6.
13. Hamdi I, Payne S, Barton D, et al. Genotype analysis in CF in relation to the occurrence of diabetes mellitus. Clin Genet 1993; 43:186-9.
14. Iannucci A, Mukai K, Johnson D, Burke B. Endocrine pancreas in cystic fibrosis: an immunohistochemical study. Hum Pathol 1984; 15:278-84.
15. Kopito LE , Schwachman H. The pancreas in CF: chemical composition and comparative morphology. Ped Res 1976; 10:742-9.
16. Lohr M, Goertchem P, Nizze H, Gould NS, GBould VE, Oberholzer M, Heitz PU, Kloppel G. CF associated islet changes may provide a basis for diabetes. Virchows Archiv A Pathol Anat 1989; 414:179-85.
17. Johnson KH, O'Brien TD, Betsholtz C, Westermark P. Islet amyloid, islet-amyloid polypeptide, and diabetes mellitus. N Engl J Med 1989; 321:513-8.

18. Laszik Z, Pap A, Farkas G, Ormos J. Endocrine pancreas in chronic pancreatitis. Arch Pathol Lab Med 1989; 113:47-51.
19. Clark A, Cooper GJS, Lewis CE, Morris JF, Willis AC, Reid KBM, Turner RC. Islet amyloid formed from diabetes-associated peptide may be pathogenic in Type-2 diabetes. Lancet 1987; 2:231-4.
20. Couce M, O'Brien TD, Moran A, Roche PC, Butler PC. Diabetes mellitus in CF is characterized by islet amyloidosis. J Clin Endocrinol Metab 1996; 81:1267-72.
21. Moran A, Diem P, Klein DJ, Levitt MD, Robertson RP. Pancreatic endocrine function in cystic fibrosis. J Pediatr 1991; 118:715-23.
22. Hartling SG, Garne S, Binder C, Heilmann C, Petersen W, Petersen KE, Koch C. Proinsulin, insulin, and C-peptide in cystic fibrosis after an oral glucose tolerance test. Diabetes Research 1988; 7:165-169.
23. Hamdi I, Green M, Shneerson JM, Palmer DR, Hales CN. Proinsulin, proinsulin intermediate and insulin in CF. Clin Endocrinol 1993; 39:21-6.
24. Lippe BM, Sperling MA, Dooley RR. Pancreatic alpha and beta cell function in cystic fibrosis. J Pediatr 1977; 90:751-5.
25. Cucinotta D, Conti Nibali S, Arrigo T, Di Benedetto A, Magazzu G, Di Cesare E, Constantino A. Beta cell function, peripheral sensitivity to insulin and islet cell autoimmunity in cystic fibrosis patients with normal glucose tolerance. Horm Res 1990; 34:33-38.
26. Meacham LR, McKean LP, Buchanan CN, Caplan DB, Pfaffle RW, Parks JS, Culler FL. Selective preservation of somatostatin secretion in CF patients with diabetes. Pediatr Pulmonol 1991; suppl 6:333.
27. Moran A, Pyzdrowski K, Weinreb MD, Kahn BB, Smith SA, Adams KL, Seaquist ER. Insulin sensitivity in cystic fibrosis. Diabetes 1994; 43:1020-6.
28. Hardin DS, LeBlanc A, Lukenbaugh S, Seilheimer DK. Insulin resistance is associated with decreased clinical status in cystic fibrosis. J Pediatr 1997; 130:948-56.
29. Holl RW, Heinze E, Wolf A, Rank M, Teller WM. Reduced pancreatic insulin release and reduced peripheral insulin sensitivity contribute to hyperglycemia in CF. Eur J Pediatr 1995; 154:356-361.
30. Lanng S, Thorsteinsson B, Roder ME, Nerup J, Koch C. Insulin sensitivity and insulin clearance in CF patients with normal and diabetic glucose tolerance. Clin Endocrinol 1994; 41:217-23.

31. Austin A, Kalhan SC, Orenstein D, Nixon P, Arslanian S. Roles of insulin resistance and b-cell dysfunction in the pathogenesis of glucose intolerance in cystic fibrosis. J Clin Endo Metab 1994; 79:80-85.
32. Yki-Jarvinen H, Helve E, Koivisto VA. Hyperglycemia decreases glucose uptake in type I diabetes. Diabetes 1997; 36:892-9.
33. Ahmad T, Nelson R, Taylor R. Insulin sensitivity and metabolic clearance rate of insulin in cystic fibrosis. Metabolism 1994; 43:163-167.
34. Hardin DS, LeBlance A, Para L, Seilheimer DK. Hepatic insulin resistance and defects in substrate utilization in cystic fibrosis. Diabetes 1999; 48:1082-7.
35. Kien CL, Horswill CA, Zipf SB, McCoy KS. Elevated hepatic glucose production in children with cystic fibrosis. Ped Res 1995; 37:600-5.
36. Yung B, Kemp M, Hooper J, Hodson M. Diagnosis of CFRD: a selective apprach in performing the OGTT based on a combination of clinical and biochemical criteria. Thorax 1999; 54:40-3.
37. Lanng S, Hansen A, Thorsteinsson B, Nerup J, Koch C. Glucose tolerance in cystic fibrosis: a five year prospective study. BMJ 1995; 311:655-9.
38. Moran A. CFRD: an approach to diagnosis and management. Pediatric Diabetes 2000; 1:14-8.
39. Moran A, Phillips J, Milla C. Insulin and Glucose Excursion Following Pre-Meal Insulin Lispro or Repaglinide in Cystic Fibrosis Related Diabetes. Submitted for publication 2001.
40. Milla C, Doherty L, Raatz S, Schwarzenberg SJ, Regelmann W, Moran A. Glycemic response to dietary supplements in CF is dependent upon the carbohydrate content of the formula. Journal of Parenteral and Enteral Nutrition 1995; 20:182-6.
41. Bertele-Harms RM , Harms HK. Sulfonylurea in the treatment of CFRD. A 15 year experience. Pediatric Pulmonology 1996; 13:380A.
42. Culler FL, McKean LP, Buchanan CJ, Caplan DB, Meacham LR. Glipizide treatment of patients with CF and impaired glucose tolerance. in Endocrine Society Program and Abstracts. 1992. San Antonio, Texas 45A.
43. Hinds A, Sheehan AG, Parsons HG. Tobutamide causes a modest increase in insulin secretion in CF patients with impaired glucose tolerance. Metabolism: Clinical and Experimental 1995; 44:13-8.

44. Horswill CA, Zipf WB, Kien CL, McCoy KS, O'Dorisio TM. Glipizide increased insulin secretion but not growth of children with CF. FASEB 1990; 4:3272A.
45. Zipf WB, Kien CL, Horswill CA, McCoy KS, O'Dorisio T, Pinyerd BL. Effects of tolbutamide on growth and body composition of nondiabetic children with CF. Pediatr Res 1991; 30:309-14.
46. Sheppard DJ , Welsh MJ. Effect of ATP-sensitive K+ channel regulators on cystic fibrosis transmembrance conductance regulator chloride currents. J. Gen. Physiol.1992; 100:573-91.
47. Hardin DS , Moran A. Diabetes mellitus in cystic fibrosis. Endo Metab Clinics No America 1999;28:787-800.
48. Ramsey BW, Farrell P, Pencharz PB. Nutritional assessment and management in cystic fibrosis: A consensus report. Am J Clin Nutr 1992; 55:71-5.
49. Rodman HM, Doershuk CF, Roland JM. The interaction of two diseases: diabetes mellitus and cystic fibrosis. Medicine 1986; 65:389-97.
50. Sullivan MM , Denning CR. Diabetic microangiopathy in patients with cystic fibrosis. Pediatrics 1989; 84:642-646.
51. Dolan TF. Microangiopathy in a young adult with CF and diabetes mellitus (letter). N Engl J Med 1986; 314:991-2.
52. Allen JL.Progressive nephropathy in a patient with CF and diabetes (letter). N Engl J Med 1986; 315:764.
53. Figueroa V, Milla C, Parks EJ, Schwarzenberg SJ, Moran A.Abnormal Lipid Levels in Cystic Fibrosis. Submitted for publication 2001.
54. Baine S, Rosenbaum P, King S.Chronic childhood illnesses: what aspects of caregiving do parents value. Child: care, health, and develop 1995; 21:291-304.
55. FitzSimmons SC, Fitzpatrick S, Thompson B, Aitkin M, Fiel S, Winnie G, Hilman B.A longitudinal sudy of the effects of pregnancy on 325 women with CF. Pediatric Pulmonology 1996; 13:99-101.
56. Gilljam M, Antoniou M, Shin J, Dupuis A, Corey M, Tullis E.A longitudinal study of the effects of pregnancy on 325 women with CF. Pediatr Pulmonol 2000; 13:99-101.

Chapter 6
DIABETES IN THE DEVELOPING COUNTRIES

P.S.N. Menon, M.D., Anurag Bajpai, M.D.
Armed Forces Hospital, Kuwait & All India Institute of Medical Sciences, New Delhi, India

INTRODUCTION

The profile of diabetes mellitus seen in the developing countries differs from that seen in the developed world with regards to clinical, genetic and etiological features. Type 1 or insulin-dependent diabetes mellitus (type 1 DM or IDDM) and type 2 or non-insulin-dependent diabetes mellitus (type 2 DM or NIDDM) are the most common forms of diabetes encountered in the developing countries[1]. A distinct form of diabetes mellitus with characteristic features of malnutrition with or without pancreatic damage termed malnutrition-related diabetes mellitus (MRDM) is peculiar to tropical countries and is a relatively uncommon cause of diabetes mellitus. Even though MRDM has been frequently reported from the Indian subcontinent, it accounts for less than 1% of all diabetics[2]. MRDM with clinical features, which are different from the type 1 and 2 DM had generated a lot of controversies, and its study has helped in better understanding of the pathogenesis of diabetes mellitus. Economic constraints of the developing countries have important implications in management policies for diabetic children.

TYPE 1 DIABETES MELLITUS

Type 1 DM is the commonest form of childhood diabetes mellitus in developing countries. The clinical, epidemiological and genetic profile is different from developed countries.

Epidemiology

Data regarding incidence and prevalence of type 1 DM in developing countries is limited and is mostly hospital-based. Epidemiological data is now emerging through international efforts. Important among them are the Diabetes Epidemiology Research International group (DERI) and the WHO sponsored multinational program for childhood diabetes (DIAMOND), which have helped to establish the epidemiological pattern of diabetes in many countries[3,4.] Most studies indicate a lower incidence of type 1 DM compared to developed countries. This low incidence may be related to under-reporting, poor infrastructure for health services, late referrals, delay in diagnosis and non-availability of life-saving insulin leading to death of patients even before diagnosis. Type 1 DM accounts for 0.9-5% of all diabetics in these countries[5,6.] The incidence in India (10.5/100000/year) and African countries (6.4/100000/year) is substantially lower than western countries such as USA (19/100000/year) and Finland (33.5/100000/year)[4,7.] The lowest incidence of type 1 DM has been reported from Mauritius (2.1/100000/year). The recent global trend for an increase in type 1 DM has also been observed in some of these countries[8.] This may be actually due to better recognition of the disease in these countries.

Etiology

Genetic and autoimmune factors are strongly associated with type 1 DM in the developed countries. These factors are equally important in developing countries as well. Environmental factors such as malnutrition and recurrent infections may modulate the presentation and clinical features of type 1 DM.

Autoimmunity

Evidence of autoimmunity in the pathogenesis of type 1 DM is substantial in the developed countries. Association with HLA antigens and antibodies directed against components of pancreas including GABA decarboxylase (GADA), islet cells (ICA) and insulin (anti-insulin antibodies) and high incidence of concurrent autoimmune diseases point towards an autoimmune basis for the development of type 1 DM. Previous studies indicated that autoimmunity might be less important in the pathogenesis of type 1 DM in the developing countries[9]. A low incidence of antibodies directed against the islet cell, GABA decarboxylase and insulin was observed in a study from south India[10] and autoantibodies remained positive for a shorter duration. These observations led to the hypothesis that lower incidence of autoimmunity was responsible for the decreased prevalence of type 1 DM in these countries. Studies on immigrant Indians residing in England and South Africa have demonstrated that the incidence of these antibodies is comparable to Caucasians[11,12.] Recent Indian studies have confirmed these observations[13.] The prevalence of autoimmune diseases such as hypothyroidism and pernicious anemia in children with type 1 DM is also similar to western countries[14,15.] These observations indicate that autoimmunity is equally important in the pathogenesis of type 1 DM in developing countries. Malnutrition by influencing immunity may alter the course and progression of the disease. In particular slower progression of type 1 DM may be related to depressed immunity due to malnutrition.

Genetic predisposition

Genetic influences in type 1 DM appear to be important in developing countries. In a study from India on pediatric diabetics, 11.2% parents had some form of diabetes[16]. Factors involved in the genetic predisposition to type 1 DM however are different compared to the developed countries. HLA studies in Caucasians have demonstrated positive correlation with DR3-DQ2 and DR4-DQ8 antigens[17]. Studies from the developing countries have confirmed the association with HLA DR3-DQ2 antigens, while association with HLA DR4-DQ8 has not been demonstrated[18,19]. This may have an important role in the slow progression of type 1 DM in these countries. It has been postulated that the combination of HLA DR3-DQ2 and HLA DR4-DQ8 is associated with rapid progression of type 1 DM. On the other hand, HLA DR3-DQ2 without HLA DR4-DQ8 is associated with slower pancreatic damage and slower course of type 1 DM[20]. The relative risk of HLA-DR3 with type 1 DM is much higher in Indian population compared to developing countries[21]. Non-MHC genetic associations with type 1 DM are also different from Caucasians. Insulin gene and IL-1 receptor locus, important in type 1 DM in western countries, are not associated with type 1 DM in these populations[22]. Genes telomeric to the IL-1 receptor (D2S308 and D2S363) and related to vitamin D receptors have been implicated in the pathogenesis of type 1 DM[23,24].

Environmental influences

The role of infections and toxins in the pathogenesis of type 1 DM appears to be similar to developed countries. Malnutrition is an important environmental factor in type 1 DM that modulates its clinical course. Its role in autoimmunity has already been alluded to. Low fat stores and carnitine levels may explain the lower tendency of these patients to progress to diabetic ketoacidosis (DKA).

Clinical features

Most children with type 1 DM in developing countries present with classical symptoms of diabetes or DKA. In a study of adolescent Nigerian patients with type 1 DM, 80% presented with symptoms of diabetes or DKA[25]. The acute presentation of DKA in children is often unrecognized and there is an extremely high short-term mortality[26]. This is often affected by poor awareness, lack of trained staff, nonavailability of insulin, inadequate laboratory facilities, prohibitive cost of transport, treatment and monitoring equipment, cultural practices, belief in traditional medicine, socioeconomic factors and lack of education[3]. Almost 100% mortality six years after diagnosis and 60% five-year survival rates following diagnosis have been documented in tropical Africa[27,28]. The age of onset is lower and progression of type 1 DM is slower in developing countries.

A substantial number of patients are malnourished. In one of the studies from India, 70% patients with type 1 DM had body mass index (BMI) less than 19 kg/m^2 [29] Children with diabetes despite good care continue to be thin and chronically malnourished. The pubertal spurt is often delayed and they frequently remain stunted. Many children report with acute infections. Association with tuberculosis and unusual fungal infections are not uncommon[30, 31].

The profile of complications associated with diabetes is also different compared to western populations. Many diabetic children in tropics do not live long enough to develop microvascular complications, as optimal care is often not available. Cardiovascular complications such as coronary artery disease and hypertension are less common[32]. This may be related to lower levels of LDL cholesterol. The incidence of retinopathy is lower[33]. This may be the result of less sensitive diagnostic techniques used for assessment of retinopathy. In a study of Indian patients with type 1 DM using non-mydriatic retinal color photography, 31% were found to have retinopathy, a figure similar to the western countries[34]. Early development of cataracts is common. There is a high prevalence of nephropathy appearing in late adolescence. Use of nephrotoxic traditional medicines and limited availability of new generation antihypertensive agents lead to chronic renal failure, which is a cause for mortality for those who survive acute complications. Incidence of neuropathy is comparable to the developed countries. Severe brain damage and cognitive dysfunction from prolonged and repeated hypoglycemia are not uncommon.

Management issues

Type 1 DM is a major therapeutic problem in developing countries due to economic constraints. The annual cost of treatment of a patient with type 1 DM in Africa was calculated to be $287 in 1989-1990[35]. Considering the low per capita income of these countries, care of patients with type 1

DM is indeed difficult. The fact that most type 1 DM patients belong to the dependent groups of the society complicates the matter further. Many children with type 1 DM are dying in developing countries due to the lack of insulin[36,37]. Even in the developed countries, young black Americans have higher short and long term mortality with type 1 diabetes compared with their Caucasian counterparts[38]. According to estimates, 0.48% of the global production of insulin (approximately $3-5 million/year) is sufficient to fulfill the requirements of 40 highly indebted countries[39]. Contributions from the developed countries may go a long way in improving the care and management of type 1 DM in the developing countries.

TYPE 2 DIABETES MELLITUS

Type 2 DM is characterized by the presence of low to higher than normal plasma insulin responses. The major defect appears to be reduced insulin sensitivity at target tissues with variable degrees of relative insulin deficiency. It is more common in adults and rare in pediatric age groups. Type 2 DM is seen among a small percentage of young adults between the ages of 15 and 30 years especially among ethnic groups with high susceptibility to diabetes such as Pima Indians, African Americans, Arabs in Libya and Asian Indians[40]. Even in UK, type 2 DM predominates in clinics where most children are from populations with a high prevalence of this condition such as Asian Indians[41, 42]. This form of diabetes has been termed "maturity onset diabetes of the young" (MODY) or "non-insulin-dependent diabetes of the young" (NIDDY)[43]. The rising incidence is attributed to changing food pattern and the increasing rate of obesity in schoolchildren.

The incidence of type 2 DM in developing countries in general and the Indian subcontinent in particular is substantially higher compared to the developed countries[44]. Importantly patients with type 2 DM have an earlier age at onset[45]. The age at presentation of type 2 DM is 10 years less compared to the developed countries. Type 2 DM in general occurs at a younger age, usually fourth decade in Indians. About 2% of patients have onset of disease below 25 years with the youngest patient reported at 10 years. Unlike the western world, it is common in all ranges of BMI. An increased prevalence of young and non-obese type 2 DM has been reported from Cameroon[46]. Association with hypertension, dyslipidemia and acanthosis nigricans is not well described. There is a strong genetic component, but there are very few studies on transcription factors such as hepatocyte nuclear factor subtypes or glucokinase mutations. Measurement of plasma C-peptide responses can be used to differentiate type 2 from type 1 DM. β-cell reserve is fairly well preserved even after 15 years of diabetes.

Autosomal dominant MODY is common in India[29,47]. MODY has been shown to be especially common in Indians residing in India as well as emigrant Indians in South Africa and Europe[48,49]. MODY is discussed in detail a separate chapter in this book.

MALNUTRITION- RELATED DIABETES MELLITUS

Presence of a form of diabetes related to malnutrition and distinct from type 1 and 2 DM in the developing countries due to probable effect of malnutrition has been observed for a long time. The study of MRDM has provided valuable insights in the understanding of diabetes mellitus.

Historical perspective

Difference in the clinical profile of DM in the tropical countries was noted for the first time in 1907 when peculiar features of tropical diabetes were described[50]. However it was only in 1956 when Hugh-Jones described a special form of diabetes in Jamaica, that interest in tropical diabetes mellitus was generated[51]. J type diabetes (J for Jamaica), as described by Hugh-Jones, involved malnourished young individuals (15-40 years) with BMI less than 19 kg/m^2. Insulin requirements were high (>1.5 U/kg/day); ketoacidosis was however not observed after discontinuation of insulin for prolonged periods. While no pathogenic mechanism was established, malnutrition was the prime suspect. Since then the occurrence of insulin-resistant and ketosis-resistant diabetes has been observed in many malnourished residents of tropical countries. A lot of controversy has been generated due to lack of uniform diagnostic criteria and unambiguous diagnostic markers. This is reflected in the myriad nomenclature used for this condition including K type diabetes, malnutrition-related diabetes mellitus (MRDM), malnutrition-modulated diabetes mellitus (MMDM), protein deficient diabetes mellitus (PDDM) and protein deficient pancreatic diabetes (PDPD).

In 1959 Zuidema reported a variant of malnutrition-related diabetes in Indonesia with clinical and laboratory features of exocrine pancreatic dysfunction and pancreatic calcification[52]. Fibrocalcific pancreatic diabetes (FCPD) as the entity was named was believed to be secondary to tropical calcific pancreatitis (TCP), a form of non-alcoholic pancreatitis common in developing countries. Studies from various tropical countries in general and South India in particular have provided valuable insight to this interesting disease.

The enthusiasm about MRDM was at its peak when the WHO working group on diabetes elevated MRDM from a category of miscellaneous causes to an entity distinct from type 1 and 2 DM[53]. MRDM was classified into PDDM and FCPD based on the presence of pancreatic calcification and exocrine pancreatic dysfunction in the latter. Recent studies have raised doubts regarding MRDM being a distinct diagnostic entity. The American Diabetic Association (ADA) in its most recent consensus statement did not recognize MRDM as a distinct category in the schema for the classification of diabetes mellitus[54].

Classification

Clinical features allow classification of MRDM into two distinct entities (Table 1). Evidence of pancreatitis in the form of recurrent abdominal pain, pancreatic calcification and exocrine pancreatic dysfunction is characteristic of FCPD. Patients with PDDM do not have clinical, radiological or biochemical evidence of pancreatic dysfunction.

PROTEIN DEFICIENT DIABETES MELLITUS

The entity of malnutrition-related, insulin-resistant and ketosis-resistant diabetes is currently classified as PDDM.

Epidemiology

PDDM has been reported from a number of tropical countries in Asia and Africa[55-58]. It accounted for 1% of all the diabetics in a study involving patients from south India[2]. The incidence of PDDM is lower in Africa than in Asia. Large studies in Cameroon and Ethiopia have failed to identify cases of PDDM[46,59]. PDDM is declining even in countries where it was once common. This may be related to changes in the diagnostic criteria or improvement in the nutritional status.

Table 1. Comparison of PDDM versus FCPD

Feature	PDDM	FCPD
Age at onset years	10-35	15-40
Sex predisposition	M>F	M: F=3:1
Malnutrition	More	Less
Ketosis	Less	More
Insulin requirement	High	Variable
Steatorrhea	Uncommon	Common
Abdominal pain	Less	More

Autoimmunity	Present	Rare
HLA association	Common	Rare
Exocrine pancreatic dysfunction	Rare	Common
Pancreatic calcification	No	Yes
C-peptide levels	Intermediate	Intermediate

Etiopathogenesis

Malnutrition

Malnutrition was the most striking difference noticed between diabetics in the tropical countries compared to the western countries. This observation fuelled the hypothesis that malnutrition was the major factor in the pathogenesis of PDDM. The effect of malnutrition on endocrine pancreatic functions is unclear. Direct damage of the islets is possible although it has not been demonstrated in experimental models[60]. Atrophy of the pancreas and generalized thinning of the pancreatic ducts were observed in patients with PDDM in a recent study suggesting ongoing pancreatic damage[61]. Other factors such as peripheral resistance to insulin due to reduced cell mass, lower pancreatic enzyme levels and insulin antagonists play a part in the pathogenesis of PDDM[62]. Low level of gut related insulinogenic factors has also been demonstrated in malnourished subjects[63]. Derangement of glucose homeostasis has been noticed in animal models, children with kwashiorkor and adults with malnutrition; the effect however is transient[64-66]. Genetic and environmental factors appear to be significant as only a small proportion of malnourished children develop PDDM. There appears to be no specific role for micronutrient and magnesium deficiencies in the pathogenesis of PDDM[67].

Genetic factors

Familial aggregation of PDDM has been observed. This may be due to genetic predisposition or environmental factors. HLA studies conducted in Nigeria and south India in patients with PDDM have found association with HLA DR7-DQ9 and DR3[68,69]. In a recent study on the HLA profile of patients with type 1 DM, PDDM and FCPD in the eastern Indian state of Orissa, PDDM was positively associated with HLA DR3-DQ2 but not with DR4-DR8[70]. Patients with type 1 DM had similar HLA predisposition. It appears that PDDM may be a variant of type 1 DM influenced by malnutrition rather than a separate entity.

Autoimmunity

Initial studies in patients with PDDM failed to demonstrate the presence of antibodies directed against the pancreatic islets. The evidence of autoimmunity in the pathogenesis of PDDM is now emerging[70-72]. In a study regarding the incidence of GADA and ICA in north Indian patients with type 1 DM, PDDM and FCPD, 14% patients with PDDM were positive for GADA as against 40% of type 1 DM[73]. The association with HLA DR3-DQ2 and presence of autoantibodies support the hypothesis that PDDM is a variant of type 1 DM with a slow onset modulated by malnutrition.

Clinical features

Patients with PDDM manifest in the second decade of life. Males predominate; the predisposition is however less striking compared to FCPD. Malnutrition is present in majority. BMI is most often less than 19 kg/m^2 and clinical evidence of vitamin and micronutrient deficiencies are evident in most patients. Past history of malnutrition is nearly universal suggesting that malnutrition acts at an early stage of the disease[74]. PDDM has also been observed in patients without clinical evidence of malnutrition. Superficial skin infections (40%) and tuberculosis (10%) are common in these patients.

Symptoms of diabetes are the commonest presenting features of PDDM. Glucose levels are usually very high but ketoacidosis is rare[75]. The cause of ketosis resistance is unclear. Residual insulin secretion may be an important factor in preventing ketosis. A study of Ethiopian patients with type 1 DM, PDDM and type 2 DM demonstrated intermediate C-peptide levels in patients with PDDM[76]. It appears that these patients have enough insulin levels to prevent ketoacidosis but not to maintain euglycemia[77]. Glucagon plays an important role in the pathogenesis of DKA and high glucagon-insulin ratio is characteristic of DKA. Low glucagon levels in PDDM due to damage to alpha cells may thus prevent ketosis[78]. Lower glucagon levels have been found in PDDM compared to type 1 DM[79]. Low levels of ketogenic substances including free fatty acids and carnitine due to malnutrition may also be responsible for the paucity of ketosis in these patients[80]. Variability in resistance to ketosis in PDDM is increasingly becoming evident. Ketoacidosis has been observed in patients with PDDM especially after nutritional rehabilitation. Some of the J type diabetics became ketoacidotic during follow-up[81]. In a study of Indian patients with PDDM, variability in insulin dependence and ketosis resistance was observed. On follow-up some improved and were controlled with oral hypoglycemic agents (OHA) alone while others went on to develop ketoacidosis[82].

High insulin (>1.5 U/kg/days) requirement is characteristic of patients with PDDM[83]. Whether this represents genuine insulin resistance or the use of impure insulin preparations that are common is unclear[84]. Hyperinsulinemic euglycemic clamp studies showed that insulin-mediated glucose disposal in PDDM is similar to type 1 DM indicating that true insulin resistance is unlikely[85]. As described above heterogeneity in insulin requirement is common and many patients may be controlled on OHA.

The profile of complications of PDDM is different from type 1 and 2 DM. Peripheral neuropathy is particularly common[86]. Microvascular complications like nephropathy and retinopathy are similar to type 1 DM. Cardiovascular complications including hypertension and coronary artery disease are less commonly observed.

Clinical and investigational evidence of exocrine pancreatic deficiency is uncommon in PDDM, a factor helpful in distinguishing it from FCPD.

Diagnosis

Diagnostic criteria for PDDM as presented by Ahuja[87] have been superseded by a scoring system described by Tripathy and Samal[88]. This scoring schema takes into account the nutritional status, insulin requirement and ketosis resistance and provides flexibility in the diagnosis (Table 2).

Management

Insulin should be started and titrated for normoglycemia as in any other child with diabetes. Nutritional rehabilitation and careful screening for infections is an important part of management of PDDM. C-peptide estimation may be helpful in deciding about insulin requirement and possibility of control with OHA.

Table 2. Diagnostic criteria for PDDM

Ahuja (87)	Tripathy & Samal (88)	Score*
Blood glucose >200 mg/dl	Age at onset- 10-30 years	1
	Poor socioeconomic status	1
Age at onset <30 years	Leanness-	
	BMI < 16 kg/m^2	2
BMI <18 kg/m^2	<18 kg/m^2	1
	Malnutrition in childhood	2
Absence of ketosis on withdrawal of insulin	Malnutrition - Clinical features	1
	Fasting blood sugar >11 mmol/L	1
Poor socioeconomic status	Ketosis resistance	3
	Insulin requirement >60 U/day	2

History of childhood malnutrition	>2 U/kg/day	
	Unresponsiveness to OHA	2
Insulin requirement	Normal pancreatic imaging	1
>60 U/day		
>1.5 U/kg/day		

** Total- 16, Diagnostic- 13, Suggestive- 12*

PDDM - A distinct entity or variant of type 1 DM?

The enthusiasm about PDDM being a form of diabetes distinct from type 1 and type 2 DM has waned[89]. Similar HLA associations and autoantibodies point towards to a common etiology. Importantly features that were initially considered to be hallmarks of PDDM have been shown to be variable. Malnutrition is common but not universal and a large number of type 1 DM patients in developing countries are also malnourished. Ketosis resistance, once considered an essential criterion is variable. Significantly type 1 DM in developing countries has a slower onset and ketoacidosis is less common. The hypothesis that PDDM is an extreme form of slow onset type 1 DM appears plausible. It remains unclear whether in PDDM is due to malnutrition or malnutrition is secondary to diabetes. What however is evident is that some diabetic children in developing countries present at a later age with malnutrition, relatively high insulin requirements and variable resistance to ketosis.

FIBROCALCIFIC PANCREATIC DIABETES

FCPD is distinguished from PDDM by the presence of exocrine pancreatic dysfunction. It is widely believed that FCPD represents a subgroup of patients with tropical calcific pancreatitis (TCP), a form of non-alcoholic pancreatitis common in tropical countries.

Epidemiology

Subsequent to the report by Zuidema, FCPD has been widely reported from various tropical countries[90-94]. Considerable geographic variations in the incidence of FCPD have been demonstrated. Higher incidence is reported from tropical regions than sub-tropical areas. Regional differences are particularly striking in India where most of the cases have been reported from south India while the disease is rare in north India[95]. The state of Kerala in south India has the highest incidence of FCPD in the world. Large series from this state have helped a lot in understanding the pathophysiology of this disease[96]. Most of the data regarding FCPD are hospital based. In a population based prevalence study in Kerala, 0.9% prevalence of TCP was observed[97]. Recent studies have demonstrated a declining trend in the prevalence of FCPD. FCPD accounted for only 1% of all diabetics in a recent study involving south Indians compared to 26% of patients in 1960[98]. In a Nigerian study only 6% of young diabetics had FCPD[99].

Etiopathogenesis

Environmental and genetic factors have been implicated in the pathogenesis of FCPD.

Malnutrition

Effects of malnutrition on the pancreas include decreased enzyme production and atrophy[100]. Inspissations of mucus plug and fibrosis have been observed in patients with malnutrition[101]. Pancreatic calcification, the hallmark of FCPD, however is not associated with malnutrition and the association with malnutrition is less striking compared to PDDM. In FCPD patients from south India only 25% had features of malnutrition[102]. These observations have raised questions regarding the role of malnutrition in FCPD.

Toxins

McMillan and Geevarghese observed that FCPD was more common in areas where cassava ingestion was endemic. They proposed the cassava hypothesis for the etiology of FCPD[103]. Cassava, a flour obtained from Manihot *sps*, leads to the production of toxic cyanide free radicals in the human body[104]. Sulphur-containing amino acids including cystine and methionine are required for detoxification of these toxins. High intake of cassava in conjunction with low levels of these amino acids due to malnutrition may expose the pancreas to damage from high levels of these toxins. Direct toxic effect of cyanide radicals on endocrine pancreas has however not been demonstrated in animal studies[105]. The cassava hypothesis has been questioned recently based on the observation that FCPD has been found to be rare in many populations where cassava is the staple diet. Similarly, the occurrence of FCPD in areas where cassava is not consumed is against this hypothesis[106].

Genetic and autoimmune factors

Genetic influences in FCPD are less substantiated than those in PDDM. HLA studies have demonstrated an association with HLA DQ β in

20% cases[107]. The role of deficient or defective lithostatin, a protein believed to be protective against pancreatic calcification, as a predisposing factor for FCPD remains unclear[108]. Evidence of autoimmunity is scarce in FCPD. In the study by Singh *et al,* no patient with FCPD was positive for autoantibodies[73]. Environmental factors thus appear to be the primary factors in FCPD.

Defective antioxidation

Higher levels of xenobiotics including polycyclic hydrocarbons and environmental toxins in patients with TCP compared to controls indicate an etiological role for environmental toxins in FCPD[109]. Evidence regarding lower clearance of these substances due to defective antioxidation is emerging. Increased theophylline clearance, a surrogate marker of increased P_{450} activity, has been demonstrated in Indian patients with FCPD. Importantly the detoxification process was reduced as reflected by low urinary levels of D-glucaric acid[110]. Low levels of vitamin C and β-carotene may be responsible for the defective anti-oxidation in these patients[111]. Micronutrient deficiency may provide the link between malnutrition and FCPD.

Pathology

Atrophy and fibrosis of pancreatic ducts are characteristic. Multiple large pancreatic calculi composed of calcium carbonate and phosphate are observed inside large ducts. In a study involving immunohistochemistry of pancreas using markers specific to individual cell lines a relative sparing of β cells was noted[112]. This may explain residual insulin secretion and thereby resistance to ketosis in these patients.

Clinical features

The typical patient with FCPD is a malnourished male belonging to a poor socioeconomic group presenting in the second decade of life with insulin resistance and ketosis resistance. However clinical heterogeneity is common; several patients have normal BMI. Patients have been detected for the first time after the age of 30 years as well. Patients from all social groups may be involved. Striking male preponderance (male: female > 2:1) has been noted.

History of recurrent abdominal pain is common. Most patients complain of epigastric pain, which may be severe enough to require opioid analgesics. Abdominal pain precedes the onset of diabetes by around 10 years. Overt evidence of exocrine deficiency is uncommon at the time of diagnosis; fat excretion increases once fat intake is increased [113].

Patients with TCP are part of a spectrum with normal glucose tolerance on one end and insulin dependency and ketoacidosis on the other. In between the two extremes patients who can be controlled with OHA and those who require insulin but are ketosis-resistant are observed. The daily insulin requirement is often similar to type 1 DM. Development of DKA is rare even after stopping insulin for long periods[114].

Similar to PDDM cardiovascular complications of FCPD are low. Other complications have similar incidence. Mortality rate is high as a substantial number of patients die within a few years of diagnosis[115].

Investigations

Imaging

Abdominal X-ray is diagnostic. Large calculi visualized at the level of the first and second lumbar spine are characteristic. Ultrasonography and computerized tomography scans of abdomen may demonstrate anatomical changes of pancreas to a greater extent.

Exocrine pancreatic function

Steatorrhea is present only in 30% cases. However once dietary fat intake is increased, most patients demonstrate enhanced fat excretion. Defective exocrine pancreatic function has been demonstrated in FCPD by measuring levels of immunoreactive trypsin and chymotrypsin in stool[115, 116]. Importantly some patients with PDDM and type 1 DM as well as normal controls may have evidence of pancreatic dysfunction.

Insulin secretion status

C-peptide studies have demonstrated variability in the disease as reflected in the relative insulin dependence and ketosis resistance[117]. C-peptide levels are higher compared to type 1 DM patients and lower than type 2 DM.

Table 3. Diagnostic criteria for FCPD[1]

1. Occurrence in tropical countries
2. Diabetes diagnosed by WHO criteria
3. Chronic pancreatitis Pancreatic calculi or any 3 of following • Chronic abdominal pain • Steatorrhea • Abnormal pancreatic imaging • Abnormal pancreatic exocrine function tests
4. Absence of other causes of chronic pancreatitis • Alcohol abuse • Hepatobiliary stones • Primary hyperparathyroidism

Note: Clinical malnutrition, early age of onset and absence of ketosis are common clinical features but not diagnostic criteria.

Diagnosis

FCPD should be suspected in a young diabetic residing in a tropical country with clinical features of pancreatitis, insulin resistance and ketosis resistance. Pancreatic calcification in the absence of secondary causes is diagnostic. Diagnostic criteria proposed by Mohan *et al* include evidence of DM, residence in tropical countries and idiopathic pancreatic caclification1. Malnutrition and ketosis resistance, once considered to be essential features for the diagnosis of FCPD are no longer required for its diagnosis (Table 3).

Management

Treatment with insulin is effective in most cases. C-peptide status may be helpful in determining insulin requirement and role of OHA. Management of malabsorption requires pancreatic enzymes, which improve the clinical status in majority. Surgery is indicated in patients with severe abdominal pain refractory to medical management. Surgery is only palliative as endocrine and exocrine defects persist after surgery.

CONCLUSIONS

Childhood diabetes in developing countries has different clinical, etiological and epidemiological features compared to the developed countries. The study of MRDM has advanced our understanding of the genetic and environmental factors playing a role in pathogenesis of DM in the developing world. The higher incidence of MODY in these countries makes evaluation of insulin secretion status especially important in adolescents with diabetes. An awareness of these differences is critical for those dealing with childhood diabetes in these countries.

ACKNOWLEDGEMENT
The authors wish to thank Dr. Ajay Sood and Dr. Pankaj Shah for their constructive criticism and suggestions to improve the manuscript.

REFERENCES

1. Mohan V, Alberti KGMM. Diabetics in the tropics. In: International Textbook of Diabetes. Eds: Alberti KGMM, Zimmet P, DeFronzo RA. Chichester, John Wiley & Sons. 2nd Edn. Vol 1. pp 177-196, 1997.
2. Mohan V, Premalatha C. Malnutrition-related diabetes mellitus. In: Textbook of Diabetes. Eds: Pickup J, Wilhany G. London, Blackwell Science. 2nd Edn. Vol 1. pp 25.1-25.14, 1997.
3. Makame MH. Childhood diabetes, insulin, and Africa. DERI (Diabetes Epidemiology Research International) Study Group. Diabet Med 9: 571-573, 1992.
4. Kayvonen M, Tuomilehto J, Libman I, LaPorte R for the World Health Organization DIAMOND Project Group. A review of the recent epidemiological data on the worldwide incidence of type 1 (insulin-dependent) diabetes mellitus. Diabetologia 36: 883-892, 1993.
5. Keen H, Ekoe JM. The geography of diabetes mellitus. Br Med Bull 40: 339-365, 1986.
6. Lester FT. Childhood diabetes mellitus in Ethiopia. Diabet Med 3: 278-280, 1986.
7. Ramachandran A, Snehalatha C, Krishnaswamy CV. Incidence of IDDM in children in urban population in southern India. Madras IDDM Registry Group Madras, South India. Diabetes Res Clin Pract 34: 79-82, 1996.
8. Tuomilehto J, Dabee J, Karvonen M, Dowse GK, Gareeboo H, Virtala E, Tiihonen M, Alberti KG, Zimmet PZ. Incidence of IDDM in Mauritian children and adolescents from 1986 to 1990. Diabetes Care 16: 1588-1591, 1993.

9. McLarty DG, Athaide I, Bottazzo GF, Swai ABM, Alberti KGMM. Islet cell antibodies are not specifically associated with insulin-dependent diabetes in Tanzanian Africans. Diabetes Res Clin Pract 9: 219-224, 1990.
10. Ramachandran A, Rosenbloom AL, Mohan V et al. Autoimmunity in South Indian patients with IDDM. Diabetes Care 9: 435, 1985.
11. Odugbesn O, Fletcher JA, Sanders A, Bradwell AR, Botazzo GF, Barneh AH. Autoantibodies in Indian Asians with insulin dependent diabetes mellitus in UK. Postgrad Med J 64: 357, 1998.
12. Srikanta S, Malviya AN, Mehra NK, Vaidya MC, Geevarghese PJ, Ahuja MMS. Autoimmunity in type 1 (insulin dependent) diabetes mellitus in north Indians. J Clin Immun 1: 169-173, 1981.
13. Singh AK, Bhatia E, Dabadghao P, Bhatia V, Gellert SA, Colman PG. Role of islet autoimmunity in the etiology of different clinical subtypes of diabetes mellitus in young north Indians. Diabet Med 17: 275-280, 2000.
14. Cardoso C, Ohwovoriole AE, KuKu SF. A study of thyroid function and prevalence of thyroid autoantibodies in an African diabetic population. J Diabetes Complications 9:37-41, 1995.
15. Menon PSN, Vaidyanathan B, Kaur M. Autoimmune thyroid disease in Indian children with type 1 diabetes mellitus. J Pediatr Endocrinol Metab 14: 279-286, 2001.
16. Ramachandran A, Snehalatha C, Tuomilehto-Wolf E, Vidgren G, Ogunkolade BW, Vijay V, Hitman GA. Type 1 diabetes in the offspring does not increase the risk of parental type 2 diabetes in south Indians. Diabetes Metab Res Rev 15: 328-331, 1999.
17. Cruikshanks KJ, Jobin LF, Lawlerhevner J et al. Ethnic differences in human leukocyte antigen markers of susceptibility to insulin dependent diabetes mellitus. Diabetes Care 17: 132-137, 1994.
18. Srikanta S, Ahuja MMS, Malviya AN, Mehra NK, Vaidya MC. HLA antigens in type 1 (insulin dependent) diabetes mellitus in north India. Metabolism 30: 992-993, 1981.
19. Bhatia E, Mehra NK, Taneja V, Vaidya MC, Ahuja MMS. HLA DR antigen frequency in a north Indian type I diabetic population. Diabetes 34: 565-567, 1985.
20. Serjenston SW, Ranford PR, Kiri RL et al. HLA DR and DQ DNA genotyping in insulin dependent diabetes mellitus in south Indians. Dis Markers 5: 101, 1982.

21. Bhatia E, Mehra NK, Malviya AN, Ahuja MMS. HLA and autoimmunity in north Indian type I (insulin- dependent) diabetic multiplex families. Horm Metab Res 18: 331-334, 1986.
22. Metcalfe KA, Hitman GA, Pociot F etal. An association between type 1diabetes and the interleukin-1 receptor gene. Hum Immunol 51: 41-48, 1996.
23. Ogunkolade WB, Ramachandran A, McDermott MF, Kumarajeewa TR, Curtis D, Snehalatha C, Mohan V, Cassell PG, Eskdale J, Gallagher G, Hitman GA. Family association studies of markers on chromosome 2q and type 1 diabetes in subjects from south India. Diabetes Metab Res Rev 16: 276-280, 2000.
24. McDermott MF, Ramachandran A, Ogunkolade BW, Aganna E, Curtis D, Boucher BJ, Snehalatha C, Hitman GA. Allelic variation in the vitamin D receptor influences susceptibility to IDDM in Indian Asians. Diabetes Metab Res Rev 16: 276-280, 2000.
25. Akanji AO. Clinical experience with adolescent diabetes in a Nigerian teaching hospital. J Natl Med Assoc 88: 101-105, 1996.
26. Rwiza HT, Swai ABM, McLarty DG. Failure to diagnose diabetic ketoacidosis in Tanzania. Diabet Med 3: 181-183, 1986.
27. Castle WM, Wicks ACB. A follow-up of 93 newly diagnosed African diabetics for 6 years. Diabetologia 18: 121-123, 1980.
28. McLarty DG, Kinabo L, Swai ABM. Diabetes in tropical Africa: a prospective study, 1981-7.II. Course and prognosis. Br Med J 300: 1107-1010, 1990.
29. Ramachandran A, Mohan V, Snehalatha C, Bharani G, Chinnikrishnudu M, Mohan R, Viswanathan M. Clinical features of diabetes in the young as seen at a diabetes center in south India. Diabetes Res Clin Pract 4: 117-125, 1988.
30. Feleke Y, Abdulkadir J, Aderaye G. Prevalence and clinical features of tuberculosis in Ethiopian diabetic patients. East Afr Med J 76: 361-364, 1999.
31. Passi GR, Menon PSN, Gupta DK, Lodha R. Recovery from pulmonary mucormycosis and candidiasis in diabetic ketoacidosis. Indian Pediatr 33: 1047-1050, 1996.
32. Ramachandran A, Snehalatha C, Sasikala R, Satyavani K, Vijay V. Vascular complications in young Asian Indian patients with type 1 diabetes mellitus. Diabetes Res Clin Pract 48: 51-56, 2000.
33. Klein R, Klein BEK, Mose SE, Davis MD, DeMets DL. The Wisconsin epidemiology study of diabetic retinopathy. Prevalence and

risk of diabetic retinopathy when age at diagnosis is less than 30 years. Arch Ophthalmol 102: 520-526, 1984.
34. Sridhar GR, Satish K, Ahuja MMS. Nonmydriatic retinal color photography in young Indian diabetic patients. Ann Ophthalmol 25: 187-190, 1993.
35. Chale SS, Swai AB, Mujinja PG, McLarty DG. Must diabetes be a fatal disease in Africa? Study of costs of treatment. Br Med J 304: 1215-1218, 1992.
36. Alberti KGMM. IDDM: a lethal disease in the developing countries. Br Med J 309: 754-755, 1994.
37. Savage A. Diabetes in the developing world. Lancet 341: 900, 1993.
38. Tull ES, Barinas E, the Pittsburgh DERI Mortality Study Group. Twofold excess mortality among black compared with white IDDM patients in Allegheny County, Pennsylvania. Diabetes Care 19: 1344-1347, 1996.
39. Yudkin JS. Insulin for the world's poorest countries. Lancet 355: 919-921, 2000.
40. Rosenbloom AL, Joe JR, Young RS, Winter WE. Emerging epidemic of type 2 diabetes in youth. Diabetes Care 22: 345-354, 1999.
41. Hattersley AT. Diagnosis of maturity-onset diabetes of the young in the pediatric diabetes clinic. J Pediatr Endocrinol Metab 13 (Suppl 6): 1411-1417, 2000.
42. Ehtisham S, Barrett TG, Shaw NJ. Type 2 diabetes mellitus in UK children--an emerging problem. Diabet Med 17: 867-871, 2000.
43. Tattersall RB. Mild familial diabetes with dominant inheritance. Q J Med 24: 44-53, 1974.
44. Ramachandran A, Jali MV, Mohan V et al. High prevalence of diabetes in an urban population in south India. Br Med J 297: 587, 1988.
45. Asmal AC, Dayal B, Jialal I, Leary WP, Omar MAK, Pilay NL, Thandaroyen FT. Non- insulin dependent diabetes mellitus with young age of onset in blacks and Asians. S Afr Med J 60: 93-96, 1981.
46. Ducorps M, Ndong W, Jupkwo B, Belmejdoub G, Poirier JM, Mayaudon H, Bauduceau B. Epidemiological aspects of diabetes in Cameroon: what is the role of tropical diabetes? Diabetes Metab 23: 61-67, 1997.
47. Mohan V, Ramachandran A, Snehalatha C, Mohan R, Bharani G, Viswanathan M. High prevalence of maturity onset diabetes of the young (MODY) among Indians. Diabetes Care 8: 371-374, 1985.

48. Mohan V, Snehalatha C, Ramachandran A, Viswanathan M. Abnormalities of Insulin secretion in healthy offspring of Indian patients with maturity onset diabetes of the young. Diabetes Care 9: 53-56, 1986.
49. Mohan V, Ramachandran A, Snehalatha C, Jayashree R, Viswanatrhan M. C peptide response to glucose load in maturity onset diabetes of young patients (MODY). Diabetes Care 8: 69-72, 1985.
50. Diabetes in the tropics: Br Med J 1: 1051, 1907.
51. Hugh-Jones P. Diabetes in Jamaica. Lancet 2: 891-897, 1955.
52. Zuidema PJ. Cirrhosis and disseminated calcification of pancreas in patients with malnutrition. Trop Geogr Med 11: 70-74, 1959.
53. WHO Study Group Report on Diabetes Mellitus. WHO Technical Report Series 727. Geneva: WHO 1985.
54. American Diabetes Association Expert Committee. Report of the expert committee on the diagnosis and classification of diabetes mellitus. Diabetes Care 20: 1183, 1997.
55. Ekoe JM. Diabetes and nutrition in developing countries. Bull Deliv Health Care Diabetes Devel Countries 6: 3-9, 1985.
56. Franco LJ. Specifities of nutritional, pancreatic and other forms of diabetes. Bull Deliv Health Diabetes Devel Countries 2: 10-13, 1985.
57. West KM. Epidemiology of diabetes and its vascular lesions. New York, Elsevier. pp 324-331, 1978.
58. Ajgaonkar SA. Epidemiology of Diabetes in the tropics. An overview. In: Diabetes. Eds: Waldhausl WK. 1979 Excerpta Med Int Congr Ser no 500. Amesterdam, Excerpta Medica. pp 219-223, 1980.
59. Lester FT. A search for malnutrition-related diabetes mellitus among Ethiopian patients. Diabetes Care 16: 187-192, 1993.
60. Gupta OP, Joshi MH, Dare SK. Prevalence of diabetes in India. Adv Metab Dis 8: 147-165, 1978.
61. Saraya A, Acharya SK, Vashisht S, Mittal A, Tandon RK. Is protein-deficient diabetes mellitus a pancreatitis? J Gastroenterol Hepatol 14: 705-708, 1999.
62. James WPI, Coore HG. Peripheral impairment of insulin secretion and glucose tolerance in protein-calorie malnutrition. Am J Clin Nutr 21: 386-389, 1970.
63. Smith SR, Edgar PJ, Pozefsky R, Chetri MK, Prout TE. Insulin secretion and glucose tolerance in adults with protein-calorie malnutrition. Metabolism 24: 1073-1083, 1978.
64. Baig A, Edozien JC. Carbohydrate metabolism in kwashiorkor. Lancet 2: 662-665, 1965.

65. Becker DJ, Pimstone BL, Hansen JDL, Hendricks S. Insulin secretion in protein energy malnutrition. Quantitative abnormalities and response to treatment. Diabetes 20: 542-551, 1969.
66. Becker DJ, Pimstone BL, Hansen JDL, MacHuschon B, Drysdale A. Patterns of Insulin response to glucose in protein-calorie malnutrition. Am J Clin Nutr 52: 299-305, 1972.
67. Khan LA, Alam AM, Ali L, Goswami A, Hassan Z, Sattar S, Banik NG, Khan AK. Serum and urinary magnesium in young diabetics in Bangladesh. Am J Clin Nutr 69: 70-73, 1999.
68. Abdulkadir J, Worku Y, Schreuder GM, D'Amaro J, de Vries RR, Ottenhoff TH. HLA-DR and -DQ antigens in malnutrition-related diabetes mellitus in Ethiopians: a clue to its etiology? Tissue Antigens 34: 284-289, 1989.
69. Sanjeevi CB, Seshiah V, Moller E, Olirup O. Different genetic background for type 1 diabetes and malnutrition related diabetes in south Indians. Diabetologia 35:283-286, 1992.
70. Sanjeevi CB, Kanungo A, Shtauvere A, Samal KC, Tripathi BB. Association of HLA class II alleles with different subgroups of diabetes mellitus in eastern India identify different associations with IDDM and malnutrition-related diabetes. Tissue Antigens 4: 83-87, 1999.
71. Wiyono P, Morimoto Y, Taniguchi H. The presence of islet cell antibodies in malnutrition-related diabetes mellitus. Diabetes Res Clin Pract 6: 75-78, 1989.
72. Huh KB, Lee HI, Kin HM, Cho YW, Kim YH, Lee KW et al. Immunogenetics and nutritional profile in insulin using youth onset diabetes in Korea. Diabetes Res Clin Pract 16: 630, 1992.
73. Singh AK, Bhatia E, Dabadghao P, Bhatia V, Gellert SA, Colman PG. Role of islet autoimmunity in the aetiology of different clinical subtypes of diabetes mellitus in young north Indians. Diabet Med 17: 275-280, 2000.
74. Chattopadhyay PS, Gupta SK, Chattopadhyay R, Kundu PK, Chakraborti R. Malnutrition-related diabetes mellitus (MRDM), not diabetes-related malnutrition. A report on genuine MRDM. Diabetes Care 18: 276-277, 1995.
75. Menon PSN, Virmani A, Shah P, Raju R, Sethia S, Bicha RP, Joshi M, Kouchupillai N, Ahuja MMS. Childhood onset diabetes mellitus in India: an overview. Int J Diabetes Developing Countries 10: 11-16, 1990.

76. Abdulkadir J, Mengesha B, Welde Gebriel Z, Keen H, Worku Y, Gebre P, Bekele A, Urga K, Taddesse AS. The clinical and hormonal (C-peptide and glucagon) profile and liability to ketoacidosis during nutritional rehabilitation in Ethiopian patients with malnutrition-related diabetes mellitus. Diabetologia 33: 222-227, 1990.
77. Mohan V, Snehalatha C, Ramachandran A, Jayashree R, Visawnathan M. Pancreatic B-cell function in tropical pancreatic diabetes. Metabolism 32: 1091-1092, 1983.
78. Rao RH, Vigg BL, Rao KSJ. Suppressible glucagon secretion in young ketosis resistant type 'J' diabetic patients in India. Diabetes 32: 1168-1171, 1983.
79. Yajnik CS, Shelgikar KM, Naik SS et al. The ketosis resistance in fibrocalcific pancreatic diabetes. Clinical observations and endocrine metabolism measures during oral glucose tolerance test. Diabetes Res Clin Pract 15: 145-156, 1992.
80. Ahuja MMS. Epidemiological studies in diabetes mellitus in India. In: Epidemiology of diabetes mellitus in developing countries. Eds: Ahuja MMS. New Delhi, Interprint, 1979.
81. Tulloch JA, MacIntosh D. 'J' type diabetes. Lancet 2: 19-121, 1961.
82. Ahuja MMS, Talwar GP, Varma VM, Kumar A. Diabetes mellitus in young Indians. Indian J Med Res 53: 1138-1143, 1965.
83. Narendranathan M. Chronic calcific pancreatitis in the tropics. Trop Gastroenterol 2: 40-45, 1981.
84. Rao RH. The role of undernutrition in the pathogenesis of diabetes mellitus. Diabetes Care 6: 595-601, 1984.
85. Garg MK, Tripathy D, Shah P. Patients with malnutrition related diabetes mellitus are as insulin sensitive as insulin dependent diabetics. J Assoc Physicians India 47: 1145-114, 1999.
86. Sutjahjo A, Taniguchi H, Hendromartono, Tjokroprawiro A, Baba S. High frequency of autonomic as well as peripheral neuropathy in patients with malnutrition-related diabetes mellitus. Diabetes Res Clin Pract 5: 197-200, 1988.
87. Ahuja MM. Diabetes- special problems in developing countries. Bull Deliv Health Care diabetes Devel Countries 1: 5-6, 1980.
88. Tripathy BB, Samal KC. Protein deficient diabetes mellitus (PDDM) in India. Int J Diabetes Developing Countries 13: 3-13, 1993.
89. Abu Bakre A, Taylor R, Gill GV, Alberti KGMM. Tropical or malnutrition-related diabetes mellitus: a real syndrome? Lancet 1: 1135-1138, 1986.

90. Shaper AG.Chronic pancreatic disease and protein malnutrition. Trop Geogr Med 11:70-7, 1959.
91. Osuntokun BO, Akinkugbe FM, Francis TI, Reddy S, Osuntokun O, Taylor GOL. Diabetes mellitus in Nigerians: a study of 832 patients. W Afr Med J 20: 295-312, 1971.
92. Viswanathan M. Pancreatic diabetes in India: an overview. In: Secondary diabetes. The spectrum of the diabetic syndromes. Eds: Podolsky S, Viswanathan M. New York, Raven Press. pp 105-116, 1980.
93. Hegde JS, Jituri KH, Channapa NK. Pancreatic diabetes in Hubli area (N Karnataka). J Assoc Phys India 24: 305-307, 1976.
94. Tripathi BB. Diabetes with exocrine pancreatic disease. In: Diabetes in developing countries. Ed: Bajaj JS. New Delhi, Interprint. pp 135-142, 1984.
95. Ahuja MMS, Sharma GP. Serum C-peptide content in nutritional diabetes. Horm Metab Res 17: 267-268, 1985.
96. Geevarghese PJ. Calcific Pancreatitis. Bombay, Varghese Publication House. 1985.
97. Balaji LN. The problem of chronic calcific pancreatitis. PhD Thesis. New Delhi, All India Institute of Medical Sciences. 1988.
98. Geevarghese PJ. Pancreatic diabetes. Bombay; Popular Prakashan. 1968.
99. Akanji AO. Malnutrition-related diabetes mellitus in young adult diabetic patients attending a Nigerian diabetic clinic. J Trop Med Hyg 93: 35-38, 1990.
100. Cook GC. Glucose tolerance after kwashiorkor. Nature 215: 1295-1296, 1967.
101. Pitchumoni CS. Pancreas in primary malnutrition disorders. Am J Clin Nutr 26:374-379, 1973.
102. Mohan V, Mohan R, Susheela L, Snehalatha C, Bharani G, Mahajan VK, Ramachandran A, Viswanathan M, Kohner EM. Tropical pancreatic diabetes in south India: heterogeneity in clinical and biochemical profile. Diabetologia 28: 229-232, 1985.
103. McMillan DE, Geevarghese PJ. Dietary cyanide and tropical malnutrition diabetes. Diabetes Care 2: 202-208, 1979.
104. Pitchumoni CS, Jain NK, Lowenfels AB, DiMagno EP. Chronic cyanide poisoning: unifying concepts for alcoholic and tropical pancreatitis. Pancreas 3: 220-230, 1988.

105. Pitchumoni CS. 'Tropical' or 'Nutritional pancreatitis' – an update. In: Pancreatitis – Concepts and Classification. Eds: Gyp KE, Singer MV, Sarles H. Amsterdam, Elsevier. pp 359-363, 1984
106. Teuscher T, Rosman JB, Balliod P, Teuscher A. Absence of diabetes in rural west African population with a high carbohydrate/cassava diet. Lancet 1: 763-767, 1987.
107. Kambo PK, Hitman GA, Mohan V et al. The genetic predisposition to fibrocalcfic pancreatic diabetes. Diabetologia 32: 45-51, 1989.
108. Sarles H, Dagron JC, Giorgi D, Bernard JP. Renaming pancreatic stone protein as "lithostatin". Gastroenterology 99: 900-905, 1990.
109. Chaloner C, Sandle LN, Mohan V et al. Evidence for induction of cytochrome P-450 in patients with tropical chronic pancreatitis. Int J Clin Pharmacol Ther Toxicol 28: 235-240, 1990.
110. Mohan V, Braganza JM. Xenobiotics in tropical pancreatic diabetes. In: The pathogenesis of Pancreatitis. Ed: Braganza JM. New York, Manchester University Press pp 115-128, 1991.
111. Braganza JM, Schofeild D, Snehalatha C, Mohan V. Micronutrient anti-oxidant status in tropical compared to temperate zone pancreatitis. Scand J Gastroenterol 20: 1048, 1993.
112. Govindrajan M, Mohan V, Deepa R, Ashok S, Pitchumoni CS. Histopathology and immunohistochemistry of pancreatic islets in fibrocalculous pancreatic diabetes. Diabetes Res Clin Pract 51: 29-38, 2001.
113. Olurin EO, Olurin O. Pancreatic calcification. Br Med J 4:534-539, 1969.
114. Yajnik CS, Shelgikar KM. Fibrocalculous pancreatic diabetes in Pune, India. Clinical features and follow-up for 7 years. Diabetes Care 16: 916-921, 1993.
115. Yajnik CS, Sahasrabudhe RA, Naik SS, Katrak A, Shelgikar KM, Kanitkar SV, Narayanan VA, Dandona P. Exocrine pancreatic function (serum immunoreactive trypsin, fecal chymotrypsin, and pancreatic isoamylase) in Indian diabetics. Pancreas 5: 631-638, 1990.
116. Bhatia E, Baijal SS, Kumar KR, Choudhuri G. Exocrine pancreatic and beta-cell function in malnutrition-related diabetes among north Indians. Diabetes Care 18: 1174-1178, 1995.
117. Mohan V, Ramachandran A, Viswanathan M. Diabetes secondary to tropical pancreatopathy. In: Diabetes secondary to pancreatopathy. Eds: Tiengo A, Alberti KGMM, Delprato S, Vranic M. Amesterdam, Elsevier. Pp 215-216, 1988.

Chapter 7
DIABETES IN SOUTH EAST ASIA

Louis C. K. Low, M.B.Ch.B., FHKAM (Paediatrics), F.R.C.P.C.H., F.R.C.P. (Lond., Edin., Glasg.)
The University of Hong Kong, ***Department of Paediatrics***

Diabetes mellitus is the second most common chronic disease in childhood in the Western world, after childhood asthma. For reasons that are not entirely clear, childhood type I diabetes is relatively uncommon in Asian populations. On the contrary, type 2 diabetes in the older population is just as common in Asia as in the West. Recent assessment of global trends in the frequency of diabetes mellitus by different authors suggests that Asia is the major site of a rapidly emerging epidemic of diabetes, with both China and India leading the field. China and India are estimated to contribute 38 million and 51 million respectively to the global burden of diabetes in the year 2025. This emerging epidemic of diabetes is not restricted to the adult population and increasing incidence of type 2 diabetes in children or adolescents have been documented in many countries in recent years. It is very likely that lifestyle changes resulting in decreased physical activity due to increasing mechanization and excessive calorie intake underlie the present epidemic.

THE EPIDEMIOLOGY OF CHILDHOOD TYPE I DIABETES MELLITUS IN THE ASIA PACIFIC REGION.

The etiology of type I diabetes mellitus has remained elusive despite intense research in the past 30 years, but both genetic and environmental factors contribute to the development of the disorder. Genetic factors play a major role in the susceptibility to type I diabetes mellitus and environmental factors trigger the autoimmune process which leads to progressive destruction of pancreatic beta cells and the onset of diabetes. Standardized collection of data on the incidence of type I diabetes in the 1980s (Diabetes Epidemiology Research International Group) and the 1990s (World Health Organization Project, the Multinational Project for Childhood Diabetes) provided information and suggested wide geographic differences in the incidence of this disease. The lowest incidence is found in Asia while the highest incidence is found in Northern Europe, and there is a nearly 60-fold difference in incidence between different populations[1]. The geographic variations in incidence very likely reflect different degrees of genetic susceptibility to the development of type I diabetes among different ethnic groups; higher incidence in Caucasians than in Mongoloid races. The overall age-adjusted incidence of type I diabetes varies from 0.23-1.4/100,000 children per year in different parts of China, 1.4-2.2/100,000 children per year in Japan, 14.5-21.9/100,000 children/year in Australia and New Zealand, 11.7-17.8/100,000 children/year in the United States, 36.5/100,000 children/year in Finland and 36.8/100,000 children/year in Sardinia. However, information on the incidence of type I diabetes in Asian countries remains scanty (Table 1). This lack of information hinders the ability of the medical community to understand the financial burden of the disease or to develop effective public health measures.

Table 1. Incidence of childhood type I diabetes mellitus in Asia Pacific Region.

Country		Incidence (cases/100,000 children <15 yrs/year)	Male/female Ratio
Singapore [1]	Malay	1.23	
	Chinese	2.25	0.54
	Indian	5.78	
Thailand [2]		0.3	0.5
Korea [3]		0.7	0.74
China	Hong Kong [4]	1.4	0.3
	Shanghai	0.7	1.0
	Beijing	0.9	0.6
India [5]		10.5	1.3
Pakistan		0.7	0.6
Japan	Hokkaido	1.7	1.0
	Chiba	1.4	0.8
Australia		14.5	0.8
New Zealand	Auckland	12.9	0.9
	Canterbury	21.9	1.2

([1] Lee WW 1998; [2] Panamota O 2000; [3] Ko KW 1994; [4] Huen KF 2000; [5] Ramachandran A 1996; Karvonen M 2000)

Apart from variation in the incidence of type I diabetes mellitus in the Asia Pacific region, there is also variation within countries especially in countries with large populations like China and Japan[2] (Figure I). The variation in incidence in different parts of a large Asian country like China can be due to different genetic background in different ethnic minority groups within the country or to very different eating habits and lifestyles. Accurate incidence data is not available from quite a number of countries in the Asia Pacific region like Philippines, Malaysia, Indonesia and the Pacific Islands. In the Philippines, the cases of type I diabetes admitted to hospitals in Metro Manila in the period 1950-1980 were few, 77 cases over 30 years[3]. From the records of 9 government teaching hospitals and 3 private hospitals, 196 new cases of type I diabetes were detected between 1995 and 1999 in Indonesia. Based on a survey in 1989, the prevalence of type I diabetes among 6-10 year old children was 0.07% and 11-15 year old children was 0.2% in Indonesia, a country with a population of more than 190 million people. In Fiji, a recent survey revealed 26 diabetic children among 295, 902 children under the age of 15 years. In Papua and New Guinea, only one case of childhood diabetes was diagnosed before 1996 over a period of 30 years. Between 1996 and 2000, 6 cases of diabetes mellitus was diagnosed with 2 deaths. Only 3 cases of childhood diabetes were under the care of tertiary institution in Tonga[4].

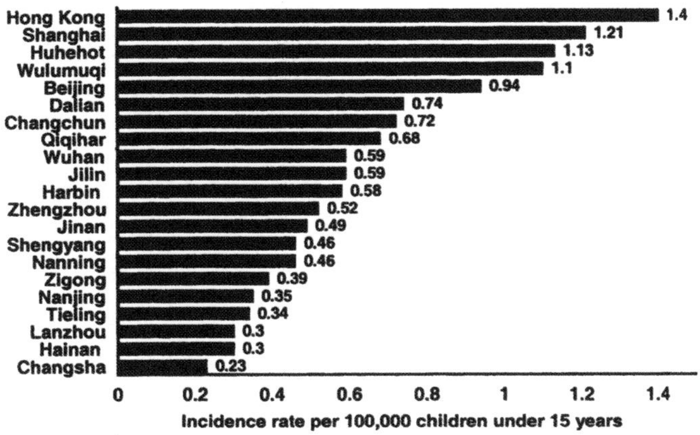

Figure 1. Geographical Variation of incidence of type 1 diabetes in China(*Adapted from Yang Z et al. Diabetes Care 1998; 21:525*)

There is a global trend in the increase in the incidence of type I diabetes over the recent years. A statistical significant increase in incidence has been found in 65% of the populations and the mean annual increase in incidence has been estimated to be 2.5% after correction for the number of cases in each individual study[5]. The relative increase is more evident in populations with a low incidence of the disease. In Shanghai where the incidence was 0.61/100,000 children/year between 1980-1991, there had been an increase of 7.4% in incidence per year to 0.83/100,000 children/year between 1989-1993 and 1.4/100,000 children/year between 1994-1996. In Hokkaido Japan, the increase in incidence has been 5.9% per year. In Hong Kong, we have also noticed a progressive increase in incidence between 1984 and 1996 (Figure 2). Despite this increase, the incidence rates in Asian countries will still be low in the coming ten to twenty years. In New Zealand, an increasing trend is only reported among the Caucasian population but not among the Maoris or Polynesians. Although Type I diabetes mellitus is common in children under the age of 15 years, the majority of the patients are diagnosed after this age. There is presently no means to ascertain whether the observed increase in incidence of childhood type I diabetes is the result of an earlier onset of the disease or a true rise in incidence. This recent rise in incidence may also reflect the association with environmental factors like diet, lifestyle changes and exposure to chemicals and viral infections. However specific environmental factors have not been identified as the cause of the continuous global increase in the incidence of type I diabetes.

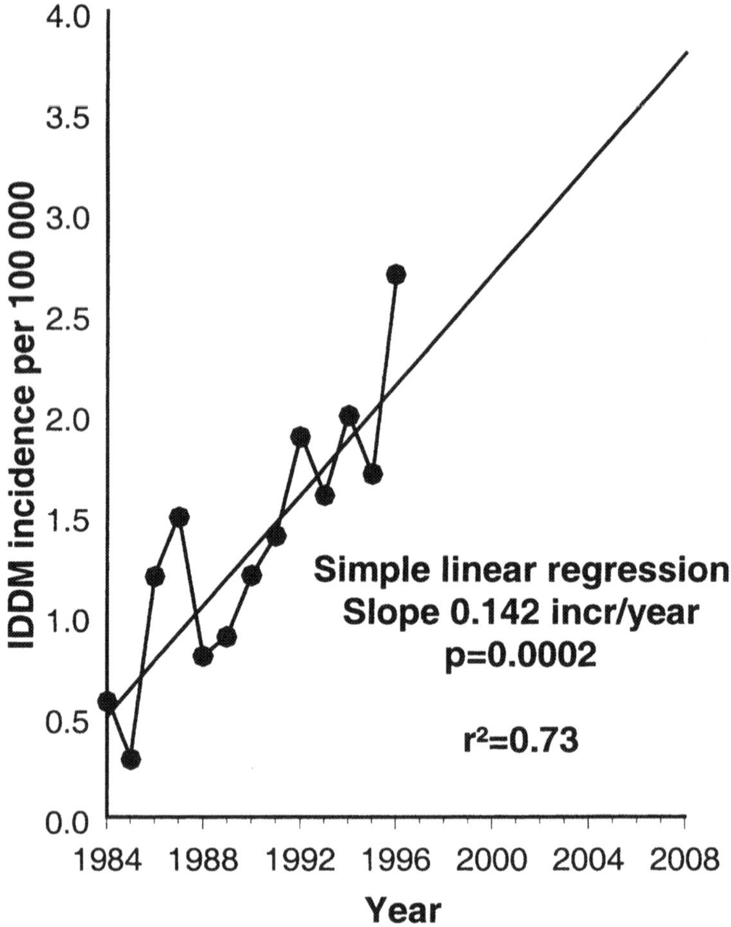

Figure 2. Annual Incidence of IDDM/100,000 persons from 1984 to 1996 and the projected incidence rate by simple linear regression. ***(Reproduced with permission from Huen KF et al. J Pediatr Endocrinol Metab 2000; 13:297)***

Transmigratory studies also provide evidence for the importance of environmental factors in the development of type I diabetes. Ethnic groups with low incidence of the disease take on a higher incidence when they immigrate to another country where the incidence of diabetes is higher. Such a phenomenon has been documented in Japanese who have emigrated to Haiwai and the Mainland of the United States and also in Chinese who have immigrated to Australia. The incidence of childhood type I diabetes in Chinese children is 7.7/100,000/year in New South Wales, Australia as compared to 1.4/100,000 children/year in Hong Kong and 0.9/100,000 children/year in Beijing. Offsprings of a transmigratory Asian population in the British Midlands had rising incidence of childhood diabetes from 3.1/100,000 children per year in 1978-81 to 11.7/100,000 children per year in 1988-1990, whereas that for other children remained constant at 10.5/100,000 children per year[6].

Seasonal variation in the incidence has been reported from countries with clearly defined warm and cold seasons and there is a tendency for a lower incidence during the warmer months. Some studies suggested that seasonal variation in the incidence of childhood is more pronounced among males and those with onset in later childhood and adolescence[7]. No seasonal variation in incidence has been documented in Asian countries where this problem has been looked at[8]. However a lower incidence of type I diabetes in the summer months has been reported in Korea[9]. With the realization that the autoimmune destruction of beta cells in diabetic individuals is a prolonged process, the seasonal variation is interpreted to mean that some infectious agents serve to precipitate the disease in the autumn and winter months.

GENETIC SUSCEPTIBILITY TO TYPE I DIABETES MELLITUS

More than 15 loci have been identified in the human genome that confers genetic susceptibility to the development of type I diabetes mellitus. One of the main genes associated with a predisposition to type I diabetes is the major histocompatibility complex on chromosome 6 and this locus contributes to 42 percent of the familial clustering of type 1 diabetes. Insulin dependent diabetes mellitus is positively associated with HLA-DR3 and DR4 in Caucasians whereas it is associated with DR3, DR4 and DR9 in Chinese and DR4 and DR9 in Japanese. Susceptibility to type I diabetes also correlates with the absence of aspartic acid at position 57 of the DQβ chain[10] and the presence of a DQ α chain bearing an arginine in position 52[11]. Susceptibility to type I diabetes is increased in individuals bearing DQ alleles that could form multiple diabetogenic dimers through the association of DQ chains encoded on the same chromosome (in cis) or on separate chromosomes (in trans). It is likely that the configuration of the DQ molecule influences susceptibility to a greater extent than any of the individual allele on the α- or β chains. Another important HLA association is the dominant protection conferred by the DQ molecules DQA1*0102-DQB1*0602 carried on DR2 haplotype[12].

In Caucasians, high risk class II molecules include DQA1*0501-DQB1*0201 associated with DR3 and DQA1*0301-DQB1*0302 associated with DR4. Individuals carrying both the DR3 and DR4 haplotypes have the highest risk of developing type I diabetes. Although the presence of an amino acid other than aspartate at position 57 of DQβ confers a strong risk of developing type I diabetes in Caucasians, this association has not been found in Japanese, Koreans or consistently in Chinese[13,14]. In Koreans, DQB1*0201 is the only DQB1 allele positively associated and DQB1*0601, DQB1*0602 and DQB1*0301 are negatively associated with type I diabetes mellitus. The DRB1*0405–DQB1*0302 and DRB1*0401–DQB1*0302 haplotypes are positively associated with type I diabetes mellitus and the lack of association of DQB1*0302 allele with disease is due to its strong linkage disequilibrium with the protective DRB1*0403 and *0406 alleles[13]. In Chinese, the DRB1*0301 – DQB1*0201 haploytype confers susceptibility to type 1 diabetes. DRB1*0405 – DQB1*0302 also confers strong susceptibility to the disease (RR of 33.7) but the strong linkage disequilibrium observed between DQB1*0302 and the two protective alleles DQB1*0403 and *0406 can explain why the frequency of DQB1*0302 is not significantly increased in Chinese type I diabetic patients[14,15]. In our study of 50 Chinese children with type I diabetes, we did not find a significant increase in non-aspartate 57 allele frequency as compared to that of 250 control subjects[16]. In our Chinese diabetic children from Hong Kong, DRB1 alleles 0301, 0901 and 0405 occurred with increased frequency as compared to controls. The susceptible haplotypes include DRB1*0301-DQA1*0501-DQB1*0201 and DRB1*0901-DQA1*0301/02-DQB1*0303. In Chinese, DR3/DR9 heterozygotes are the only DR9-containing genotype that is significantly increased in diabetic patients compared to controls probably due to the 0301/0201 DQαβ transdimer[14]. Eleven of the 14 DR4-bearing patients carried the DRB1*0405 allele which was associated with DQ4 (DQA1*0301/02–DQB1*04) similar to what is found in Japanese patients with type 1 diabetes. In other studies on Chinese diabetic patients, the frequency of DQA1*0301 and DQA1*0302 and DQB1*0201 and DQB1*0302 was found to be significantly higher in diabetic patients as compared to control individuals[17]. The inconsistent association of non-asparate 57 DQB allele with type 1 diabetes reported in the literature could be partly accounted by the small number of control individuals included in the studies.

In Japanese, the frequency of DR9-DQA1*0302-DQB1*0303 haplotype is higher in the younger type I diabetic children whereas the frequency of DR4-DQA1*0303-DQB1*0401 is higher in the older age group with type I diabetes[18]. DRB1*0802-DQA1*0301-DQB1*0302 also confers susceptibility while DRB1*1501-DQA*0102-DQB1*0602 and DRB1*1502-DQA1*0103-DQB1*0601 are the major resistance haplotypes. The hypothesis that alleles encoding non aspartic acid at the DQB1 position 57 contributes to type I diabetes susceptibility is not applicable in Japanese because HLA-DQB1*0303 and *0401 which encode aspartic acid at position 57 are strongly associated with susceptibility to type I diabetes in Japanese. It has also been demonstrated that only HLA-DR4 and DQA1*0301-DQB1*0401 were associated with the slowly progressive group of type I diabetes while three diabetogenic HLA-DQ haploytypes DQA1*0301-DQB1*0401, DQA1*0301-DQB1*0302 and DQA1*0301-DQB1*0303 were associated with the acute onset group in Japanese[19]. In Japanese, the DR3 haplotype is very uncommon contrary to what is found in Chinese and Caucasians. In Chinese and Japanese, the increased frequency of DQB1*0401 among diabetic patients may be due to strong linkage disequilibrium with the strong susceptible DRB1*0405 allele. The absence of significant association between DQB1*0302 and type 1 diabetes in Chinese, Japanese and Koreans is likely to be due to linkage disequilibruin of this allele with the protective DRB1*0403 and DRB1*0406 alleles.

In the Indo-Aryan population, DRB1*04-DQA1*03-DQB1*0302 haplotype has been found to be transmitted preferentially to the diabetic probands. The DRB1*03-DQA1*05-DQB1*02 haplotype also occurs in a higher frequency (78%) in diabetic children than in normal children (22.6%). It thus appears that the haplotypes associated with type I diabetes mellitus in the Indo-Aryan population are similar to that observed in Anglo-Europeans[20]. In limited reports from other parts of Asia, Arginine 52-DQA1 and non-Aspartate 57 DQB1 alleles confer susceptibility to type I diabetes in children from Thailand[21].

Using both association and linkage studies, a 4.1Kb genomic region spanning the human insulin gene on chromosome 11p15.5 has been shown to confer susceptibility to type I diabetes and this locus contributes to 10 percent of the familial clustering of this disorder. The most important insulin gene 5' flanking polymorphism associated with type I diabetes is the polymorphic variable number of tandem repeats (VNTR) region located 365 bp upstream from the start site of insulin gene transcription. In Caucasians, the short 5' flanking polymorphism averaging 40 repeats (class 1 allele) is positively associated with type 1 diabetes while the long allele averaging 157 repeats is regatively associated with the disease[22]. Approximately 95% of Japanese population are homozygous for the class I allele and no association has been demonstrated between the insulin gene polymorphic region with type I diabetes[23]. In our study of 71 type I diabetic patients presenting before the age of 15 years, 44 type I diabetic patients presenting after age 15 years and 67 non-diabetic control subjects, the patients had a frequency of class I VNTR alleles which was not different from that of controls[24]. Similar to Japanese, greater than 95% of Chinese patients and controls (1 of 77 controls and 5 of 111 diabetic patients had class I/III VNTR genotype) had the class I allele. The distribution of the class I VNTR repeat number in our patients was different from those reported in Caucasian (approximately 60% in Chinese vs. less than 15% of Caucasian subjects with 28-37 repeats) but similar to that reported in Japanese[25]. In Japanese, the homozygous short class I allele (25-38 repeats) frequency was significantly increased in type I patients relative to controls suggesting that class I allele subset may have a role in type I diabetes susceptibility in Japanese[25]. In summary then, the variation of the incidence of type I diabetes mellitus in different population can be partly explained by the frequencies of different HLA genes and their linkage disequilibrium between highly susceptible DR and protective DQ alleles or vice versa. Given that Chinese have a low incidence of type I diabetes mellitus and a predominant class I VNTR allele, the class 1 VNTR allele could not be a simple universal risk conferring factor in all ethnic groups.

TYPE 2 DIABETES MELLITUS

Type 2 diabetes mellitus is the most prevalent form of diabetes which results from insulin resistance together with an insulin secretory defect. It is a polygenic disorder with a strong hereditary component. Until recently type 2 diabetes has never been regarded as a paediatric disease because it has been reported to account for only 2-3% of childhood diabetes. Increasing incidence of type 2 diabetes has been reported in ethnic minorities like Pima Indians, Mexican-Americans, First Nation People in Canada and African Americans [26]. The incidence of type 2 diabetes has also been on the rise in pediatric populations not belonging to the minority groups[27]. In a report from Cincinnati, there was an increase in the percentage of diabetic children with type 2 diabetes from 4% in 1982 to 16% in 1994 and among the 10 to 19 age group, type 2 diabetes accounted for 33% of newly diagnosed cases of diabetes in 1994[28]. In addition to the ethnic risk factor, other factors increasing the likelihood of the development of type 2 diabetes include obesity, family history of diabetes, fetal hyperinsulinemia from maternal gestational diabetes, intrauterine growth retardation, puberty, and the presence of acanthosis nigricans on physical examination[29,27].

Type 2 diabetes as an emergent paediatric problem is not limited to ethnic minorities and the North American continent (vide infra). This rise in incidence of type 2 diabetes worldwide may be associated with increasing obesity, decreasing activity and "Westernized" lifestyle. The trends in childhood obesity worldwide should be closely monitored because of their public health importance. It is difficult to make comparisons of trends internationally because of a lack of an internationally accepted definition and standard for childhood obesity.

The International Obesity Task Force developed a body mass index (BMI) standard constructed from data drawn from 6 nationally representative data sets (Brazil, Great Britain, Hong Kong, Netherlands, Singapore and United States)[30]. The cutoffs for overweight and obesity are based on extrapolation of BMI at 18 years of 25 and 30 on to the age and sex specific BMI charts. Using this international standard, the prevalence of overweight varies from 6.3% to 30.5% in Hong Kong, Singapore, Taiwan and Japan [31-33]. The percentage of total overweight adolescent boys are 10.3%, 15.3%, 20% and 30.5% in Hong Kong, Singapore, Japan and Taiwan respectively. The percentage of total overweight adolescent girls are 6.3%, 11.4%, 15.7% and 21.1% in Hong Kong, Singapore, Japan and Taiwan respectively. The prevalence of overweight and obesity is higher in males than in females in Asian populations contrary to the female dominance of obesity in Caucasian populations.

Although urine testing with a glucose dipstick is easy to perform, this method has not been widely used for screening for diabetes because of its poor sensitivity. However the method of screening has been used to screen for childhood diabetes in Asia. In order to detect type 2 diabetes mellitus and slow onset type 1 diabetes in childhood, urine screening for glycosuria using glucose oxidase test has been performed on school children age 6 to 15 years in Japan since 1974. The mean incidence rates increased from 2.8 per 100,000 children under the age of 15 years per year during the period 1975 to 1980 to 4.61 per 100,000 children per year between 1981- 1990[35]. This 1.5 fold increase in type 2 diabetes has been attributed to a similar increase in the prevalence of obesity in school children in Japan. In another report on Tokyo school children, the incidence of newly diagnosed type 2 diabetes increased from 0.2 to 2 per 100,000 population per year in primary school children and from 7.3 to 13.9 per 100,000 population per year in junior high school children between 1976 to 1995. This increase in incidence of type 2 diabetes correlated with an increase the prevalence of childhood obesity from 5% to 8% and an increase in the consumption of animal protein and fat in the Japanese population during this period but the total caloric intake by the Japan population had not significantly increased during this period[35]. A more marked increase in incidence of type 2 diabetes was seen after 12 years of age. There is a female predominance in adolescents with type 2 diabetes.

Another population-based screening for diabetes in school children (grade 1 to grade 12) was performed in Taiwan in 1997[36]. About 3 million school children were screened for glycosuria in a first void morning urine sample. Fasting blood glucose was performed if glycosuria persisted in a second urine sample and they used the diagnostic criteria recommended by the American Diabetes Association of a fasting blood sugar concentration equal to or greater than 7mmol/L as diabetes and a level of between 6 and 6.9 mmol/L as impaired fasting glycaemia (IFG). The prevalence of type 2 diabetes in school children age 6-18 years was 14.2 per 100,000 population in boys and 20.4 per 100,000 population in girls. The prevalence of IFG was 19.97 per 100,000 children. Body mass index was the strongest predictor of childhood type 2 diabetes in a multivariate analysis with an odds ratio of 2.2 (CI 1.78-2.81) for a BMI of 20-25 kg/m^2 and 8.31 (CI 6.38-10.85) for a BMI of > than 25 kg/m^2 as compared to children with a BMI of <20 kg/m^2. The risk of type 2 diabetes was 7.1 folds (CI 5.56-9.62) higher in children with a family history of type 2 diabetes than those without such a history. Type 2 diabetes now accounts for about 30% of the patients with diabetes attending a tertiary centre in Taipei. 3515 students in Madras India were screened for diabetes with a standard oral glucose tolerance test. A family history of diabetes was present in 8.2% of the children. No case of diabetes was detected[37]. In another study where 10,513 students between 3 and 20 yeas of age were screened for glycosuria, two children with a clinical course suggestive of maturity onset diabetes of youth were detected[38]. This would suggest that type 2 diabetes is not a problem in south India at this point in time although type 2 diabetes is a very common problem in the adult Indian population.

Less well documented rising trend of childhood type 2 diabetes and childhood obesity have also been noted in Singapore and the Hong Kong SAR. We have recently performed screening using oral glucose tolerance test in a target group of 83 obese adolescents (age 16.8 ±2.8 years) attending our clinic with a mean BMI of 31.4 ± 4.3. 85% of the adolescents had acanthosis nigricans and 88% had a family history of type 2 diabetes mellitus. Asymptomatic type 2 diabetes mellitus was detected in 4 patients (4.8%), impaired glucose tolerance in 13 (15.7%) and abnormal haemoglobin A_{1C} in 5 (6%). Impaired fasting glycaemia was found 3 subjects all of whom were diagnosed as suffering from asymptometic type 2 diabetes mellitus based on a blood sugar of >11.1 mmol/L 2 hour after a standard glucose load[39]. The American Diabetes Association recommended that only a single fasting plasma glucose greater than or equal to 7.0 mmol/L should be used for diagnosing diabetes in epidemiological studies and a value of between 6 and 6.9 mmol/L denotes impaired fasting glycaemia. (The expert committee on the diagnosis and classification of diabetes mellitus 1997). However in an analysis of 11 population-based studies, 6 preselected hyperglycaemic cohorts, and one suspected diabetic cohort involving Asian patients, it was found that more than half the diabetic subjects had post challenge hyperglycaemia in isolation and 75% of the subjects with impaired glucose tolerance according to the 2 hour glucose criteria were normal according to fasting glucose criteria[40]. Our results in obese adolescents concur with the conclusion of this study that it would be inappropriate to use the fasting glucose criteria alone in screening for diabetes in Asian populations. Furthermore, data collected in Europe, Mauritius, Fiji, and Nauru indicated that 2-hour post-load plasma glucose level was a better predictor of mortality[41]. In Hong Kong, a territory-wide effort has been initiated to screen for diabetes using the 2 hour blood glucose post glucose challenge in obese children with a family history of diabetes and other cardiovascular risk factors and the presence of acanthosis nigricans on physical examination.

CLINICAL ASPECTS OF CHILDHOOD AND ADOLESCENT TYPE I DIABETES MELLITUS

In most populations, the peak age of onset of type I diabetes mellitus coincides with puberty in both males and females and there is another peak between 5 and 7 years of age. In recent years, there is a tendency for a rising incidence in the less than 5 years of age cohort[42]. In many studies in Caucasians there is little evidence for a marked sex difference in incidence although a modest excess of males have been noticed in some studies. An excess of males among type I diabetic patients with an age of onset below 5 years had been reported in some populations[43]. On the contrary, in most countries in Asia where the incidence of type I diabetes is low, there is a predominance of girls among the diabetic children. (Table 1) The reason for this difference is not immediately apparent.

In Pittsburgh, children with type 1 diabetes mellitus diagnosed before puberty were taller than normal children whereas those who were diagnosed after puberty were shorter than normal children of the same age and sex. In Japan, there was no such association between age at onset and relative height[44]. In south India, the urban and high income patients had a peak age of onset of diabetes at 11 years as opposed to a peak age of onset of disease at 18 years in the rural and lower income group. The patient from the low income group had poorer nutritional status and lower body weight than the urban children from high income families[45]. No difference was observed in the heights of 250 Indian diabetic children at the onset of disease as compared to an age and sex matched control population[46]. In a study from Hong Kong, the mean height standard deviation score at diagnosis was +0.76 for boys and –0.07 for girls. The mean final height was +0.14 SDS for boys and –0.57SDS for girls suggesting that there is a sex difference in the growth of diabetic children[47].

In some Asian populations and especially in Japanese, patients with type I diabetes mellitus can present with abrupt onset of symptoms or take on a slow onset and progression course of the disease[48]. In a review, 14% of type 1 Japanese children with diabetes presented with coma and 12% of the cases were asymptomatic at diagnosis[34]. This suggests that slow onset type I diabetes is common in Japan but this could partly be due to the detection of cases early by the annual screening for glycosuria in school children in this country. There is no difference in the frequency of anti-GAD or ICA positivity in the slow-onset and the abrupt onset groups[48,49]. A subtype of non-autoimmune fulminant type I diabetes has been recently reported in 11 of 56 consecutive Japanese adult patients with type I diabetes, characterized by absence of pancreatic autoantibodies, abrupt disease onset, low HbA_{1c} and C-peptide and evidence of exocrine pancreatic damage[50]. However as stated in the accompanying editorial, the non-immune etiology of this subtype could not been regarded as a certainty as 8 of the 11 patients had the HLA DRB1*0405 – DQA1*0303-DQB1*0401 and HLA DR0901–DQA1*0302–DQB1*0303 haplotypes common in Japanese diabetic patient and that T-cell infiltration of the exocrine pancreas could be demonstrated in some of the patients.

CLASSIFICATION OF DIABETES

Although type I diabetes mellitus is characterized by absolute insulin requirement for survival, increasing evidence is available to show that it is clinically and immunologically a heterogeneous disorder. In Caucasians, the predominant autoimmune nature of type I diabetes is reflected by the presence of circulating antibodies to pancreatic β cell autoantigens [islet cell antibody (ICA), antibodies to glutamic acid decarboxylase (antiGAD) and tyrosine phosphatase-like protein (IA-2) and insulin autoantibody (IAA)] in up to 90% of cases at the time of disease onset[51]. These antibodies may occur very early in life and precede the clinical onset of the disease by years. In Asian populations, a significant proportion of type I diabetic patients have no evidence of an autoimmune disorder and these patients are now classified as "type I idiopathic" diabetes in the new WHO classification[52]. ICA and anti-GAD were found to be present in 41.5% of newly diagnosed patients from Singapore. In Japanese, the frequency of anti-GAD in newly diagnosed type I diabetic children varies between 58% and 73.1% in recent studies[49,53,54]. The IA-2 autoantibody was found to be present in 47% of newly diagnosed Japanese type I diabetic patients and the positivity decreased with increasing age of onset of diabetes. In combination, IA-2 and GAD65 antibodies improved the test sensitivity for IDDM to 92% in Japanese patients[53]. Others have found that measurement of IA-2 and anti-GAD in combination is no more sensitive than the assay of anti-GAD alone[55]. In Korea, about 40% of the newly diagnosed type I paediatric patients were positive for the 64k autoantibody[56]. This suggests that multiple pancreatic autoantigens may be involved in the type I diabetes autoimmune process or genetic differences within and between ethnic groups that contribute to the heterogeneous autoimmune response to glutamic acid decarboxylase or both. Alternatively some cases of type I diabetes have an etiology unrelated to autoimmunity.

With increasing frequency of type 2 diabetes and the prevalence of idiopathic slow onset type I diabetes in Asian populations, it becomes increasingly important to classify the diabetes correctly in patients so that appropriate treatment can be instituted. Pancreatic autoantibodies can help to distinguish autoimmune type 1 diabetes from the idiopathic type 1 or type 2 diabetes. Anti-GAD antibodies have been detected in 9% of Finns, 16% of Singaporeans, 4.3% of Japanese, 8.3% of Thai and 1.7% of Korean patients with type 2 diabetes mellitus[57]. A high C-peptide concentration taken either fasting (>0.6 ng/ml or 0.2 nmol/L) or in response to oral Sustacal (Mead Johnson) challenge (>1.5 ng/ml or 0.5 nmol/L) two years after diagnosis is also helpful. Clinically 85% of the type 2 diabetic patients presenting in adolescence are obese but as many as 24% of type I diabetic patients are also obese at presentation. Although ketoacidosis has usually been regarded as the hallmark of type I diabetes 33% of obese type 2 diabetic patients have ketonuria and 5-25% have ketoacidosis at presentation or at times of severe physiological stress[27]. There was a predominance of female children developing type 2 diabetes in Japan (female: male ratio of 1.3). Only 23.6% of the female and 3.4% of the male adolescents with type 2 diabetes were non-obese. The children and adolescents with type 2 diabetes were on the whole taller than their peers[35]. There is a high frequency of patients with positive family history for diabetes. Diet and exercise may result in remission of the diabetes in newly diagnosed patients. Insulin and oral hypoglycaemic agents are frequently required.

The classic type 2 diabetes in childhood should be differentiated from syndromal disorders associated with diabetes and monogenic type 2 diabetes. Maturity-onset diabetes of youth (MODY) is a dominantly inherited monogenic subtype of diabetes mellitus with an early age of onset characterized by a primary defect in insulin secretion. At least six distinct defects have been identified so far with varying severity of symptoms of diabetes. The patients are not obese and serum markers of pancreatic autoimmunity are not present. Mutation in the hepatocyte nuclear factor-1 alpha and glucokinase gene account for 5% and 3% respectively of young onset type 2 diabetic Chinese patients with a positive family history[58]. Similar low prevalence of MODY gene mutations has been found among type 2 Asian diabetic patients in other studies[59]. Among Asian Indians living in India and Africa, 5-10% of all diabetes may be of the MODY type[60]. Polymorphism of the Neuro D/BETA 2 gene encoding a transcription factor for the insulin gene and beta-cell differentiation may play a role in the pattern of onset and clinical course of diabetes as NeuroD/BETA2 may affect the ability of regeneration of beta cells[61].

The most common mitochondrial diabetes syndrome results from a mutation in nt 3243 of the mitochondrial gene for leucine tRNA but other mutations like deletions or G to A mutation at nt 3316 in the ND-1 gene of the mitochondrial DNA have also been described[62,63].

These mutations only account for 0.9%-2.4% of patients with type 2 diabetes[63,64] and can also account for a small number of cases diagnosed as type I diabetes in childhood[65]. A history of maternal transmission and hearing defect may improve the yield.

Two forms of diabetes due to disease of the pancreas have a higher prevalence in the Asia Pacific region than in Europe and North America. Transfusion dependent thalassaemia major is a common inherited haematological disorder in the Indian subcontinent and in Southeast Asia. Progressive accumulation of iron in different endocrine glands from repeated blood transfusions and increased absorption of iron from the gut leads to many endocrinopathies in the second and third decade of life. The prevalence of insulin dependent diabetes among 1861 patients with thalassemia major was 4.9% with all but one of the patient diagnosed after the age of 10 years[66]. A higher prevalence of diabetes mellitus of 15%-16% is observed with increasing age. The mean age of diagnosis of the patients is 17 to 18 years of age. The clinical presentation can vary from asymptomatic glycosuria to ketoacidosis[67]. The majority of patients with diabetes are also affected by hypogonadism and hypothyroidism. The insulin requirement in thalassaemic patients is not very different from that of other diabetic children. Impaired glucose tolerance could be present in these patients for months or up to 5 years before the onset of overt diabetic symptoms. The prognosis of patients has improved in recent years with 34% being still alive 8 years after the diagnosis of diabetes mellitus[66].

A brief mention should also be made about fibrocalculous pancreatic diabetes which was first described from Indonesia and subsequently reported in a lot of tropical developing countries in the Indian subcontinent, Thailand and some areas of the Asia Pacific region. It is a rare form of diabetes and accounts for about 1% of the cases of diabetes seen in the developing tropical countries. The condition is characterized by a young age of onset, low BMI, high insulin dosage requirement and evidence of pancreatic calcification on plain x-ray of the abdomen or on ultrasonography. Although these patients require insulin therapy, most do not suffer from diabetic ketoacidosis even when insulin treatment is interrupted for a long time. The two pathognomonic complaints of abdominal pain and steatorrhoea are not always present[68]. Also many patients do not fulfill the accepted criteria of malnutrition-related diabetes.

CRITICAL ISSUES IN DIABETES CARE IN THE ASIA PACIFIC REGION

Despite marked differences in the gross national product and annual expenditure on health care and health care delivery, representatives of different countries in the Asia Pacific region participating in the International Diabetes Federation Leadership Needs

Assessment Workshop on Childhood and Adolescent Diabetes held in Sydney Australia in March 1996 identified common critical issues for action in the region. With the exception of the more developed countries like Australia, Japan and New Zealand, reliable epidemiological data on incidence, morbidity, mortality and diabetes complications are needed to facilitate health care planning and finance. Much work would be needed to promote education and awareness processes on childhood diabetes involving patients, their families, health care professionals, people in the community and government agencies. In the less developed countries in the Asia Pacific region, availability and accessibility of insulin and testing materials remain a problem because of financial reasons. The ISPAD Consensus Guidelines for the Management of Type I Diabetes Mellitus in Children and Adolescents published in 2000 is a most valued resource in most countries lacking protocols and guidelines for diabetes care. The number of paediatric diabetic patients attending the different centres in the region is small because of a low incidence of disease, thus making it difficult to justify the establishment of centres with the necessary critical mass of multi-disciplenary team of doctors, nurses, educators, dietitians, social workers and psychologists. Elimination of social discrimination on patients with diabetes mellitus remains high on the priority list in some developing countries more than others. Collaboration between countries to promote research and collection of epidemiological data on diabetes as well as sharing of expertise through twinning programmes (between centres of developing and well developed countries) are now actively pursued in the Asia Pacific region. Members of the IDF-WPR Working Group on Childhood and Adolescent Diabetes have volunteered to undertake representation and advocacy of issues relevant to care of diabetic children and adolescents at regional and international level.

REFERENCES

1. Karvonen M, Viik-Kajander M, Moltchanova E et al.. Incidence of childhood type I diabetes worldwide. Diabetes Care 2000; 23:1516-26.
2. Yang Z, Wang K, Li J et al.. Childhood diabetes in China. Diabetes Care 1998; 21:525-9.
3. Fernando RE, Panelo AA. A report from the Philippines on diabetes among the young. In Mimura G (ed) Childhood and juvenile diabetes mellitus. Amsterdam: Excepta Medica 1985: pp33-42.
4. Presentations by country representatives. IDF-WPR Workshop on Childhood and Adolescent Diabetes, Kuala Lumpur, Malaysia 16-19 August 2000.

5. Onkamo P, Vaananen S, Karvonen M, Tuomilehto J. Worldwide increase in incidence of type 1 diabetes – the analysis of the data on published incidence trends. Diabetologia 1999; 42:1395-1403.
6. Bodansky HJ, Staines A, Stephenson C, Haigh D, Cartwright R. Evidence from an environmental effect in the etiology of insulin dependent diabetes in a transmigratory population. BMJ 1992; 304:1020-2.
7. Mustonen A, Honen J, Tiilikainen A, Kataja M, Akerblom HK. An analysis of epidemiological data in HLA-typed diabetic children. Diabetologia 1985; 28:397-400.
8. Kida K, Mimura G, Ito T, Murakami K, Ashkenazi I, Laron Z. Incidence of type I diabetes mellitus in children aged 0-14 in Japan, 1986-1990, including an analysis for seasonally of onset and month of birth: JDS study. The Data Committee for Childhood Diabetes of the Japan Diabetes Society (JDS). Diabetic Med 2000; 17:59-63.
9. Ko KW, Yang SW, Cho NH. The incidence of IDDM in Seoul from 1985 to 1988. Diabetes Care 1994; 17:1473-5.
10. Todd JA, Bell JI, McDevitt HO. HLA-DQ-beta gene contributes to susceptibility and resistance to insulin in dependent diabetes mellitus. Nature 1987; 329:599-604.
11. Khalil I, d' Auriol L, Gobet M et al.. A correlation of HLA-DQ beta Asp 57-negative and HLA-DQ alpha Arg 52 confers susceptibility to insulin dependent diabetes mellitus. J Clin Invest 1990; 85:1315-9
12. Baisch JM, Weeks T, Giles R et al.. Analysis of HLA genotypes and susceptibility in insulin dependent diabetes mellitus. N Engl J Med 1990; 322:1836-41.
13. Park YS, Wang CY, Ko KW, Yang SW, Park M, Yang MC, She JX. Combinations of HLA DR and DQ molecules determine the susceptibility to insulin independent diabetes mellitus in Koreans. Hum Immunol 1998; 59:794-801.
14. Huang HS, Peng JY, She JY, Zhang LP, Chao CC, Liu KH, She JX. HLA-encoded susceptibility to insulin-dependent diabetes mellitus is determined by DR and DQ genes as well as their linkage disequilibrium in a Chinese population. Hum Immunol 1995; 44:210-9.
15. Hu CY, Allen M, Chuang LM, Lin BJ, Gyllensten U. Association of insulin-dependent diabetes mellitus in Taiwan with HLA class II DQB1 and DRB1 alleles. Hum Immunol 1993; 38:105-14.
16. Cheung PT, Chang YW, Kwan EYW, Low LCK, Hawkins BR. Higher restrictive distribution of class II HLA alleles in type 1 diabetes of early onset in Chinese. Abstract in 79th Annual Meeting of Endocrine Society Minneapolis USA, 11-14 June 1997.
17. Chen BH, Chiang CH, Liu SR, Chao MG, Tsai ST. The influence of age at onset and gender on HLA-DQA1, DQB1 association in

Chinese children with insulin dependent diabetes mellitus. Hum Immunol 1999; 60:1131-7.

18. Sugihara S, Sakamaki T, Konda S et al. Association of HLA-DR, DQ genotype with different beta-cell functions at IDDM diagnosis in Japanese children. Diabetes 1997; 46:1893-7.
19. Kobayahsi T, Tamemoto K, Nakanishi K et al. Immunogenetic and clinical characterization of slowly progressive IDDM. Diabetes Care 1993;16:780-8.
20. Kelly MA, Alvi NS, Croft NJ, Mijovic CH, Bottazzo GF, Barnett AH. Genetic and immunological characterisation of type I diabetes mellitus in Indo-Aryan population. Diabetologia 2000; 43:450-6.
21. Sujirachato K, Chiewsilp P, Tsuji K, Panyim S, Inoko H, Tuchinda C, Vannasaeng S. HLA Class II polymorphism in Thai insulin dependent diabetes mellitus. Tokai J Exp Clin Med 1994; 19:73-81.
22. McGinnis RE, Spielman RS. Insulin gene 5' flanking polymorphism. Length of class 1 alleles in number of repeat units. Diabetes 1995; 44:1296-1301.
23. Matsumoto C., Awata T, Iwamoto Y, Kuzuya T, Saito T, Kanazawa Y. Lack of association of the insulin gene region with type I (insulin-dependent) diabetes mellitus in Japanese subjects. Diabetologia 1994; 37:210-3.
24. Cheung PT, Low LCK, Hawkins BR, Tan KCB, Kwan EYW, Lam KSL, Chan V. Genetic predisposition to IDDM at the insulin gene linked polymorphic region IDDM2 is different between Chinese and Caucasian. Abstract in 81st Annual Meeting of Endocrine Society, San Diego, USA, 12-15 June, 1999.
25. Awata T, Kurihara S, Kikuchi C et al. Evidence for association between class I subset of the insulin gene minisatellite (IDDM2 locus) and IDDM in the Japanese population. Diabetes 1997; 46:1637-42.
26. Dabelea D, Pettitt DJ, Jones KL, Arslanian SA. Type 2 diabetes mellitus in minority children and adolescent. Endocrinol Metab Clin N Am 1999; 28:709-29.
27. American Diabetes Association. Type 2 diabetes in children and adolescents. Pediatrics 2000; 105:671-80.
28. Pinhas-Hamiel O, Dolan LM, Daniel SR et al. Increased incidence of non-insulin dependent diabetes mellitus among adolescents. J Pediatr 1996; 128:608-15.
29. Glaser NS. Non-insulin-dependent diabetes mellitus in childhood and adolescence. Pediatr Clin N Am 1997; 44:307-37.
30. Cole TJ, Bellizzi MC, Flegal KM, Dietz WH. Establishing a standard definition for child overweight and obesity worldwide: international survey. BMJ 2000; 320:1-6.
31. Naiu-Feng C, Rimm EB, Wang DJ, Liou HS, Sheh SM. Clustering of cardiovascular disease risk factors among obese school children : the Taipei children heart study. Am J Clin Nutr 1998; 67:1141-6.

32. Rajan U. Obesity among Singapore students. Int J Obesity 1994; 18(Suppl 2):27.
33. Leung SSF, Cole TJ, Tse LY, Lau JT. Body anass index reference curves for Chinese children. Ann Hum Biol 1998; 25:169-74.
34. Kitagawa T, Owada M, Urakami T, Tajima N. Epidemiology of type 1 (insulin dependent) and type 2 (non-insulin dependent) diabetes mellitus in Japanese children. Diabetes Res and Clin Pract 1994; 24 Suppl: S7-13.
35. Kitagawa T, Owada M, Urakami T, Yamauchi K. Increased incidence of non-insulin dependent diabetes mellitus among Japanese school children correlates with an increased intake of animal protein and fat. Clin Pediatr 1998; 37:111-5.
36. Chuang LM, Sung JFC, Liu CC, Lin RS. Population-based diabetes screening in school children and adolescents in Taiwan. Proceedings of meeting "Emerging Health Problems in Childhood and Adolescents: Obesity and Diabetes 3 June 2001, Taipei: 4-5.
37. Bai PV, Krishnaswami CV, Chellamariappan M, Kumar GV, Subramaniam JR, Srivatwa A, Subramanyam B, Rao MB. Prevalence of diabetes in the young in South India. Indian Paediatr 1995; 32:1173-6.
38. Bai PV, Krishnaswami CV, Chellamariappan M, Kumar GV, Subramaniam JR. Glycosuria and diabetes mellitus in children and adolescents in South India. Diabetes Res Clin Pract 1991; 13:131-5.
39. Kwan EYW, Cheung PT, Yeung LPK, Low LCK. The assessment of glucose tolerance and insulin resistance in overweight and obese Chinese children. Abstract of the 23rd International Congress of Pediatrics, Beijing, 10-15 September 2001.
40. Qiao Q, Nakagami T, Tuomilehto J et al.. Comparison of the fasting and the 2-h glucose criteria for diabetes in different Asian Cohorts. Diabetologia 2000; 43:1470-5.
41. Shaw JE, Hodge AM, de Courten M, Chitson P, Zimmet PZ. Isolated post-challenge hyperglycaemia confirmed as a risk factor for mortality. Diabetologia 1999; 42:1050-4.
42. Huen KF, Low LCK, Wong GWK et al.. Epidemiology of diabetes mellitus in children in Hong Kong. The Hong Kong Childhood Diabetes Register. J Pediatr Endocrinol Metab 2000; 13:297-302.
43. Laron Z, Kamp M, Modan M. The incidence of insulin dependent diabetes mellitus – Israeli children adolescents 0-20 years of age, a retrospective study. Diabetes Care 1985; 8(Suppl 1):24-8.
44. Anonymous. Height at onset of insulin-dependent diabetes mellitus in high- and low-risk countries. Japan and Pittsburgh Childhood Diabetes Research groups. Diabetes Res Clin Pract 1989; 6:173-6.
45. Ramachandran A, Snehalatha C, Joseph TA, Vijay V, Viswanathan M. Delayed onset of diabetes in children of low economic stratum – a story from southern India. Diabetes Res Clin Pract 1994a; 22:171-4.

46. Ramachandran A, Snehalatha C, Joseph TA, Vijay V, Viswanathan M. Height at onset of insulin-dependent diabetic children in South India. Diabetes Res Clin Pract 1994b; 23:55-7.
47. Wong GW, Cheng PS, Leung F. Sex differences in the growth of diabetic children. Diabetes Res Clin Pract 2000; 50:187-93.
48. Urakami T, Miyamoto Y, Fujita H, Kitagawa T. Type I (insulin-dependent) diabetes in Japanese children is not a uniform disease. Diabetologia 1989; 32:312-5.
49. Kasuga A, Falorni A, Maruyama T et al. HLA class II is associated with the frequency of glutamic acid decarboxylase M(r)65,000 autoantibodies in Japanese patient with insulin-dependent diabetes mellitus. Acta Diabetologica 1996; 33:108-13.
50. Imagawa A, Hanafusa T, Miyasama JI, Matsuzawa Y for the Osaka. IDDM study group. A novel subtype of type I diabetes mellitus characterized by a rapid onset and an absence of diabetes-related antibodies. N Engl J Med 2000; 342:301-7.
51. Bonifacio E, Genovese S, Braghi S et al. Islet autoantibody markers in insulin-dependent diabetes: risk assessment strategies yielding high sensitivity. Diabetologia 1995; 38:816-22.
52. Alberti KGMM, Zimmet PZ for the WHO Consultation. Definition, diagnosis and classification of diabetes mellitus and its complications. Part I: Diagnosis and classification of diabetes mellitus. Provisional report of a WHO consultation. Diabetic Med 1998; 15:539-53.
53. Kasuga A, Ozawa Y, Maruyama T, Ishihara T, Amemiva S, Surata T. Autoantibody against IA-2 improve the test sensitivity for insulin-dependent diabetes mellitus in Japanese patients of child onset. Endocr J 1997; 44:485-91.
54. Kida K, Mimura G, Kobayashi T et al. ICA and organ-specific autoantibodies among Japanese patients with early-onset insulin-dependent diabetes mellitus – the JDS study. Diabetes Res Clin Pract 1994; 23:187-93.
55. Lee YS, Ng WY, Thai AC, Liu KF, Loke KY. Prevalence of ICA and GAD antibodies at initial presentation of type I diabetes mellitus in Singapore children. J Pediatr Endocrinol Metab 2001; 14:767-72.
56. Lee HC, Cha BS, Nan MS et al. Relationships among 64k autoantibodies, pancreatic beta-cell function, HLA-DR antigens and HLA-DQ genes in patients with insulin-dependent diabetes mellitus in Korea. Korean J Int Med 1995; 10:1-9.
57. Thai AC, WY Ng, Loke KY, Lee WR, Liu KE, Cheah JS. Anti-GAD antibodies in Chinese patients with youth and adult-onset IDDM and NIDDM. Diabetologia 1997; 40:1425-30.
58. Ng MC, Cockburn BN, Lindner TH et al. Molecular genetics of diabetes mellitus in Chinese subjects: identification of mutations in glucokinase and hepatocyte nuclear factor-1 alpha genes in patients

with early-onset type 2 diabetes mellitus/MODY. Diabetic Med 1999; 16:956-63.
59. Nishigori H, Yamada S, Kohama T, Utsugi T, Shimizu H, Takeuchi T, Takeda J. Mutations in the hepatocyte nuclear factor-1 alpha gene (MODY 3) are not a major cause of early-onset non-insulin dependent (type 2) diabetes mellitus in Japanese. J Hum Genet 1998; 43:107-10.
60. Mohan V, Ramachandran A, Snehalatha C, Mohan R, Bharani G, Viswanathan M. High prevalence of maturity-onset diabetes of the young (MODY) among Indians. Diabetes Care 1985; 8:371-4.
61. Yamada S, Motoshashi Y, Yanagawa T et al. NeuroD/BETA2 gene G→A polymorphism may affect onset pattern of type I diabetes in Japanese. Diabetes Care 2001;24:1438-41.
62. Odawara M, Sasaki K, Yamashita K. A G to A substitution at nucleotide position 3316 in mitochondrial DNA is associated with Japanese non-insulin dependent diabetes mellitus. Biochem Biophys Res Comm 1996; 227:147-51.
63. Otabe S, Sakura H, Shimokawa K et al. The high prevalence of the diabetic patients with a mutation in the mitochondrial gene. J Clin Endocrinol Metab 1994; 79:768-71.
64. Xiang K, Wang Y, Wu S et al. Mitochondrial tRNA [Leu (UUR)] gene mutation diabetes mellitus in Chinese. Chinese Med J 1997; 110:372-8.
65. Smith PR, Dronsfield MJ, Mijovic CH et al. The mitochondrial RNA [Leu (UUR)] A to G 3243 mutation is associated with insulin dependent and non-insulin dependent diabetes in a Chinese population. Diabetic Med 1997; 14:1026-31.
66. Italian Working Group on Endocrine Complications in non-endocrine disease. Multicentre study in prevalence of endocrine complications in thalassaemia major. Clin Endocrinol 1995; 42:581-6.
67. Low LCK. Growth, puberty and endocrine function in beta-thalassaemia major. J Pediatr Endocrinol Metab 1997; 10:175-84.
68. Yajnik CS, Shelgikar KM. Fibrocalculous pancreatic diabetes in Pune, India. Clinical fetures and follow-up for 7 years. Diabetes Care 1993; 16:916-21.

Chapter 8
LIPOATROPHIC DIABETES MELLITUS

Elif Arioglu Oral[1] and Stephanie Moran[2]
1. University of Michigan, Department of Internal Medicine, Division of Endocrinology and Metabolism
2. Diabetes Branch, National Institute of Diabetes, Digestive and Kidney Diseases, National Institutes of Health, Bethesda, Maryland

Millions of Americans are afflicted by obesity and type 2 diabetes mellitus. Obesity is characterized by increased body adiposity and leads to insulin resistance. Paradoxically, some conditions that are characterized by a paucity of fat also cause insulin resistance, namely the syndromes of lipoatrophy (Figure 1). The resemblance between the metabolic abnormalities of these two extreme states of adiposity emphasizes the

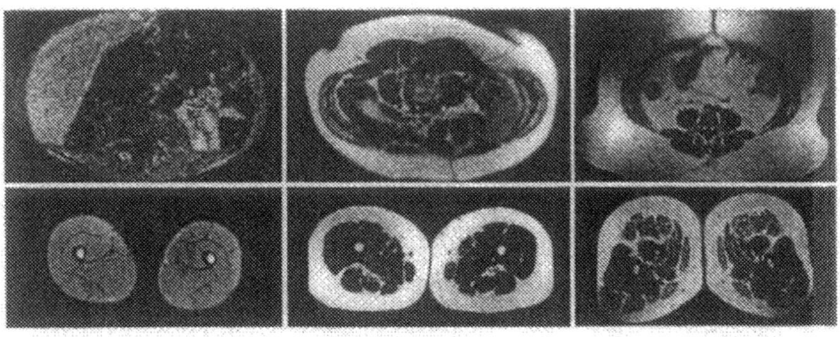

Figure 1. Clinical spectrum of adiposity. T1-weighted magnetic resonance images in which lipid appears white. Transverse sections of the torso at the level of the fifth lumbar vertebra (top panels) and mid-thigh (bottom panels) are shown. Generalized lipoatrophy (left panels), normal individual with body mass index of 24 kg/m^2 (middle panels), an obese individual with body mass index of 38 kg/m^2 (right panels) Note the marked absence of all fat depots in the patient with generalized lipoatrophy, with preservation of marrow fat, and a lipid filled liver. Also, the bright color of the muscle is reflective of lipid-filled myocytes.

importance of fat tissue in energy homeostasis. This chapter focuses on the syndromes of lipodystrophy and lipoatrophy that are at the lean extreme of the spectrum and which are characterized by near-complete absence of fat.

A definition of lipodystrophy, lipoatrophy, and lipoatrophic diabetes

Lipoatrophy syndromes comprise a heterogeneous cluster of disease states having in common a lack of fat tissue [1]. The deficiency of adipose tissue can be partial or generalized, and these abnormalities may be congenital or acquired [1]. The characteristic loss of fat is known as "lipoatrophy" whereas an abnormal distribution of fat is "lipodystrophy". The term "lipoatrophic diabetes" refers to patients who have diabetes mellitus in association with lipoatrophy. It is important to realize that lipodystrophy is a generalized term that encompasses lipoatrophy and other abnormalities of adipose tissue such as lipedema or lipomatosis. In this review, we focus on syndromes characterized primarily by adipocyte deficiencies throughout the body. Although it is important to describe the amount and distribution of adipose tissue, there is also a distinction between the actual insufficiency of adipocytes and preadipocytes that results in metabolic disturbances and those states of total body fat deficiency caused by decreased triglyceride storage. In the latter state, the adipocytes are still basically normal, but are chronically forced to mobilize their stored triglycerides (e.g. under conditions of chronic caloric depletion, intense exercise or increased sympathetic drive [2-5]). Furthermore, we now know from rodent models that genetic defects that interfere with triglyceride storage alone and result in "empty" adipocyte syndrome, do not lead to the metabolic consequences so long as the other functional capabilities (like endocrine function) of the adipocytes are not altered[6]. In all cases of lipoatrophy there is adipocyte insufficiency and the metabolic consequences are peripheral insulin resistance and hypertriglyceridemia. It is also interesting to note that experimental approaches that completely ablate white adipose tissue lead to the metabolic syndrome regardless of the strategy. These observations underscore the importance of the adipocyte not only as storage site for triglycerides; but also as a cell which is capable of sensing nutrient availability and abundance and responding with signals that play a regulatory role in energy storage and partition.

MECHANISMS OF DISEASE

Lipodystrophy and lipoatrophy syndromes are characterized by decreased adipose tissue. The congenital forms demonstrate a reduction in adipose tissue throughout life. The proposed mechanism for these forms of lipodystrophy/lipoatrophy results from defects in adipocytes differentiation and function. In the acquired syndromes there is evidence of normal adipocyte development but then a loss of adipose tissue later in life which implies a mechanism of adipocyte destruction. The reduction of adipocytes may occur via decreased growth and differentiation, increased apoptosis, or enhanced destruction as may occur in autoimmune destruction.

In order to better understand possible etiologies of congenital lipodystrophy/lipoatrophy it is important to understand normal adipocyte growth and differentiation. Normal adipose tissue develops in multiple sites throughout the body from embryonic mesenchymal cells. Over the last decade, there have been great advances in understanding the differentiation program of adipocytes. Precursor cells are committed to adipogenesis through transient expression of certain transcription factors such as the CCAAT/enhancer binding proteins (C/EBPs) and Perioxisome proliferator activating receptors (PPARs). Other transcription factors are also involved either in activating these key factors or controlling the synthesis of their ligands (for example SREBP1/ADD1 may regulate synthesis of ligands for PPARγ).

Through expression of these nuclear transcription factors, the cell differentiates into an adipocyte and develops the ability to store triglycerides, repress cell-cycle genes and secrete adipocyte-specific hormones. Recently, a novel molecule called lipin has been cloned as a result of positional cloning efforts to identify the genetic etiology of a naturally occurring mouse model with partial lipoatrophy and fatty liver. This novel protein has nuclear localization and is induced during adipocyte differentiation [7]. Its exact role in the adipocyte differentiation pathway remains to be identified.

Defects in adipocyte differentiation commitment steps may lead to adipocyte deficiency; however, the exact control of normal adipocyte growth and cell cycle are not yet fully understood. Furthermore, as we will discuss later on in this chapter, identification of some of the genes responsible from known human lipoatrophy syndromes did not easily fit the known pathways in adipocyte differentiation.

Another mechanism by which to lose adipocytes is through increased destruction of these cells (such as induction of apoptosis). Animal models of lipoatrophy have been engineered via either disruption of adipogenesis or induction of adipocyte-death. These models help us understand the pathophysiology of fat loss. All of these models use an adipose-specific promoter / enhancer to introduce a transgene. A review on animal models of lipoatrophy can be found elsewhere [8].

When discussing the mechanisms of disease in lipoatrophy syndromes, it is important to recognize that the primary event is adipocyte deficiency and that the metabolic problems associated with the syndromes are secondary. The circumstantial evidence for this supposition was based on the similarity of the metabolic phenotype in a wide range of human syndromes. However, the direct proof came with the demonstration that the metabolic phenotype was largely reversed upon fat transplantation in a genetically engineered rodent model of lipoatrophy[9]. Why does fat transplantation reverse metabolic phenotype of lipoatrophy? One hypothesis stresses the endocrine function of the adipocyte. The discovery of the adipocyte hormone leptin underscored the endocrine function of adipose tissue. Leptin communicates body energy stores to the neuroendocrine system to control food-intake and energy expenditure. Leptin has effects (direct or indirect) on the key organs of metabolism, including the liver, muscle and pancreas. Another molecular signal originating from the adipocytes, ACRP 30 [10](also called adipoQ [11], APM1 or Adiponectin [12]) was found to be important in inducing fat oxidation in the muscle and liver [10]. The list of endocrine signals originating from the adipocyte is growing. Lack of adipocytes results in deficiency of these signals, thus contributing to many of the abnormalities seen in these syndromes characterized by absence of fat. Thus, it is possible to view the metabolic aspects of the lipoatrophy syndromes as a consequence of the hormonal insufficiency created by the absence of the organ producing the hormone.

CLASSIFICATION OF LIPOATROPHY SYNDROMES

As mentioned above, absence of fat can be partial or generalized. and the syndrome can manifest at birth or later in life [13]. If fat loss is partial, the residual fat undergoes compensatory hypertrophy. Usually, there is a rough correlation between the severity of metabolic consequences and the degree of fat loss. There is also an entity called focal lipoatrophy where the loss of fat involves a single region in the body. One example of this are the loss of fat in the gluteal area usually following intramuscular injections [14]. Therapy with protein hormones, such as insulin [15, 16] and growth hormone [17] may lead to focal lipoatrophy. A focal lipoatrophy may also occur on the face referred to as the Romberg's syndrome [18]. There are other specifically described fat distributions reported in the literature as 'annular" or "semicircular" lipoatrophy [19, 20]. Usually, the isolated loss of fat from a limited body region is not associated with metabolic consequences, supporting the hypothesis that a crucial degree of fat loss is required to observe the metabolic abnormalities.

Table 1. Genetic Syndromes of Lipoatrophy

Syndrome	Lipoatrophy	Gene/Locus	Inheritance	OMIM[1]
Primary Lipoatrophy Syndromes				
CGL[2] (Seip-Berardinelli)	Generalized See text for details	9q34 Gene unknown[4] 11q13 Seipin gene	AR[3]	269700
Dunnigan Syndromes	Familial partial See text for details	1q21-22 Lamin A/C	AD[5]	151660
Late-onset FPLD	Familial partial See text for details	3p25 ppar-gamma	AD	604367
Others	Numerous distributions	Unknown	AD/AR	N/A
Complex Syndromes Associaed with Lipoatrophy				
Mandibuloacral dysplasia	Congenital, partial Involves extremities	Unknown	AR	248370
Werner syndrome	Congenital, partial Involves extremities	8p12 Werner's Helicase	AR	277700
Cockayne syndrome	Congenital, partial Involves extremities	5 CSA	AR	216400
Carbohydrate-deficiency glycoprotein syndrome	Transient, partial buttocks	16p.13.3 PMM1 and 2[6]	AR	212065
SHORT[7] syndrome	Generalized, congenital	Unknown	AR	269880
AREDYLD[8] syndrome	Generalized, congenital	Unknown	Unknown	207780

[1] Online-Mendelian Inhertance of Man, reference 119, data base providing information about genetic syndromes
[2]Congenital generalized lipoatrophy
[3]Autosomal recessive
[4]Evidence for genetic heterogeneity
[5]Autosomal dominant
[6]Phosphomannomutase 1 and 2
[7]Short stature, hyperextensibility, hernia, ocular depression, Rieger anomaly, and teething delay
[8]Acrorenal field defect, ectodermal dysplasia, and lipoatrophic diabetes, not clear if this is a variation of Berardinelli-Seip syndrome

GENETIC SYNDROMES OF LIPOATROPHY AND LIPODYSTROPHY

Primary Lipoatrophy Syndromes

Congenital Generalized Lipoatrophy (Figure 1). This condition is also known as Seip-Berardinelli syndrome [21, 22]. In this syndrome, children present with generalized absence of fat within the first year of life. This is followed by insulin resistance, acanthosis nigricans and diabetes mellitus before the teen-age years. Hypertriglyceridemia is severe and is accompanied by frequent bouts of pancreatitis. Affected patients have a high basal metabolic rate [23] and an increased appetite. Circulating leptin levels are usually quite low [24-26]. This syndrome has an autosomal recessive mode of inheritance, and has been described in all ethnic groups. We have observed a sexual dimorphism in the severity of metabolic complications. Female patients manifest diabetes and hypertriglyceridemia much earlier and usually more severely than the male siblings in the same family.

Although well described clinically for decades, the molecular basis for congenital generalized lipoatrophy remained a mystery until quite recently . In the 1970s Foss et.al. demonstrated the presence of a urinary lipolytic factor in cases of congenital generalized lipoatropy; however, these studies have not been reproduced [27]. Candidate gene approach did not elucidate the genetic cause for this syndrome. Genes for peroxisome-proliferator activated receptor-gamma, beta-3-adrenergic receptor, leptin, leptin receptor and lipoprotein lipase [28-30] are among genes that have been excluded. The disease has been mapped to chromosome 9q34 in some, but not all pedigrees [31]. Thus, there must be multiple causative genes involved. Maigre et. al. very recently cloned the first gene responsible from congenital generalized lipoatrophy using positional cloning and interval refining[32]. This gene is located on chromosome 11q13 and is a separate gene from the putative CGL-1 gene located on chromosome 9q34. This new gene was named Seipin as an attribute to Seip who is one of the first to describe the syndrome. The protein product of the Seipin gene is most likely a signaling molecule. It has three trans-membrane domains and the ligand is not known. The mouse orthologue of the gene is a G-protein related receptor gene[32]. Contrary to the predictions that prevailed prior to the discovery of this gene, Seipin is not abundantly expressed in the fat cells. It is expressed predominantly in the central nervous system and especially in the pituitary. Another location where it is expressed in high levels is the testes. This localization outside of adipose tissue implies a greater role for the central nervous system in energy storage and fuel metabolism than has currently been known and is likely to change our views on adipocyte differentiation mechanisms[32].

Familial partial lipodystrophy (FPLD, Dunnigan's syndrome) (Figure 2). Also referred as Kobberling-Dunnigan syndrome, this condition is inherited in an autosomal dominant fashion. It has been seen mostly in Caucasians of Northern European descent, but pedigrees of Asian descent have also been described. Although rare, pediatricians may be presented with the question whether a child of an affected parent also has the disease. It is usually impossible to distinguish affected patients from unaffected ones before the onset of puberty. Patients are born with normal fat distribution but notice loss of subcutaneous fat in the extremities and trunk with early puberty. This is followed by increased fat in the face and neck as puberty is completed [33, 34]. The visceral fat and interfascicular intramuscular fat depots are preserved [35, 36]. While the disease affects both sexes, the phenotype is much easier to discern in females leading to ascertainment bias of female

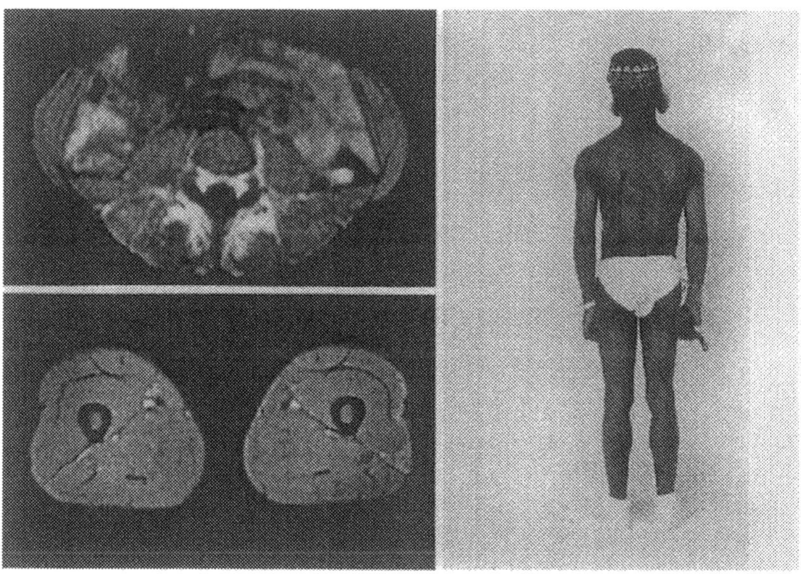

Figure 2. Congenital generalized lipoatrophy in a 16-year old girl. Picture (Right) and T1-weighted magnetic resonance images (Left). Transverse sections of the torso at the level of the fifth lumbar vertebra demonstrate markedly deficient subcutaneous and visceral fat (left upper panel). Transverse sections of the midthigh demonstrate absence of subcutaneous, deep, intrafascicular and marrow fat. Note again light-colored, lipid-filled muscle tissue (left lower panel). Note absence of fat throughout the body and the differences between these images and those presented in figures 1 and 2.

probands. Overall, female patients develop diabetes and dyslipidemia earlier and more severely. For example, from our case series, affected females develop diabetes about 73% of the time and hypertriglyceridemia 90% of the time. In contrast, these incidences are 36% and 45% respectively, in affected male individuals. Our observations are similar to recently published observations of another group [37].

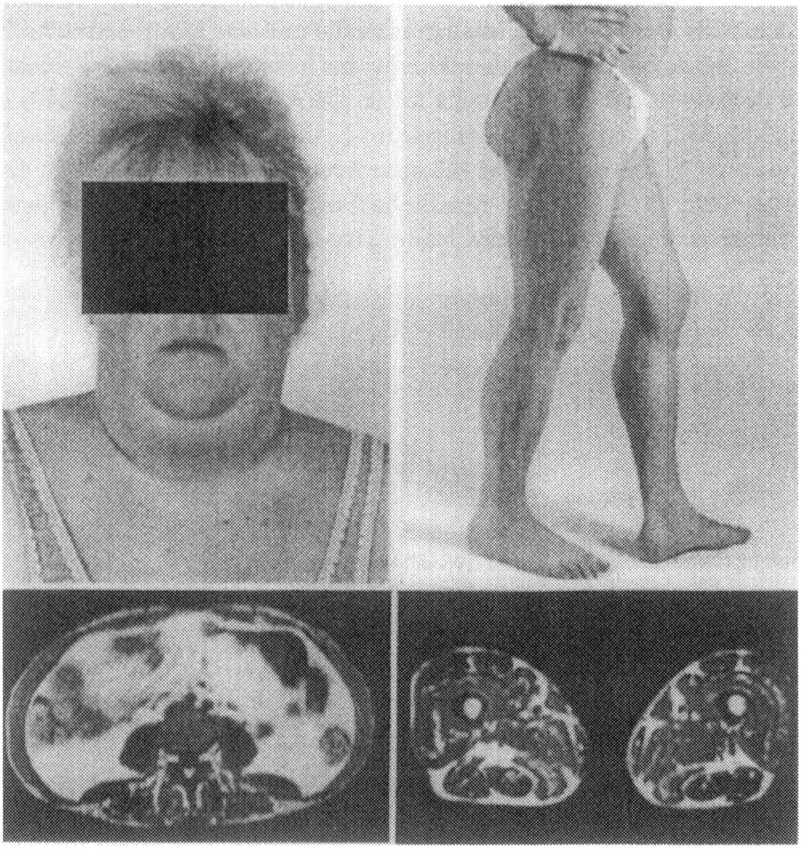

Figure 3. Dunnigan's familial partial lipodystrophy. (Top) Pictures of a 26-year old female. Note increased fat around the face/neck (left panel) and deficiency in the gluteal region and lower extremities (right panel). (Bottom) T1-weighted magnetic resonance images. Transverse sections of the torso at the level of the fifth lumbar vertebra demonstrate markedly deficient subcutaneous and increased visceral fat (left panel). Transverse sections of the midthigh demonstrate absence of subcutaneous fat with preservation of deep, intrafascicular and marrow fat (right panel).

An exciting advance in the understanding of the syndrome has been the discovery that the disease is caused by mutations in the lamin A/C gene

(LMNA) located at 1q21-23 [38-42]. Lamin A and C are alternatively spliced products of the same gene and are ubiquitously; but not equally expressed [43]. They belong to a family of intermediate filament proteins that form the nuclear matrix [44, 45], which is located just inside the nuclear membrane. Lamins dimerize and oligomerize within the structure of the nuclear matrix [45]. There is developmental regulation of the expression of lamins in humans.

Besides Dunnigan's FPLD, multiple other diseases are associated with mutations in LMNA: Emery Dreyfus muscular dystrophy (a progressive muscular dystrophy of upper and lower extremity muscles with prominent contractures of ankles and elbows, and cardiac conduction abnormalities) [46, 47], hereditary limb-girdle muscular dystrophy [48], a familial cardiomyopathy associated with conduction abnormalities [49, 50] and hereditary Charcot-Marie Tooth Neuropathy type 2[51]. The degree of overlap between these diseases and FPLD is subject of research. In addition, how the mutations in the LMNA result in multiple different diseases and how the mutations in a ubiquitously expressed gene cause various syndromes with a strong regional distribution are questions still awaiting answers. As far as FPLD is concerned, investigation of expression patterns of various lamins in different adipose depots (visceral versus subcutaneous) did not provide any clues into the mechanism of disease of FPLD[52]. Likewise, investigation of the nuclear targeting or interaction with dimerization partner emerin in a common mutant form seen in FPLD did not elucidate any abnormalities [53].

Partial Lipodystrophy Associated with Dominant Negative Mutations on PPAR-gamma gene (late-onset familial partial lipodystrophy). Barroso and colleagues described two probands with severe insulin resistance and hypertension as well as severe acanthosis nigricans[54]. Initially, no changes in body composition were reported. However, careful body composition studies revealed that these patients have significant fat loss in the lower extremities, particularly in the buttock region. The onset of fat loss is not at birth, but develops sometime in adulthood. There is also increased visceral adiposity. Agarwal and Garg described another female patient with a different mutation on ppar-gamma gene who had a similar body fat distribution without any hypertension and acanthosis nigricans[55]. These observations suggest that dominant-negative mutations of the ppar-gamma gene result in both severe insulin resistance and also an abnormality in body fat distribution that manifests later in life.

Congenital Syndrome Complexes associated with Lipoatrophy

There are also other complex monogeneic syndromes that are not characterized as primary lipodystrophy syndromes but are associated with abnormal body fat distribution among other complex abnormalities. Progeria syndromes such as Werner's (adult progeria syndrome, Figure 4a, [56] and Cockayne's Syndrome (one of the juvenile progeria syndromes) [57, 58], carbohydrate-deficient glycoprotein syndrome Type 1 [59], SHORT syndrome (an acronym for short stature, hyperextensibility, hernia, ocular depression,

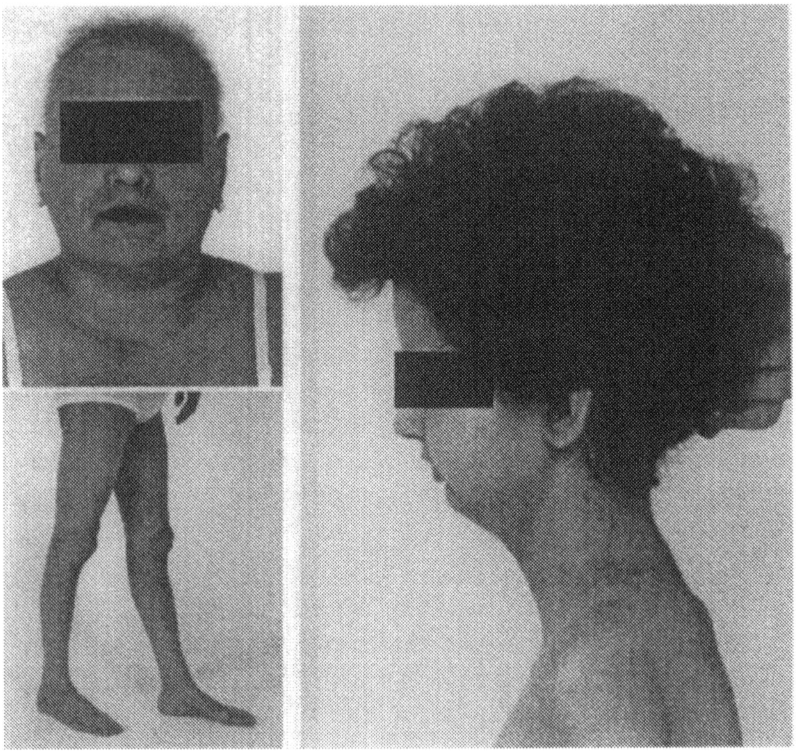

Figure 4. Left panel - Werner's Syndrome in a 37-year old woman. Clinical features evident include premature aging, allopecia, scleroderma-like changes in the skin and peripheral lipoatrophy as shown (left panels). Insulin-resistant diabetes is an associated feature. Right panel - Mandibuloacral dysplasia in a 14 year old girl. This rare recessive syndrome is characterized by acroosteolysis, widened sutures, hypoplastic mandible (shown) and clavicles (shown). Marked peripheral lipoatrophy and insulin resistance are associated features.

Rieger anomaly and teething delay) [60, 61] and mandibuloacral dysplasia (figure 4b) [62, 63] are among such syndromes. AREDYLD syndrome (acral, renal and ectodermal dysplasia in association with generalized lipodystrophy) [64] probably represents another complex progeria syndrome.

Mandibuloacral dysplasia is a genetic disorder with multi-system involvement and autosomal recessive inheritance. This extremely rare syndrome is characterized by multiple skeletal abnormalities, acroosteolysis, joint and skin problems and is also associated with lipodystrophy and metabolic abnormalities [62, 63]. The genetic etiology remains unknown. In this condition, the predominant fat loss is from the extremities and trunk with increased visceral adiposity[65]Some unusual congenital associations such as Vitamin D resistance and persistent Mullerian ducts [66], retinal pigmentation abnormalities [67] and sensorineural deafness [68] have been reported in association with lipoatrophy in isolated cases. These unusual patients present as pediatric patients or young adults.

In our case series, we have encountered an autosomal dominant form of congenital lipodystrophy (characterized by absence of fat from face, upper trunk, arms and below the knees) associated with a progressive neurodegenerative disorder (characterized by progressive spinocerebellar ataxia, pyramidal weakness and spasticity, and autonomic insufficiency) and congenital cataracts. In this small pedigree, affected individuals also have insulin resistance and dyslipidemia and both the neurodegenerative disorder and dyslipidemia are more severe in affected female members [69].

ACQUIRED SYNDROMES OF LIPOATROPHY

Syndromes of acquired generalized lipoatrophy are hard to categorize due to the apparent heterogeneity of case reports. As it is clear from the genetic syndromes, certain genetic defects do not manifest an abnormality until a certain point in life. Hence some genetic syndromes can present as so-called "acquired" syndromes. Especially, in the case of recessive disorders, the proband may be the only affected patient and it may be difficult to tease out a genetic pattern of inheritence. Though there are two epinyms used in the literature to describe acquired generalized and acquired partial lipodystrophy syndromes, we will use the descriptive names rather than the epinyms for these syndromes until a better molecular tools enable us to categorize these syndromes precisely.

Acquired Generalized Lipoatrophy

Lawrence described acquired generalized lipoatrophy with the onset of the disease during childhood [70]. His original report remains an excellent description of generalized lipoatrophy. Fat loss is usually a remarkable event leading to a dramatic change in physical features (Figure 5). The median time to develop diabetes after loss of fat tissue is about 4 years. Both basal metabolic rate and hepatic glucose output are increased. While it is known that these patients lack fully differentiated adipocytes, it is not clear whether they also lack adipocyte precursors [71]. Patients with this type of lipodystrophy may have very severe fat loss, including retroorbital fat and supportive fat in their hands, feet and genital area. Bone marrow fat is lost in some cases, while preserved in others.

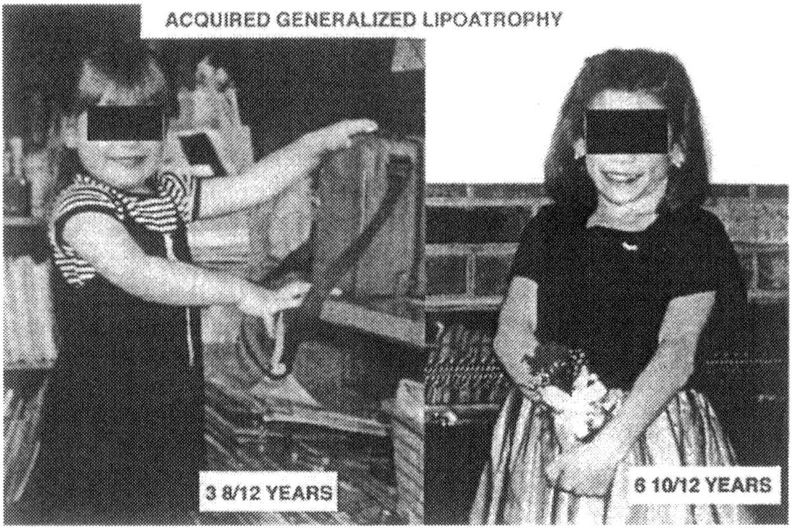

Figure 5. Acquired generalized lipoatrophy is in the differential diagnosis of congenital generalized lipoatrophy. The patient had completely normal fat distribution at age 3 8/12 years old (left) and acutely lost her body fat with a febrile illness at age around age 6 (shown on the right).

Acquired Partial Lipodystrophy

The case reports that refer to Barraquer-Simons syndrome describe a wide-range of variation with few shared features. Patients usually are women in their second or third decades, who also have a well described autoimmune disorder such as scleroderma or glomerulonephritis, presenting with partial fat loss [13], [72, 73]. Fat loss usually starts from the face and descends downward until the gluteal line. There is usually increased adiposity in unaffected fat depots (lower extremities). The prevalence of diabetes and hypertriglyceridemia is about 50% in these cases and seems to coseggragate with lower total body fat in our series.

Other Associated Conditions

Some cases of acquired lipodystrophy occur in the presence of a population of circulating autoantibodies or an association with another autoimmune disease (e.g juvenile dermatomyositis) and therefore are thought to be autoimmune in nature. There is a clear association of lipodystrophy with juvenile dermatomyositis [74-77]. These patients typically present before teen-age years. The fat loss can be both generalized or partial. There is usually increased visceral fat despite very severe preipheral fat loss and a specific asymmetric pattern of fat loss on extremities (figure 6).

Panniculitis, a chronic (as defined by lasting 3 months or longer), generalized inflammation of the subcutaneous tissue, has been observed either clinically or proven by biopsy to proceed the loss of fat in some cases of lipodystrophy[78]. The evidence for long-sought specific anti-fat cell autoantibodies or specific activated T-cell clones is still weak. A portion of

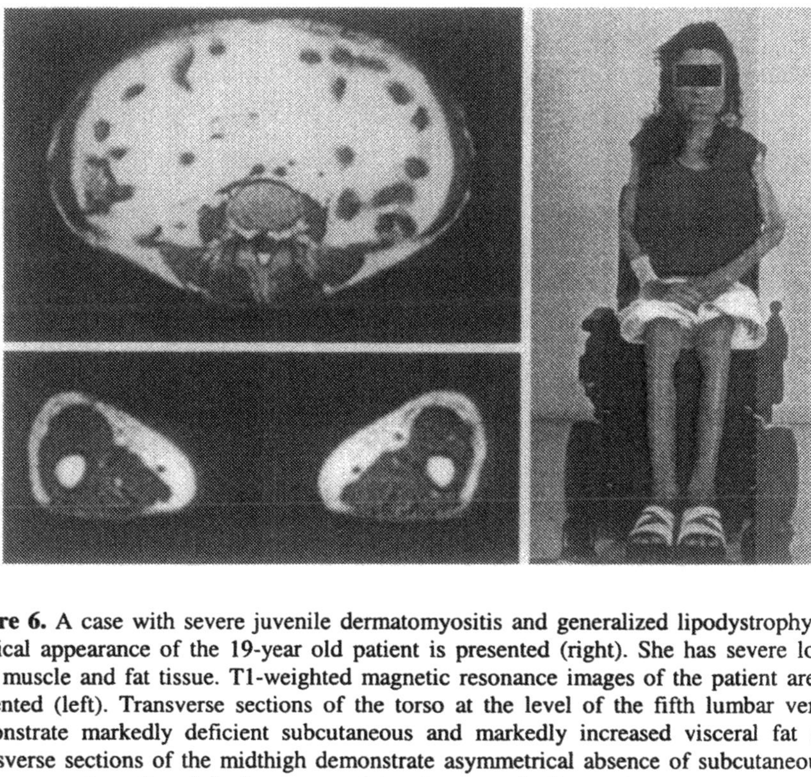

Figure 6. A case with severe juvenile dermatomyositis and generalized lipodystrophy. The physical appearance of the 19-year old patient is presented (right). She has severe loss of both muscle and fat tissue. T1-weighted magnetic resonance images of the patient are also presented (left). Transverse sections of the torso at the level of the fifth lumbar vertebra demonstrate markedly deficient subcutaneous and markedly increased visceral fat (top). Transverse sections of the midthigh demonstrate asymmetrical absence of subcutaneous fat with preservation of medial subcutaneous fat and marrow fat (bottom).

acquired lipodystrophy patients are demonstrated to have low C3 levels [79] and it was speculated that adipsin, a factor produced by fat cells was responsible for the loss of fat due to alternative activation of complement pathway. Generalized or partial fat loss has been described in association with familial [80] or acquired hypocomplementemia [81-83].

CLINICAL ABNORMALITIES OBSERVED IN LIPOATROPHY/ LIPODYSTROPHY SYNDROMES: A RECAPITULATION OF SHARED FEATURES

Table 2: Characteristics of Patients with Generalized and Partial Lipoatrophy

	Generalized	Partial	
General characteristics			
M/F(n)	2/8	4/23	
Age range (years)	6-19	26-65	
Genetic/other	4/6	10/17	
Clinical characteristics			
Diabetes/IGT[1]/IR[2]	9/1/0	15/5/3	
Acanthosis Nigricans (%)	70%	56%	
Hyperandrogenism (%)	50%	50%	
Central Hypogonadism	50%	0%	
NASH[3](%)	70%	33%	
Laboratory Characteristics			**Normal Range**
HbA1c (%)	9.9±3.5	7.2±0.8	<6.2
Triglycerides (mg/dl)[4]	2015±1463	426±164	35-155
Free fatty acids (μmol/L)	926±156	693±115	50-550
HDL-cholesterol[5]	21.4±10.3	22.7±11.9	35-85
Leptin[6] (ng/ml)	1.8±1.0	10.5±6.3	Variable
Body fat by DEXA (%)	7.7±2.6	23.8±2.5	Variable

[1] Impaired glucose tolerance
[2] Insulin resistance
[3] Non-alcoholic steatohepatitis
[4] Conversion factor to mmol/L: 0.01129X
[5] Conversion factor to mmol/L: 0.02586X
[6] Conversion factor to nmol/L: 0.08X

Some patients infected with HIV while being aggressively treated with protease inhibitors, develop a partial lipoatrophy. The characteristic loss of subcutaneous fat occurs in the face, extremities and trunk. In contrast, visceral fat increases and a "buffalo hump" like that is seen in Cushing syndrome develops [84-86]. The lipodystrophy is accompanied by the development of insulin resistance and hypertriglyceridemia. The changes in body composition and metabolic parameters are usually apparent within 3 to 6 months of therapy. There is a quicker onset of this partial lipoatrophy when more than one protease inhibitor is used. The syndrome is recognized in both sexes and in pediatric as well as adult patients. Why do treated HIV patients develop this characteristic phenotype? One hypothesis is that an aspartyl protease (like the HIV protease) may be important in the differentiation of adipocytes. In support of this hypothesis, several groups reported that protease inhibitors blocked preadipocyte differentiation in vitro [87, 88]. Interestingly, some groups have reported the development of a similar phenotype when HIV-infected patients are treated aggressively with other antiretroviral agents other than protease inhibitors (including nucleoside analogues) [89-91]. This suggests that the lipodystophy may be related to aggressively treated HIV infection rather than to a specific therapy [89, 92]. Further investigations are underway to better categorize the fat tissue changes and metabolic consequences during HIV therapy. While the HIV related lipodsytrophy is the most prevalent form of lipodystrophy, the details of this unique syndrome is not in the scope of this chapter.

Different syndromes of lipodystrophy have a heterogeneous clinical presentation; however, findings of insulin-resistance and hypertriglyceridemia are seen in all forms of lipoatrophy. A greater loss of adipose tissue is associated with an increased severity of the metabolic abnormalities (Table 2). The insulin resistance leads to hyperinsulinemia, and the associated clinical features of acanthosis nigricans and hyperandrogenism in female patients are commonly observed.

The reproductive abnormalities are more complicated than simple hyperandrogenism and polycsytic ovaries in the patients with more severe forms of lipoatrophy. About 50 % of all the patients with generalized lipoatrophy and the majority of the female patients (85%) present with very low LH levels, more consistent with hypogonadotropic hypogonadism (Table 2). This creates a paradox with the findings on ovarian imaging studies since these usually reveal enlarged, polycystic ovaries. Hence, it appears that severe hyperinsulinemia in the most severe cases of lipoatrophy is sufficient to drive the ovarian enlargement and associated hyperandrogenism without any apparent stimulation from the pituitary[93].

Patients with early-onset hyperinsulinemia (as in congenital generalized lipoatrophy) develop acromegaloid features with soft tissue hyperplasia, somatomegaly and bony abnormalities[94]. Cardiomyopathy is also described in some of these cases[95, 96].

Another notable finding in the most severely fat deficient patients is their food-seeking behavior. They may consume large amounts of food (similar to patients with bulimia) and get the urge to eat frequently. This behavior is associated with low levels of circulating leptin which may contribute to the increased appetite [26].

Diabetes will develop in the setting of long-standing hyperinsulinemia due to beta-cell failure. Diabetic retinopathy, nephropathy, neuropathy, gastroparesis as well as coronary heart disease are seen in these patients with uncontrolled and longstanding hyperglycemia.

There is a high incidence of proteinuria leading to chronic renal failure among patients with lipoatrophy syndromes. While diabetic nephropathy seem to play a role in some of these patients, it does not account for all the cases[97]. The patients with hypocomplementemia develop membranous glomerulonephritis[98]. Focal segmental glomerulosclerosis and tubular lipidosis are also among various kidney pathology that have been described in association with lipoatrophy[99].

Patients with lipoatrophy have a dyslipidemia that is primarily characterized by elevated triglycerides. This is thought to be secondary to decreased storage site for triglycerides. There is also strong evidence from animal models that lipid synthesis is paradoxically increased in the liver possibly due to decreased signal coming from the adipocyte that "sufficient " lipid storage is achieved. Leptin may be this crucial signal since this abnormality gets corrected in one animal model of lipoatrophy upon leptin replacement [100].

Most patients have a low HDL and some may have a high LDL. Particularly, the patients with one type of partial lipodystrophy, namely familial partial lipodysrophy of the Dunnigan type have elevated LDL and a markedly increased risk of coronary artery disease [101].

It is thought that due to a relative paucity of adipose tissue, there is excessive accumulation of triglycerides in multiple locations, most notably in muscle and the liver. Increased deposition of fatty acids and triglycerides in the muscle or in the beta-cell may be responsible for causing insulin resistance (lipotoxicity) [102-104]. It is possible that the accumulation of triglycerides in hepatocytes somehow causes the injury associated with non-alcoholic steatohepatitis (NASH) [105]. In patients will all types of lipoatrophy there is an increased incidence of non-alcoholic steatohepatitis (NASH) compared to both the diabetic and general population. This condition is seen in about a third of patients with lipoatrophy and may progress into end-stage liver failure.

We have previously observed that the respiratory quotient (RQ) is elevated in patients with lipoatrophy / lipodystrophy[106]. The RQ is the ratio of carbon dioxide production to oxygen consumption and reflects the relative contributions of carbohydrates and fat in providing fuel for metabolism. The elevated RQ suggests that there is an increase in fuel consumption relative to synthesis. Therefore, either the rate of fatty acid oxidation is decreased or the rate of lipogenesis is increased. Either change might contribute to the observed elevation in the levels of free fatty acids and triglycerides [107]. Furthermore, because fatty acids are known to antagonize insulin's effects upon glucose metabolism, this provides a potential mechanism to account for the state of insulin resistance [108].

TREATMENT OF LIPOATROPHY/LIPODYSTROPHY

The clinical problems requiring treatment in lipoatrophy syndromes are diabetes, hypertriglyceridemia and cosmetic problems. The cosmetic problems are quite severe especially for the female patients and can be emotionally scarring. It is important not to underestimate the cosmetic issues while taking care of the metabolic problems. In patients with lower body fat abundance and upper body fat loss, local fat implantation taken from the area of excess and implanted to the face have produced satisfying results. Facial silicon implants in a few patients with HIV-lipodystrophy have also produced successful cosmetic recovery. It is important to understand patients' expectations and wishes and referral to a plastic surgery center with academic interest in the syndromes may be valuable.

Treatment of diabetes in lipoatrophy

Although there are several classes of anti-diabetic drugs marketed in the U. S, it is difficult to achieve good glycemic control (glycated hemoglobin < 7.2%) in most of the patients with lipoatrophic diabetes. There are five groups of pharmaceuticals available to treat diabetic patients [109] all of which may be used to treat lipoatrophic patients: insulin secretagogues, biguanides (metformin), thiazoladienediones (pioglitazone, rosiglitazone), intestinal enzyme inhibitors (acarbose), and insulin itself.

Insulin. Because of their severe insulin resistance, it is frequently necessary to administer extremely high doses (e.g., in excess of 1000 units per day) in patients with various syndromes of lipoatrophy [110]. The volume of injections is more difficult to tolerate in younger patients. Nevertheless, insulin remains the only approved medication for treatment of children with diabetes.

Insulin secretagogues. The principal mechanism of action for this class of drugs is to promote insulin secretion by beta cells [111]. Because patients with isolated insulin resistance may not have an independent defect in insulin secretion, sulfonylureas are frequently ineffective in patients with lipoatrophic diabetes.

Metformin. This drug works primarily through inhibiting hepatic glucose output. We (and others) have observed that it may help to decrease insulin requirements in some patients with lipoatrophy/ lipodystrophy. To our knowledge, there are no systematic trials looking at the efficacy of this drug in lipoatrophy/lipodystrophy. While the pediatric experience with metformin is growing, it is still not approved by the U.S Food and Drug Administration to be used in children. Therefore, it needs to be administered by clinicians who have prior experience with treatment with this drug, ideally in centers specialized in treating children with unusual forms of diabetes.

Acarbose. This drug interferes with GI absorption of many carbohydrates [112]. While we are not aware of systematic studies of the efficacy of this drug in patients with lipoatrophy, it has relatively limited efficacy to decrease glucose levels in type 2 diabetes mellitus.

Thiazolidinediones. This class is the newest addition to oral hypoglycemic agents. Members of this class are agonists of peroxisome-proliferator activated receptor-gamma (PPAR-gamma); thereby, stimulating adipocyte differentiation [113]. In vivo, this class of drugs functions as insulin-sensitizers and increase insulin-stimulated glucose uptake by the muscle [114, 115]. Troglitazone was the first member to be approved by the US Food and Drug Administration. These effects of thiazolidinedione compounds seemed ideally suited to treat the problems encountered in lipoatrophy/lipodystrophy syndromes. In addition, troglitazone exerted favorable effects in an animal model of lipoatrophy [116]. We thus undertook a treatment trial in these patients with troglitazone[106]. The primary end-points were metabolic control and adipose tissue mass. Six months of troglitazone therapy led to significant improvement in metabolic control with a reduction in HbA1c, triglycerides, and free fatty acids[106]. In addition, there was a small, but statistically significant increase in body fat[106]. Interestingly, the increase was predominantly in the subcutaneous compartment. Furthermore, body weight did not change significantly and there was a decrease in liver size[106].

Despite the favorable effects of troglitazone, the FDA withdrew troglitazone from the US market in March 2000 due to concerns over hepatotoxicity. The newer members of the class, rosiglitazone and pioglitazone, remain in clinical use. The preclinical studies with these two medications suggested that they did not have the same risk of hepatotoxicity.. Since the use of thiazolidinediones requires judicious monitoring for side-effects, their use should be supervised by clinicians who are experienced in administering these medications after careful assessment of risk: benefit ratio.

Treatment of dyslipidemia in lipoatrophy

The dyslipidemia of severe lipoatrophy is difficult to treat with the currently available therapeutic interventions which still results in significant morbidity and mortality from this condition. Patients with triglyceride levels over 1000 mg/dl are at risk of developing acute pancreatitis. Recurrent episodes lead to pancreatic insufficiency. Chronically elevated triglycerides in the setting of hyperinsulinemia and low HDL increase the predisposition for coronary artery disease. Severely elevated triglycerides may lead to eruptive painful cutaneous xanthomata[117].

Troglitazone was remarkable in its ability to improve hypertriglyceridemia in addition to improving glycemia. As niacin is known to worsen glycemic control, we prefer to use fibrates and statins in these severely insulin resistant lipoatrophic patients. Both fibrates and statins may need to be used in combination with careful monitoring for side-effects. Again, the pediatric experience with these medications is extremely limited.

Limitation of caloric intake may be useful for short-term results, but is not possible to implement for long-term management as dietary fat is required for proper growth and development. Medium chain triglycerides and fish oil have not been tested in a systematic fashion, but may prove to be useful. We have attempted to use intestinal lipase inhibitors in a few of the most severely affected pediatric patients with some positive results. Finally, we have employed long-term plasmapheresis in one patient with extreme hypertriglyceridemia with moderate clinical success[117].

Leptin: from the laboratory to clinical trials

As mentioned earlier, the metabolic abnormalities of diabetes and hypertriglyceridemia in lipoatrophy may be caused by the absence of hormones produced by fat cells. Shimomura et al administered one such hormone, leptin, to lipoatrophic mice. Prior to therapy, these mice exhibited

Table 3: Efficacy of leptin in the treatment of lipodystrophy (n=9)

Parameter	Baseline	4-months of therapy	P-value
HbA1c (%)	9.1	7.2	<0.001

Triglycerides (mg/dL)	1405	348	<0.001
Free fatty acids (mcmole/L)	1540	790	<0.05
K-constant @ Insulin Tolerance Test	0.0071	0.0169	<0.04
Liver volume (cc.s)	3097	1998	<0.002

diabetes, hypertriglyceridemia, hepatic steatosis and severe leptin deficiency. Interestingly, 3 weeks of leptin therapy ameliorated all the metabolic abnormalities and also decreased the degree of steatosis in the liver [118]. These results from animal models warranted a clinical trial.

In the published portion of the trial[26], 9 female patients with various forms of lipodystrophy (4 with congenital generalized, 3 with acquired generalized and 1 with Dunnigan's familial partial lipodystrophy) were treated with 4 months of subcutaneous leptin administered to achieve physiological concentrations of leptin. Leptin levels increased from a mean of <2 ng/mL to a mean of 12 ng/mL, indicating that that the goal of leptin replacement was largely achieved. There was a remarkable decrease in both hyperglycemia and hypertriglyceridemia as well as improved total body insulin sensitivity and decreased liver volumes (Table 3). In addition, the reproductive abnormalities were studied in 7 of these patients. Leptin therapy corrected the amenorrhea seen in 4 of the 5 patients with intact reproductive systems and normalized the attenuated LH response to LHRH stimulation[93]. This leptin-replacement study is likely to inspire similar studies using replacement of adipocyte-specific hormones to treat metabolic abnormalities thus marking the era of the adipocyte as an endocrine organ, playing a conductor role in glucose and lipid metabolism.

REFERENCES

1. Foster DW. The lipodystrophies and other rare disorders of the adipose tissue. In: (*Fauci A.S. et. al* eds). Harrison's Principals of Internal Medicine. New York: McGraw-Hill:2209-2214, 1998.
2. Yura S, Ogawa Y, Sagawa N, et al. Accelerated puberty and late-onset hypothalamic hypogonadism in female transgenic skinny mice overexpressing leptin. J Clin Invest 2000; 105:749-55.

3. Aizawa-Abe M, Ogawa Y, Masuzaki H, et al. Pathophysiological role of leptin in obesity-related hypertension. J Clin Invest 2000; 105:1243-1252.
4. Waller EG, Wade AJ, Treasure J, Ward A, Leonard T, Powell-Tuck J. Physical measures of recovery from anorexia nervosa during hospitalised re-feeding. Eur J Clin Nutr 1996; 50:165-70.
5. Horska A. Use of magnetic resonance in body composition studies: applications to research on caloric restriction and exercise. Coll Antropol 1998; 22:385-92.
6. Tansey JT, Sztalryd C, Gruia-Gray J, et al. Perilipin ablation results in a lean mouse with aberrant adipocyte lipolysis, enhanced leptin production, and resistance to diet-induced obesity. Proc Natl Acad Sci U S A 2001; 98:6494-9.
7. Peterfy M, Phan J, Xu P, Reue K. Lipodystrophy in the fld mouse results from mutation of a new gene encoding a nuclear protein, lipin. Nat Genet 2001; 27:121-4.
8. Reitman ML, Arioglu E, Gavrilova O, Taylor SI. Lipoatrophy revisited. Trends Endocrinol Metab 2000; 11:410-6.
9. Gavrilova O, Marcus-Samuels B, Graham D, et al. Surgical implantation of adipose tissue reverses diabetes in lipoatrophic mice. J Clin Invest 2000; 105:271-8.
10. Fruebis J, Tsao TS, Javorschi S, et al. Proteolytic cleavage product of 30-kDa adipocyte complement-related protein increases fatty acid oxidation in muscle and causes weight loss in mice. Proc Natl Acad Sci U S A 2001; 98:2005-10.
11. Hu E, Liang P, Spiegelman BM. AdipoQ is a novel adipose-specific gene dysregulated in obesity. J Biol Chem 1996; 271:10697-703.
12. Matsuzawa Y, Funahashi T, Nakamura T. Molecular mechanism of metabolic syndrome X: contribution of adipocytokines adipocyte-derived bioactive substances. Ann N Y Acad Sci 1999; 892:146-54.
13. Taylor SI, Arioglu E. Syndromes associated with insulin resistance and acanthosis nigricans . J Basic Clin Physiol Pharmacol 1998; 9:419-39.
14. Kayikcioglu A, Akyurek M, Erk Y. Semicircular lipoatrophy after intragluteal injection of benzathine penicillin. J Pediatr 1996; 129:166-7.
15. Reeves WG, Allen BR, Tattersall RB. Insulin-induced lipoatrophy: evidence for an immune pathogenesis. Br Med J 1980; 280:1500-3.
16. Murao S, Hirata K, Ishida T, Takahara J. Lipoatrophy induced by recombinant human insulin injection. Intern Med 1998; 37:1031-3.

17. Buyukgebiz A, Aydin A, Dundar B, Yorukoglu K. Localized lipoatrophy due to recombinant growth hormone therapy in a child with 6.7 kilobase gene deletion isolated growth hormone deficiency. J Pediatr Endocrinol Metab 1999; 12:95-7.
18. Rees TD. Facial atrophy. Clin Plast Surg 1976; 3:637-46.
19. Hodak E, David M, Sandbank M. Semicircular lipoatrophy--a pressure-induced lipoatrophy? Clin Exp Dermatol 1990; 15:464-5.
20. Rongioletti F, Rebora A. Annular and semicircular lipoatrophies. Report of three cases and review of the literature. J Am Acad Dermatol 1989; 20:433-6.
21. Berardinelli W. An undiagnosed endocrinometabolic syndrome: report of two cases. Journal of Clinical Endocrinology 1954; 14:193-204.
22. Seip M, Trygstad O. Generalized lipodystrophy, congenital and acquired (lipoatrophy). Acta Paediatr Suppl 1996; 413:2-28.
23. Copeland KC, Nair KS, Kaplowitz PB, Robbins DC, Calles-Escandon J. Discordant metabolic actions of insulin in extreme lipodystrophy of childhood. J Clin Endocrinol Metab 1993; 77:1240-5.
24. Jaquet D, Khallouf E, Levy-Marchal C, Czernichow P. Extremely low values of serum leptin in children with congenital generalized lipoatrophy. Eur J Endocrinol 1999; 140:107-9.
25. Pardini VC, Victoria IM, Rocha SM, et al. Leptin levels, beta-cell function, and insulin sensitivity in families with congenital and acquired generalized lipoatrophic diabetes. J Clin Endocrinol Metab 1998; 83:503-8.
26. Oral EA, Simha V, Ruiz E, et al. Leptin-replacement therapy for lipodystrophy. N Engl J Med 2002; 346:570-8.
27. Foss I, Trygstad O. Lipoatrophy produced in mice and rabbits by a fraction prepared from the urine from patients with congenital generalized lipodystrophy. Acta Endocrinol (Copenh) 1975; 80:398-416.
28. Vigouroux C, Khallouf E, Bourut C, et al. Genetic exclusion of 14 candidate genes in lipoatropic diabetes using linkage analysis in 10 consanguineous families. J Clin Endocrinol Metab 1997; 82:3438-44.
29. Vigouroux C, Fajas L, Khallouf E, et al. Human peroxisome proliferator-activated receptor-gamma2: genetic mapping, identification of a variant in the coding sequence, and exclusion as the gene responsible for lipoatrophic diabetes. Diabetes 1998; 47:490-2.

30. Silver K, Walston J, Plotnick L, Taylor SI, Kahn CR, Shuldiner AR. Molecular scanning of beta-3-adrenergic receptor gene in total congenital lipoatrophic diabetes mellitus. J Clin Endocrinol Metab 1997; 82:3395-8.
31. Garg A, Wilson R, Barnes R, et al. A gene for congenital generalized lipodystrophy maps to human chromosome 9q34. J Clin Endocrinol Metab 1999; 84:3390-4.
32. Magre J, Delepine M, Khallouf E, et al. Identification of the gene altered in Berardinelli-Seip congenital lipodystrophy on chromosome 11q13. Nat Genet 2001; 28:365-70.
33. Dunnigan MG, Cochrane MA, Kelly A, Scott JW. Familial lipoatrophic diabetes with dominant transmission. A new syndrome. Q J Med 1974; 43:33-48.
34. Kobberling J, Willms B, Kattermann R, Creutzfeldt W. Lipodystrophy of the extremities. A dominantly inherited syndrome associated with lipotrophic diabetes. Humangenetik 1975; 29:111-20.
35. Wildermuth S, Spranger S, Spranger M, Raue F, Meinck HM. Kobberling-Dunnigan syndrome: a rare cause of generalized muscular hypertrophy. Muscle Nerve 1996; 19:843-7.
36. Garg A, Peshock RM, Fleckenstein JL. Adipose tissue distribution pattern in patients with familial partial lipodystrophy (Dunnigan variety). J Clin Endocrinol Metab 1999; 84:170-4.
37. Garg A. Gender differences in the prevalence of metabolic complications in familial partial lipodystrophy (Dunnigan variety). J Clin Endocrinol Metab 2000; 85:1776-1782.
38. Cao H, Hegele RA. Nuclear lamin A/C R482Q mutation in Canadian kindreds with Dunnigan- type familial partial lipodystrophy. Hum Mol Genet 2000; 9:109-12.
39. Shackleton S, Lloyd DJ, Jackson SN, et al. LMNA, encoding lamin A/C, is mutated in partial lipodystrophy . Nat Genet 2000; 24:153-6.
40. Speckman RA, Garg A, Du F, et al. Mutational and Haplotype Analyses of Families with Familial Partial Lipodystrophy (Dunnigan Variety) Reveal Recurrent Missense Mutations in the Globular C-Terminal Domain of Lamin A/C. Am J Hum Genet 2000; 66:1192-1198.
41. Peters JM, Barnes R, Bennett L, Gitomer WM, Bowcock AM, Garg A. Localization of the gene for familial partial lipodystrophy (Dunnigan variety) to chromosome 1q21-22. Nat Genet 1998; 18:292-5.

42. Jackson SN, Pinkney J, Bargiotta A, et al. A defect in the regional deposition of adipose tissue (partial lipodystrophy) is encoded by a gene at chromosome 1q. Am J Hum Genet 1998; 63:534-40.
43. Wilson KL. The nuclear envelope, muscular dystrophy and gene expression. Trends Cell Biol 2000; 10:125-9.
44. Heald R, McKeon F. Mutations of phosphorylation sites in lamin A that prevent nuclear lamina disassembly in mitosis. Cell 1990; 61:579-89.
45. Clements L, Manilal S, Love DR, Morris GE. Direct interaction between emerin and lamin A. Biochem Biophys Res Commun 2000; 267:709-14.
46. Bonne G, Di Barletta MR, Varnous S, et al. Mutations in the gene encoding lamin A/C cause autosomal dominant Emery-Dreifuss muscular dystrophy. Nat Genet 1999; 21:285-8.
47. Raffaele Di Barletta M, Ricci E, Galluzzi G, et al. Different Mutations in the LMNA Gene Cause Autosomal Dominant and Autosomal Recessive Emery-Dreifuss Muscular Dystrophy. Am J Hum Genet 2000; 66:1407-1412.
48. Kitaguchi T, Matsubara S, Sato M, et al. A missense mutation in the exon 8 of lamin A/C gene in a Japanese case of autosomal dominant limb-girdle muscular dystrophy and cardiac conduction block. Neuromuscul Disord 2001; 11:542-6.
49. Brodsky GL, Muntoni F, Miocic S, Sinagra G, Sewry C, Mestroni L. Lamin A/C gene mutation associated with dilated cardiomyopathy with variable skeletal muscle involvement. Circulation 2000; 101:473-6.
50. Morris GE, Manilal S. Heart to heart: from nuclear proteins to emery-dreifuss muscular dystrophy . Hum Mol Genet 1999; 8:1847-51.
51. De Sandre-Giovannoli A, Chaouch M, Kozlov S, et al. Homozygous Defects in LMNA, Encoding Lamin A/C Nuclear-Envelope Proteins, Cause Autosomal Recessive Axonal Neuropathy in Human (Charcot- Marie-Tooth Disorder Type 2) and Mouse. Am J Hum Genet 2002; 70:726-36.
52. Lelliott CJ, Logie L, Sewter CP, et al. Lamin expression in human adipose cells in relation to anatomical site and differentiation state. J Clin Endocrinol Metab 2002; 87:728-34.
53. Holt I, Clements L, Manilal S, Brown SC, Morris GE. The R482Q lamin A/C mutation that causes lipodystrophy does not prevent nuclear targeting of lamin A in adipocytes or its interaction with emerin. Eur J Hum Genet 2001; 9:204-8.

54. Barroso I, Gurnell M, Crowley VE, et al. Dominant negative mutations in human PPARgamma associated with severe insulin resistance, diabetes mellitus and hypertension. Nature 1999; 402:880-3.
55. Agarwal AK, Garg A. A novel heterozygous mutation in peroxisome proliferator-activated receptor-gamma gene in a patient with familial partial lipodystrophy. J Clin Endocrinol Metab 2002; 87:408-11.
56. Yu CE, Oshima J, Wijsman EM, et al. Mutations in the consensus helicase domains of the Werner syndrome gene. Werner's Syndrome Collaborative Group. Am J Hum Genet 1997; 60:330-41.
57. Henning KA, Li L, Iyer N, et al. The Cockayne syndrome group A gene encodes a WD repeat protein that interacts with CSB protein and a subunit of RNA polymerase II TFIIH. Cell 1995; 82:555-64.
58. Cotton RB, Keats TE, McCoy EE. Abnormal blood glucose regulation in Cockayne's syndrome. Pediatrics 1970; 46:54-60.
59. Petersen MB, Brostrom K, Stibler H, Skovby F. Early manifestations of the carbohydrate-deficient glycoprotein syndrome. J Pediatr 1993; 122:66-70.
60. Schwingshandl J, Mache CJ, Rath K, Borkenstein MH. SHORT syndrome and insulin resistance. Am J Med Genet 1993; 47:907-9.
61. Aarskog D, Ose L, Pande H, Eide N. Autosomal dominant partial lipodystrophy associated with Rieger anomaly, short stature, and insulinopenic diabetes. Am J Med Genet 1983; 15:29-38.
62. Freidenberg GR, Cutler DL, Jones MC, et al. Severe insulin resistance and diabetes mellitus in mandibuloacral dysplasia. Am J Dis Child 1992; 146:93-9.
63. Cutler DL, Kaufmann S, Freidenberg GR. Insulin-resistant diabetes mellitus and hypermetabolism in mandibuloacral dysplasia: a newly recognized form of partial lipodystrophy. J Clin Endocrinol Metab 1991; 73:1056-61.
64. Breslau-Siderius EJ, Toonstra J, Baart JA, Koppeschaar HP, Maassen JA, Beemer FA. Ectodermal dysplasia, lipoatrophy, diabetes mellitus, and amastia: a second case of the AREDYLD syndrome. Am J Med Genet 1992; 44:374-7.
65. Simha V, Garg A. Body fat distribution and metabolic derangements in patients with familial partial lipodystrophy associated with mandibuloacral dysplasia. J Clin Endocrinol Metab 2002; 87:776-85.
66. Van Maldergem L, Bachy A, Feldman D, et al. Syndrome of lipoatrophic diabetes, vitamin D resistant rickets, and persistent

Mullerian ducts in a Turkish boy born to consanguineous parents. Am J Med Genet 1996; 64:506-13.
67. Davis TM, Holdright DR, Schulenberg WE, Turner RC, Joplin GF. Retinal pigment epithelial change & partial lipodystrophy.Postgrad Med J 1988; 64:871-4.
68. Spranger S, Spranger M, Tasman AJ, Reith W, Voigtlander T, Voigtlander V. Barraquer-Simons syndrome (with sensorineural deafness): a contribution to the differential diagnosis lipodystrophy syndromes.Am J Med Genet1997;71:397-400.
69. Berger JR, Arioglu Oral E, Taylor SI. Familial lipodystrophy associated with neurodegeneration and congenital cataracts. Neurology 2002; 58:43-7.
70. Lawrence RD. Lipodystrophy and hepatomegaly with diabetes, lipaemia, and other metabolic disturbances: a case throwing new light on the action of insulin. Lancet 1946; I:724-731 and 773-775.
71. Hubler A, Abendroth K, Keiner T, et al. Dysregulation of insulin-like growth factors in a case of generalized acquired lipoatrophic diabetes mellitus (Lawrence Syndrome) connected with autoantibodies against adipocyte membranes. Exp Clin Endocrinol Diabetes 1998; 106:79-84.
72. Perrot H, Delaup JP, Chouvet B. [Barraquer and Simons lipodystrophy. Complement anomalies and cutaneous leukocytoclasic vasculitis]. Ann Dermatol Venereol 1987; 114:1083-91.
73. Biasi D, Caramaschi P, Carletto A, Bambara LM. A case of acquired partial lipodystrophy associated with localized scleroderma and undifferentiated connective tissue disease. Rheumatol Int 1999; 19:75-6.
74. Quecedo E, Febrer I, Serrano G, Martinez-Aparicio A, Aliaga A. Partial lipodystrophy associated with juvenile dermatomyositis: report of two cases. Pediatr Dermatol 1996; 13:477-82.
75. Kavanagh GM, Colaco CB, Kennedy CT. Juvenile dermatomyositis associated with partial lipoatrophy. J Am Acad Dermatol 1993; 28:348-51.
76. Sasaki T, Ono H, Nakajima H, Sugimoto J. Lipoatrophic diabetes. J Dermatol 1992; 19:246-9.
77. Commens C, O'Neill P, Walker G. Dermatomyositis associated with multifocal lipoatrophy. J Am Acad Dermatol 1990; 22:966-9.
78. Peters MS, Winkelmann RK. Localized lipoatrophy (atrophic connective tissue disease panniculitis). Arch Dermatol 1980; 116:1363-8.

79. Sissons JG, West RJ, Fallows J, et al. The complement abnormalities of lipodystrophy. N Engl J Med 1976; 294:461-5.
80. McLean RH, Hoefnagel D. Partial lipodystrophy and familial C3 deficiency. Hum Hered 1980; 30:149-54.
81. Fontaine M, Daveau M, Lebreton JP, Dumouchel L, Vannier JP, Godin M. Evidence that an autoantibody of IgG3 subclass against C3b discloses a C3 Nef activity in a patient with partial lipodystrophy and glomerulonephritis. Ann Immunol (Paris) 1980; 131C:39-53.
82. Jasin HE. Systemic lupus erythematosus, partial lipodystrophy and hypocomplementemia. J Rheumatol 1979; 6:43-50.
83. Wakefield MA. The interrelationship between hypocomplementaemia, partial lipodystrophy and mesangiocapillary glomerulonephritis. Postgrad Med J 1976; 52:651-2.
84. Carr A, Samaras K, Burton S, et al. A syndrome of peripheral lipodystrophy, hyperlipidaemia and insulin resistance in patients receiving HIV protease inhibitors. Aids 1998; 12:F51-8.
85. Yanovski JA, Miller KD, Kino T, et al. Endocrine and metabolic evaluation of human immunodeficiency virus-infected patients with evidence of protease inhibitor-associated lipodystrophy. J Clin Endocrinol Metab 1999; 84:1925-31.
86. Viraben R, Aquilina C. Indinavir-associated lipodystrophy. Aids 1998; 12:F37-9.
87. Wentworth JM, Burris TP, Chatterjee VK. HIV protease inhibitors block human preadipocyte differentiation, but not via the PPARgamma/RXR heterodimer. J Endocrinol 2000; 164:R7-R10.
88. Zhang B, MacNaul K, Szalkowski D, Li Z, Berger J, Moller DE. Inhibition of adipocyte differentiation by HIV protease inhibitors. J Clin Endocrinol Metab 1999; 84:4274-7.
89. Vigouroux C, Gharakhanian S, Salhi Y, et al. Adverse metabolic disorders during highly active antiretroviral treatments (HAART) of HIV disease. Diabetes Metab 1999; 25:383-92.
90. Vigouroux C, Gharakhanian S, Salhi Y, et al. Diabetes, insulin resistance and dyslipidaemia in lipodystrophic HIV-infected patients on highly active antiretroviral therapy (HAART). Diabetes Metab 1999; 25:225-32.
91. Christeff N, Melchior JC, de Truchis P, Perronne C, Nunez EA, Gougeon ML. Lipodystrophy defined by a clinical score in HIV-infected men on highly active antiretroviral therapy: correlation

between dyslipidaemia and steroid hormone alterations. Aids 1999; 13:2251-60.
92. Saint-Marc T, Partisani M, Poizot-Martin I, et al. Fat distribution evaluated by computed tomography and metabolic abnormalities in patients undergoing antiretroviral therapy: preliminary results of the LIPOCO study. Aids 2000; 14:37-49.
93. Oral EA, Ruiz E, Andewelt A, et al. Effect of leptin replacement on pituitary hormone regulation in patients with severe lipodystrophy. J Clin Endocrinol and Metabolism 2002; In Press.
94. Brunzell JD, Shankle SW, Bethune JE. Congenital generalized lipodystrophy accompanied by cystic angiomatosis. Ann Intern Med 1968; 69:501-16.
95. Bjornstad PG, Semb BK, Trygstad O, Seip M. Echocardiographic assessment of cardiac function and morphology in patients with generalised lipodystrophy. Eur J Pediatr 1985; 144:355-9.
96. Rheuban KS, Blizzard RM, Parker MA, Carter T, Wilson T, Gutgesell HP. Hypertrophic cardiomyopathy in total lipodystrophy. J Pediatr 1986; 109:301-2.
97. Eisinger AJ, Shortland JR, Moorhead PJ. Renal disease in partial lipodystrophy. Q J Med 1972; 41:343-54.
98. Meyrier A. The patient with glomerulonephritis and lipodystrophy. Nephrol Dial Transplant 1997; 12:226-7.
99. Casali RE, Resnick J, Goetz F, Simmons RL, Najarian JS, Kjellstrand C. Renal transplantation in a patient with lipoatrophic diabetes. A case report. Transplantation 1978; 26:174-7.
100. Shimomura I, Matsuda M, Hammer RE, Bashmakov Y, Brown MS, Goldstein JL. Decreased IRS-2 and increased SREBP-1c lead to mixed insulin resistance and sensitivity in livers of lipodystrophic and ob/ob mice. Mol Cell 2000; 6:77-86.
101. Hegele RA. Premature atherosclerosis associated with monogenic insulin resistance. Circulation 2001; 103:2225-9.
102. Unger RH. Lipotoxicity in the pathogenesis of obesity-dependent NIDDM. Genetic and clinical implications. Diabetes 1995; 44:863-70.
103. Wang MY, Lee Y, Unger RH. Novel form of lipolysis induced by leptin. J Biol Chem 1999; 274:17541-4.
104. Unger RH, Zhou YT, Orci L. Regulation of fatty acid homeostasis in cells: novel role of leptin. Proc Natl Acad Sci U S A 1999; 96:2327-32.

105. James OF, Day CP. Non-alcoholic steatohepatitis (NASH): a disease of emerging identity and importance. J Hepatol 1998; 29:495-501.
106. Arioglu E, Duncan-Morin J, Sebring N, et al. Efficacy and safety of troglitazone in the treatment of lipodystrophy syndromes. Ann Intern Med 2000; 133:263-74.
107. Jequier E, Felber JP. Indirect calorimetry. Baillieres Clin Endocrinol Metab 1987; 1:911-35.
108. Lillioja S, Bogardus C. Obesity and insulin resistance: lessons learned from the Pima Indians. Diabetes Metab Rev 1988; 4:517-40.
109. Clark CM, Jr. The National Diabetes Education Program: changing the way diabetes is treated [editorial]. Ann Intern Med 1999; 130:324-6.
110. Meyer L, Hadjadj S, Guerci B, Delbachian I, Ziegler O, Drouin P. Lipoatrophic diabetes mellitus treated by continuous subcutaneous insulin infusion. Diabetes Metab 1998; 24:544-6.
111. Nathan DM, Roussell A, Godine JE. Glyburide or insulin for metabolic control in non-insulin-dependent diabetes mellitus. A randomized, double-blind study. Ann Intern Med 1988; 108:334-40.
112. Bressler R, Johnson DG. Pharmacological regulation of blood glucose levels in non-insulin- dependent diabetes mellitus. Arch Intern Med 1997; 157:836-48.
113. Tontonoz P, Hu E, Spiegelman BM. Stimulation of adipogenesis in fibroblasts by PPAR gamma 2, a lipid- activated transcription factor [published erratum appears in Cell 1995 Mar 24;80(6):following 957]. Cell 1994; 79:1147-56.
114. Inzucchi SE, Maggs DG, Spollett GR, et al. Efficacy and metabolic effects of metformin and troglitazone in type II diabetes mellitus [see comments]. N Engl J Med 1998; 338:867-72.
115. Maggs DG, Buchanan TA, Burant CF, et al. Metabolic effects of troglitazone monotherapy in type 2 diabetes mellitus. A randomized, double-blind, placebo-controlled trial. Ann Intern Med 1998; 128:176-85.
116. Burant CF, Sreenan S, Hirano K, et al. Troglitazone action is independent of adipose tissue. J Clin Invest 1997; 100:2900-8.
117. Bolan C, Oral EA, Gorden P, Taylor S, Leitman SF. Intensive, long-term plasma exchange therapy for severe hypertriglyceridemia in acquired generalized lipoatrophy. J Clin Endocrinol Metab 2002; 87:380-4.

118. Shimomura I, Hammer RE, Ikemoto S, Brown MS, Goldstein JL. Leptin reverses insulin resistance and diabetes mellitus in mice with congenital lipodystrophy. Nature 1999; 401:73-6.

119. 2002 Online Mendelian Inheritence in Man. McKusick-Nathans Institute for Genetic Medicine, Johns Hopkins University (Baltimore, MD) and National Center for Biotechnology Information, National Library of Medicine (Bethesda, MD). http://www.ncbi.nlm.nih.gov/OMIM

Chapter 9

NEONATAL DIABETES

Mark A. Sperling, M.D.
Children's Hospital of Pittsburgh, University of Pittsburgh School of Medicine

INTRODUCTION

Neonatal Diabetes Mellitus (NDM) is defined as persistent hyperglycemia occurring in the first months of life, lasting for more than two weeks and requiring insulin for management[1]. It is considered distinct from autoimmune type 1 DM which manifests after the first three to six months of life[2]. Whereas type 1 DM in the first year of life is characterized by markers of autoimmunity such as ICA, GAD_{65}, or IA_2 antibodies, neonatal DM does not share these characteristics. Rather, NDM is increasingly recognized as a genetic disorder with disturbances in the genes regulating islet organogenesis and function, including insulin secretion[3,4]. The tools of molecular biology have permitted remarkable progress in delineating the defects responsible for transient and permanent NDM, providing a rational basis for classification, prognosis and management[3,4]. Moreover, the identified defects in genes during islet organogenesis or insulin secretion are being investigated as potential contributors to diabetes mellitus in later life[3-5]. Thus, although NDM is rare, with an incidence of approximately 1:500,000 births[1], it has been quite instructive for providing insight on the regulation of insulin secretion and action[3,4]. Neonatal diabetes mellitus must be distinguished from the much more common hyperglycemia affecting immature infants under stress (e.g., sepsis or respiratory distress syndrome) and who simultaneously receive intravenous therapy with glucose[6]. Hyperglycemia in these ill prematures reflects immaturity of gluco-regulatory mechanisms, and other hormone-effector systems that resolve in time[6].

GENETIC REGULATION OF PANCREATIC ISLET DEVELOPMENT

During embryonal development, pancreatic islets differentiate from pancreatic ducts under the influence of a number of differentiation, transcriptional, and growth factors as well as hormones and cell adhesion molecules[7-9]. Newer genes specifically expressed in pancreatic β-cells but not fully identified or characterized also are involved. Among the transcriptional factors, the homeodomain protein PDX-1(*Pancreas and*

Duodenum homeoboX), a known regulator of insulin gene transcription, is uniformly expressed in the early pancreatic bud. Null mutation of PDX-1, also known as IDX-1, STF-1, and IPF-1 (*Insulin Promoter Factor*), introduced in the mice result in failure of growth and differentiation of the pancreatic bud (i.e., pancreatic agenesis). A homozygous point deletion in this gene in humans has been described in a person with pancreatic agenesis, suggesting that this gene is critical for human pancreas development[10]. Clinical presentation of this entity, subsequently described, clearly involves absence of both exocrine as well as endocrine pancreatic function with documented absence of pancreatic tissue on abdominal imaging studies[10]. Heterozygosity for PDX-1 mutation is associated with a later onset of DM, as occurs in Maturity-Onset Diabetes of Youth (MODY)[11,12]. Other heterozygous mutations in transcription factors known to be associated with MODY include hepatic nuclear factor-4α, hepatic nuclear factor 1α, hepatic nuclear 1β, and neurogenic differentiation factor 1 (Neuro D1), also known as beta-cell E-box transactivator (BETA 2)[12]. Heterozygous mutation in the glycolytic enzyme glucokinase also causes MODY. Homozygous mutations in glucokinase result in neonatal DM[13]. The regulation of endocrine pancreatic cell differentiation and its genetic control are extensively detailed in recent reviews[7-9, 14-16]. Several gene families involving homeobox genes, differentiation factors, transcription factors, growth factors, or hormones and their signaling proteins act in a temporal specific fashion to coordinate pancreatic endocrine cell development. Although the mouse has been the primary model for these studies, the insights gained have found rapid application to humans[7-9, 14-16].

MATURATION OF INSULIN SECRETION

Regulation of insulin secretion in the fetus and newborn differs from that of the adult. For example, glucose is a relatively weak stimulus for insulin secretion in fetal and immediate neonatal life, whereas amino acids such as arginine evoke brisk insulin secretion. It is not clear whether these differences result from maturational patterns of noninsulin-dependent glucose transport into fetal/neonatal islets by the glucose transporter GLUT-2 or from delay in the maturation of glucokinase, the rate-limiting enzyme for glucose metabolism and hence insulin secretion in fetal/neonatal pancreatic islets[17]. There is some evidence for a maturational delay of the adenyl cyclase-cyclic adenosine monophosphate (cAMP) system in islets as a consequence of delayed maturity of the enzyme adenyl-cyclase or its more rapid destruction by an overactive cAMP phosphodiesterase system[18]. These tentative conclusions were inferred from physiologic manipulation through intramuscular injection of caffeine benzoate, which evoked considerable insulin secretion at a time when intravenous administration of the sulfonylurea, tolbutamide, failed to elicit any significant insulin release in a case of transient DM in the newborn. Such findings were considered to be exaggerations of the normally impaired insulin response to intravenous glucose and tolbutamide usually seen in both full-term and premature infants, suggesting the possibility that some cases of neonatal DM are the result of a quantitative rather than qualitative difference in the regulation of perinatal insulin secretion[18].

INSULIN ACTION

The number or affinity of insulin receptors in the cell membranes of tissues such as liver, peripheral blood leukocytes, and red blood cells is higher in fetal/neonatal preparation than in corresponding adult tissues[19]. Functional linkage of these fetal/neonatal receptors is suggested by their ability to phosphorylate tyrosine kinase with endogenous or exogenous substrate in proportion to the increased number of insulin receptors[20-22]. Moreover, the mitogen-activated protein (MAP) kinase signaling pathway is functional[22]. By contrast, insulin's ability to enhance glycogen synthase activity or whole-body glucose turnover is impaired in fetal tissues compared with corresponding adult tissues until late in gestation. The switch to more adult-like patterns occurs close to term, probably under the influence of glucocorticoid secretion, which increases near term. These distinctions in insulin action suggest that growth-promoting effects of insulin through the tyrosine kinase/MAP kinase pathways are functional earlier in development than insulin's glucose-regulating actions. Indeed, there is convincing evidence from states of fetal insulin excess, fetal insulin deficiency, or genetic defects in insulin receptors that insulin is an important determinant of fetal growth[22]. Thus, most of the entities associated with neonatal DM are characterized by being small for gestational age (SGA) at birth[23-26]. Mutations in insulin receptors responsible for fetal growth retardation syndromes such as leprechaunism or Rabson-Mendenhall syndrome are discussed elsewhere[27].

CLINICAL MANIFESTATIONS AND COURSE

Intrauterine growth retardation, a reflection of deficient insulin secretion *in utero*, is a prominent feature of infants with neonatal DM. In addition to being SGA, these infants have hyperglycemia with glycosuria, osmotic polyuria, and consequent failure to thrive, plus severe dehydration. Keotacidosis, when it occurs, is generally mild. Diagnosis is established by demonstrating hyperglycemia; insulin (and insulin-like growth factor-1) levels, when measured, are low and respond poorly to oral or intravenous glucose. Apart from SGA and dehydration, dysmorphic features are not usually present, although macroglossia has been reported[23-26]; epiphyseal dysplasia plus renal impairment and DM are the hallmarks of the Wolcott-Rallison syndrome (see below).

Therapy with insulin administered subcutaneously twice daily at a dose of 0.5 to 1.0 U/kg/day corrects hyperglycemia and results in dramatic catch-up growth. In some infants, insulin treatment can be withdrawn after several weeks to months when it is observed that the exogenous insulin induces hypoglycemia and omission of insulin is not associated hyperglycemia. Such cases constitute typical transient neonatal DM. However, hyperglycemia and insulin dependency has been reported to persist for up to 5 years with subsequent resolution[1]. Thus, the course of neonatal DM is highly variable[1, 23-26]. Onset in most is in the first month of life, but in approximately 15% to 20% of reported cases, onset was between 1 and 3 months of life[1]. Approximately one third of patients with neonatal DM have transient disease that resolves after several months, with no further recurrence even after many years of follow-up. Anti-insulin or anti-islet cell antibodies are not found. Approximately one fourth of affected infants have transient neonatal DM followed by recurrence from 7 to 20 years later[1]. The remainder, almost one half of the patients with neonatal DM, have permanent DM with no remission[1]. A genetic basis for some of these cases was suggested by the occurrence of neonatal DM in twins and several pairs of triplets or siblings, not including cases of pancreatic agenesis or Wolcott-Rallison syndrome. A long-term survivor has become a parent of a boy with transient DM[1]. These variable patterns for neonatal DM suggest differing underlying mechanisms, some of which are described below. Although the presence of human leukocyte antigen haplotypes commonly associated with type 1 DM has been reported in cases of neonatal DM, they are not necessarily indicative of type 1 DM due to autoimmune mechanism. In view of the variable course of neonatal DM, and its recurrence in siblings, prognostic counseling to parents should be guarded[1].

GENETIC ENTITIES

Transient Neonatal Diabetes

About one half of the cases of NDM constitute the transient form for which the majority map to a locus on 6q24[3,4]. As mentioned, some of these transient neonatal forms ameliorate, only to recur in later life, with characteristics of type 2 DM[3,4]. At birth, these infants are small, reflecting the important role of insulin for intrauterine growth and suggesting that insulin secretion is impaired *in utero*. A few have macroglossia. Markers of autoimmunity are absent.

Clues to the genetic basis of this entity were obtained from two clinical observations. First, in several familial with an apparent autosomal pattern, the transmission was always from the father, himself affected[4]. Second, an unaffected father sired three affected infants by three different wives[28]. The serendipitous discovery of NDM in an infant with an inborn error of metabolism due to a homozygous mutation of a gene on 6p21 led to the discovery that the mother was entirely normal, whereas the father was heterozygous[29]. Hence, uniparental disomy (UPD) was suspected, and confirmed by demonstrating only paternal alleles in a stretch of bases around the mutation. Uniparental disomy, in each case of paternal origin, was then confirmed in several sporadic cases of NDM, suggesting that the paternal familial cases must have arisen from a gain of function mutation when the paternal gene was duplicated and transmitted by the father[30,31]. Eventually, the gene was localized to 6q24, a region in which the ZAC gene (*Zinc-finger protein regulating Apoptosis and Cell cycle*) was located[32-35]. This zinc-finger transcription factor regulates a protein involved in insulin secretion. The expression of the ZAC gene was found to be imprinted and exclusively paternal. Imprinting in this case is rendered by methylation of the maternal copy thereby explaining how paternal duplications cause disease. There have now been cases of TNDM described in which uniparental disomy or duplication are absent but in which there is under methylation of the maternal copy, in effect resulting in expression of two activated genes[35]. It remains to be explained how this genetic imprint impairs insulin secretion leading to neonatal diabetes mellitus, why it is transient allowing recovery in certain instances, and why it may recur in later life with a type 2 diabetes mellitus phenotype.

PERMANENT NEONATAL DIABETES

MODY Syndrome Genes

In the largest series of neonatal diabetes reported in recent years, about half the affected infants had permanent neonatal diabetes[1]. As in the transient form, genetic defects are increasingly recognized as responsible for these permanent forms. Two of these involved genes now known to be responsible in the heterozygous state for two distinct Maturity-Onset of Diabetes in Youth (MODY) syndromes.

MODY 4 is known to be due to a heterozygous mutation in the gene encoding the insulin-promoter factor 1 (*IPF1*) also called *PDX1* (***P**ancreas and **D**uodenum Homeobo**x***) located on 13q12.1[12]. *IPF1* is a pancreas-specific transcription factor which regulates the development of both endocrine and exocrine cells and its expression persists in mature beta and delta cells for the respective regulation of insulin and somatostatin gene transcription[7-9]. Knowledge of these effects led to the discovery of a homozygous inactivating mutation in this gene in a child with both neonatal diabetes and exocrine pancreatic insufficiency in the first days of life; ultrasonography suggested absence of a pancreas[10]. As anticipated, carriers on both the paternal and maternal families had MODY. Only a handful of these cases have been described indicating their rarity as a cause of NDM. However, it has been suggested that other missense mutations in *IPF1* may be involved in type 2 diabetes in adults[3,11].

The glucokinase gene (GCK) on 7p15-p13 is expressed in hepatocytes and pancreatic beta cells where it phosphorylates glucose, a rate-limiting step which has resulted in this enzyme being termed the "glucose sensor" of the beta cell. Heterozygous mutation in this enzyme is responsible for MODY2, one of the two most common types of MODY syndromes[3]. As might be predicted, homozygosity for similar GCK mutations should result in more severe diabetes and this has been described as the cause of permanent neonatal-onset diabetes in two siblings[3].

Wolcott-Rallison Syndrome

The Wolcoltt-Rallison syndrome is a disorder characterized by the appearance of diabetes mellitus within three months of birth, associated with multiple epiphyseal or spondylo epiphyseal dysplasia, renal impairment and poor prognosis. The responsible gene has been mapped to 2p12 and identified as being *E1F2AK3 (Eukaryotic translation-Initiation Factor 2-Alpha Kinase 3*), a translation-initiation factor[36].

Another rare, x-linked disease associated with neonatal diabetes mellitus occurs with phosphoribosyl adenosine triphosphate pyrophosphate overactivity, in which hyperurycemia is a major clue. In this entity, affected patients have considerable periods in which insulin was not required; severe physical and developmental delay was noted[1].

The IPEX Syndrome (Immunodysregulation, Polyendocrinopathy, and Enteropathy, X-linked)

This rare, x-linked disease is characterized by autoimmunity, susceptibility to infection and universal fatal outcome. Insulin-dependent diabetes is a frequent aspect. The responsible gene was initially mapped to the Xp11.23-q13.3 and the responsible gene identified as *JM2*, also called *FOXP3 (Forkhead Box P3)*. Here, the diabetes may be autoimmune but absent islets have been reported at autopsy in several cases suggesting that other mechanisms may also be involved[37,38]. These genetic entities are summarized in the table.

Table 1. Neonatal Diabetes: Genetic Entities

	Fraction of all Neonatal Diabetes	Gene Locus	Gene	Mechanism
Transient Usually ameliorate by 3-6 months of life; may recur as type 2 DM in later life	About 60%	6q24	ZAC*	Imprinted Paternal Uniparental disomy Paternal duplication Maternal under methylation
Permanent a. Pancreas/Duodenum homeobox Homozygous inactivating	10%	13q12.1	PDX-1(IPF-1) §(‡)	Absence of pancreas-specific transcription factor. Absent pancreas.
b. Glucokinase	10%	7p15-13	GCK†	Absence of key enzyme for glucose-stimulated insulin secretion
c. Wolcott-Rallison Syndrome Diabetes mellitus Epiphyseal/spondylo Epiphyseal dysplasia Renal defects/failure	10%	2p12	EIF2AK3∞	Mutated translation initiation factor
d. IPEX Syndrome	10%	Xp11.23-q 13.3	FOXP3#	Autoimmune Absent islets

*=ZAC. Zinc-finger protein regulating Apoptosis and Cell cycle
§=PDX-1. Pancreas and Duodenum homeoboX
‡=IPF-1. Insulin Promoter Factor
†=GCK. Glucokinase
∞=EIF2AK3. Eukaryotic Translation-Initiation Factor 2-Alpha Kinase 3
#=FOXP3. Forkhead boX P3

CONCLUSION

Diabetes mellitus in the newborn is a rare entity for which the etiologic mechanisms are still incompletely understood, and whose course is highly variable. Almost all affected neonates are SGA, reflecting the critical role of insulin for intrauterine growth. By definition, neonatal DM manifests in the first weeks of life, usually failure to thrive with osmotic polyuria, dehydration, and hyperglycemia, but only mild keotacidosis. Antibodies to insulin or islet cells and other markers of autoimmune type 1 DM are absent. Such markers of type 1 DM may be present in those who initially present with DM after 3 to 6 months of life. In neonatal DM, evidence of renal impairment not corrected by rehydration suggests the possibility of the Wolcott-Rallison syndrome, which can be confirmed by radiologic demonstration of epiphyseal dysplasia. If there are signs are symptoms of malabsorption, pancreatic agenesis may be confirmed by abdominal ultrasonography; homozygous deletions in the IFP1 gene have been described in this entity. Other gene mutations have emerged as factors regulating islet development. The response to exogenous insulin is dramatic and rewarding, with catch-up growth a prominent feature. The subsequent course of neonatal DM is highly variable; approximately one third of patients have a transient form that spontaneously resolves after several months, a phenomenon that remains poorly understood. Another one fourth have a transient form that resolves, only to reemerge years later as permanent DM. For the transient forms, the genetic basis has been ascribed to the ZAC gene on chromosome 6q24. The remainder of patients with neonatal DM have a permanent form of the disease from the outset. This variable course requires appropriate caution in providing counseling to parents of an affected neonate.

REFERENCES

1. von Muhlendahl KE, Herkenhoff H. Long-term course of neonatal diabetes. NEJM 1995;333:704-708.
2. Hathout EH, Sharkey J, Racine M, et al. Diabetic autoimmunity in infants and pre-schoolers with type 1 diabetes. Pediatric Diabetes 2000;1:131-134.
3. Shield JPH, Temple IK. Neonatal diabetes mellitus. Pediatric Diabetes 2002;3:109-112.
4. Temple IK, Gardner RJ, MacKay DJG, et al. Transient neonatal diabetes mellitus: widening our understanding of the aetiopathogenesis of diabetes. Diabetes 2000;49:1359-1366.
5. Stoffers DA, Stanojevic V, Haberer JF. Insulin promoter factor-1 gene mutation gene linked to early-onset type 2 diabetes mellitus directions expression a dominant negative isoprotein. J Clin Invest 1998;102:232 -241.
6. Cowett RM, Farrag HM. Neonatal glucose metabolism. In: Cowett RM, ed. *Principles of perinatal-neonatal metabolism*. New York Springer –Verlag 1998:663.

7. Humphrey RK, Smith MS, Tuch BE, et al. Regulation of the pancreatic cell differentiation and morphogenesis. Pediatric Diabetes 2002;3:46-63.
8. Sander M, German MS. The beta cell transcription factors and development of the pancreas. J Mol Med 1997;75:327-340.
9. Kemp DM, Thomas MK, Habener JF. Developmental aspects of the endocrine pancreas. Reviews in Endocrine and Metabolic Disorders, in press.
10. Stoffers DA, Zinkin NT, Stanojevic V, et al. Pancreatic agenesis attributable to a single nucleotide deletion in the human IPFI gene coding sequence. Nat Genet 1997; 1997:15-106.
11. Habener JF, Stoffers DA. A newly discovered role of transcription factors involved in pancreas development and the pathogenesis of diabetes mellitus. Proc Assoc Am Physicians 1998;110:12-21.
12. Fajans SS, Bell GI, Polonsky KS. Molecular mechanisms and clinical pathophysioloyg of maturity-onset diabetes of the young. NEJM 2001;345:971-980.
13. Njolstad PR, Sovik O, Cuesta-Munoz A, et al. Neonatal diabetes mellitus due to complete glucokinase deficiency. NEJM 2001;344:1588-1592.
14. Arava Y, Adamsky K, Ezerzer C, et al. Specific gene expression in pancreatic beta cells cloning and characterization of differentially expressed genes. Diabetes 1999;48:552 - 556.
15. Jiang FX, Cram DS, DeAizpurua HJ, et al. Laminin-1 promotes differentiation of fetal mouse pancreatic beta-cells. Diabetes 1999;48:772 -730.
16. Yamaoka T, Itakura M. Development of pancreatic islets. In J Mol Med 1999;3:247-261.
17. Menon RK, Sperling MA. Carbohydrate metabolism is neonatal adaptation: the transition to post-natal life. Semin Perinatol 1988;12:157 -162.
18. Pagliara AS, Karl IE, Kipnis DB. Transient neonatal diabetes: delayed maturation of the pancreatic beta-cell. J Pediatr 1973;82:97-101.
19. Chernausek SD, Beach DC, Banach W, et al. Characteristics of hepatic receptors for somatomedin-C/insulin-like growth factor-1 and insulin in the developing human. J Clin Endocrinol Metab 1987;64:737 -743.
20. Menon RK, Chernausek SF, Sperling MA. Ontogeny of insulin-like growth factor1 and insulin receptor kinase activity in rat liver. J Dev Physiology 1991;16:87.-97

21. Sperling MA, Ganguli S. Pre and post-natal development of insulin glucagon receptors: potential role in energy storage and utilization. J Pediatr Gastroenterol Nutr 1983;2[Suppl 1]:S46-S51.
22. Menon RK, Sperling MA. Insulin as a growth factor. Endocrinol Metab Clin North Am 1997;25:633-647.
23. Ferguson AW, Milner RDG. Transient neonatal diabetes mellitus in sibs. Arch Dis Child 1970;45:80 -83.
24. Schiff D, Colle E, Stern L. Metabolic and growth patterns in transient neonatal diabetes NEJM 1972;287:119-122.
25. Blethen SL, White NH, Santiago JV, et al. Plasma somatostatins, endogenous insulin secretions, and growth in transient neonatal diabetes mellitus. JCEM 1981;52:144 -147.
26. Salerno MC, Gasparini N, Sandomerico ML, et al. Two interesting cases of transient neonatal diabetes mellitus. Journal of Pediatric Endocrinology 1994;7:47-52.
27. Longo N, Wang Y, Smith SA, et al. Genotype-phenotype correlation in inherited severe insulin resistance. Hum Mol Genet 2002;11:1465-1475.
28. Coffey Jr. JD, Killelea DE. Transient neonatal diabetes mellitus in half sisters. A sequel. Am J Dis Child 1982;136:626-627.
29. Abramowicz MJ, Andriien M, Dupont E, et al. Isodisomy of chromosome 6 in a newborn with methylmalonic acidemia and agenesis of pancreatic beta cells causing diabetes mellitus. J Clin Invest 1994;94:418-421.
30. Das S, Lese CM, Song M, et al. Partial paternal uniparental disomy of chromosome 6 in an infant with neonatal diabetes, macroglossia, and craniofacial abnormalities. Am J Hum Genet 2000;57:1586-1591.
31. Gardner RJ, Robinson DO, Lamont L, et al. Paternal uniparental disomy of chromosome 56 and transient neonatal diabetes mellitus. Clin Genet 1998;54:522-525.
32. Varrault A, Bilanges B, MacKay DJ, et al. Characterization of the methylation-sensitive promoter of the imprinted ZAC gene supports its role in transient neonatal diabetes mellitus. J Biol Chem 2001;276:18653-18656.
33. Gardner RJ, MacKay DJG, Mungall AJ, et al. An imprinted locus associated with transient neonatal diabetes mellitus. Hum Mol Genet 2000;9:589-596.
34. MacKay DJG, Coupe A-M, Shield JPH, et al. Relaxation of imprinted expression of ZAC and HYMAI in a patient with transient neonatal diabetes mellitus. Hum Genet 2002:110:139-144.

35. Arima T, Drewell RA, Arney KL, et al. A conserved imprinting control region at the HYMAI/ZAC domain is implicated in transient neonatal diabetes mellitus. Hum Mol Genet 2001;10:1475-1483.
36. Delepine M, Nicolino M, Barrett T, et al. EIF2AK3, encoding translation initiation factor 2-alpha kinase 3, is mutated in patients with Wolcott-Rallison syndrome. Nat Genet 2000;25:406-409.
37. Chatila TA, Blaeser F, Ho N, et al. JM2, encoding a fork head-related protein, is mutated in X-linked autoimmunity-allergic disregulation syndrome. J Clin Invest 2000;106:R75-81.
38. Wildin RS, Ramsdell F, Peake J, et al. X-linked neonatal diabetes mellitus, enteropathy and endocrinopathy syndrome is the human equivalent of mouse scurfy. Nat Genet 2001;27:18-20.

Chapter 10
DIABETIC KETOACIDOSIS

Ram K. Menon, M.D. and Mark A. Sperling, M.D.
Children's Hospital of Pittsburgh, University of Pittsburgh School of Medicine

Diabetic ketoacidosis (DKA) is a potentially life-threatening medical emergency that reflects a state of metabolic decompensation in patients with insulin-dependent diabetes mellitus (IDDM).[1-6] It should be distinguished from non-ketotic hyperglycemic-hyperosmolar syndrome with which it shares some similarities in pathophysiology and treatment.[1] 25-50% of children and adolescents with new onset diabetes mellitus type 1, will present in ketoacidosis[2]. Whereas circumstances such as infection and emotional problems can trigger decompensation to DKA, the most common cause for DKA in patients with established diabetes is inadvertent or deliberate omission of insulin.[1-7] In this Chapter we provide an overview of the pathogenesis and management of DKA with particular reference to the unique features of DKA in children and adolescents.

DEFINITION

DKA is characterized by hyperglycemia, ketonemia with total ketones (beta-hydroxybutyrate and acetoacetate) in serum exceeding 3 mM, and acidosis with blood pH lower than 7.3 or a serum bicarbonate lower than 15 mEq/L.[1-7] Blood glucose concentration over 300 mg/dl is usually present in DKA. However, hyperglycemia is not a *sine qua non* for its diagnosis because DKA can occur with blood glucose less than 300 mg/dl and, rarely, even with normal blood glucose concentrations if, for example, vomiting with resulting reduced carbohydrate assimilation ensues while insulin administration is continued.[8] Ketonemia is usually diagnosed by demonstrating a positive sodium nitroprusside reaction (Acetest; Ketostix; Chemstrips UGK) with 1:2 dilution of serum or undiluted urine. Acidosis in DKA is predominantly due to accumulation of ketoacids and is thus characterized by an increased anion gap.[9] Other mechanisms contributing to the acidosis include lactic acidosis from tissue hypoperfusion and hyperchloremic acidosis, particularly during therapy with intravenous fluids.[9-10] The spectrum of acidosis encountered in DKA usually extends from pure ketoacidosis to a mixture of keto, lactic, and hyperchloremic acidosis.[1-4,9,10] However, a patient may present with predominant hyperchloremic acidosis and, hence, normal anion gap[9]. Some suggest that patients with pure hyperchloremic acidosis may experience a slower recovery from their metabolic decompensation[9]. It should also be emphasized that the degree of acidosis bears no relation to the degree of hyperglycemia.

In addition to non-ketotic hyperglycemic hyperosmolar coma, DKA should be distinguished from lactic acidosis, another metabolic condition that may be confused with DKA, which is characterized by blood lactate values (<more than>7 mM) rarely encountered in DKA.[9,10]

BIOCHEMICAL PATHOPHYSIOLOGY

Actions of insulin and glucagon

The cardinal hormonal alteration that triggers the metabolic decompensation of DKA is insulin deficiency with concomitant excess of glucagon and the stress hormones epinephrine, norepinephrine, cortisol, and growth hormone.[2,3,6] Insulin stimulates anabolic processes in liver, muscle, and adipose tissues and thereby permits glucose utilization and storage of the energy as glycogen, protein, and fat (Table 1). Concurrently with these anabolic actions, insulin inhibits catabolic processes such as glycogenolysis, gluconeogenesis, proteolysis, lipolysis, and ketogenesis. Insulin deficiency curtails glucose utilization by insulin-sensitive tissues, disinhibits lipolysis in adipose tissue, and enhances protein breakdown in muscle. Glucagon acting unopposed by insulin causes increased glycogenolysis, gluconeogenesis, and ketogenesis.

Although insulin and glucagon may be considered as the primary hormones responsible for the development of DKA, increased levels of the stress hormones epinephrine, nor-epinephrine, cortisol, and growth hormone play critical auxiliary roles. Epinephrine and nor-epinephrine activate glycogenolysis, gluconeogenesis, and lipolysis and inhibit insulin release by the pancreas. Cortisol elevates blood glucose concentration by decreasing glucose utilization in muscle and by stimulating gluconeogenesis. Growth hormone increases lipolysis and impairs insulin's action on muscle. The catabolic and metabolic effects of each of these counter-regulatory hormones are accentuated during insulin deficiency.[2,3,6] Under experimental conditions, the hyperglycemic effect of all these counter-regulatory hormones infused together is greater than the sum of the effects of the individual hormones; i.e., the effects are synergistic and not merely additive. Even in normal persons, high concentrations of these counter-regulatory hormones can induce hyperglycemia and ketonemia, a phenomenon that may explain the rapid development of DKA during stress induced by infection, vomiting, trauma, and infarction (in patients with IDDM).[1] Acute psychological stress induced by anger and rage may also precipitate DKA in some patients.[2,11] Indeed, there is consensus that although insulin deficiency *per se* is a prerequisite for the development of DKA, the complete features of metabolic decompensation characteristic of DKA are the result of the elevated levels and actions of the stress counter-regulatory hormones.[1-7]

Ketogenesis

The keto acids relevant to DKA are beta-hydroxybutyric acid and acetoacetic acid[2,3,6]. The primary mode of keto acid generation is from free fatty acids (FFAs). Released from triglycerides in adipose tissue, FFAs are transported to the liver, where they are converted to acyl-CoA derivatives in the cytosol of hepatocytes. These acyl-CoA derivatives enter the mitochondria as carnitine esters via a process catalyzed by carnitine acyl transferase I (CAT I) (Fig. 1). In the mitochondria, acyl-CoA is regenerated and subsequently oxidized to acetyl-CoA. Acetyl-CoA condenses with acetoacetyl-CoA to form beta-hydroxy-beta-methylglutaryl-CoA (HMGCoA), which then splits to form acetoacetate and acetyl-CoA. Acetoacetate is converted to beta-hydroxybutyrate in the presence of NADH. The net metabolic effect of ketone formation is accumulation of keto anions and the formation of three hydrogen ions for every triglyceride molecule metabolized to ketones.[3]

Low insulin and elevated glucagon concentrations facilitate the release of FFA from adipose stores; the opposite hormonal milieu of elevated insulin and low glucagon concentrations inhibits keto acid production. In the whole animal, keto acid generation is to the greatest extent regulated by substrate, i.e., FFA availability.[3] The rate of accumulation of keto acids is dependent on the ability of the tricarboxylic acid (TCA) cycle to utilize acetyl-CoA and the rate at which acetyl-CoA is generated. Evidence indicates that overproduction of acetyl-CoA and not reduced TCA cycle activity is the major mechanism for the increase in keto acids in DKA.[3]

Acetone is a neutral compound with no effect on blood pH; it is formed by the nonenzymatic decarboxylation of acetoacetate. Acetone is metabolically of little importance, but it provides an important bedside clinical clue to the diagnosis of DKA because of its characteristic odor and excretion via expired air and urine.

In the normal fasting state, the ratio of serum beta-hydroxybutyrate to acetoacetate is of the order of 3:1. The rate of interconversion of acetoacetate and beta-hydroxybutyrate depends on the cellular redox state (Fig. 2). A reduced redox state, as encountered in DKA, favors the formation of beta-hydroxybutyrate, whereas an increase in the redox state associated with recovery from DKA favors the conversion of beta-hydroxybutyric acid to acetoacetic acid. Thus, in severe DKA the ratio of beta-hydroxybutyric acid to acetoacetic acid is usually about 7:1 and may even increase to 15:1.[1-6] The nitroprusside reaction used in the semiquantitative and qualitative tests (Acetest; Ketostix; Chemstrips UGK) for ketonemia and ketonuria does not measure beta-hydroxybutyric acid, reacts weakly with acetone, and predominantly measures acetoacetic acid. About 80% of the color reaction in the nitroprusside test is due to acetoacetate, and acetoacetate comprises only one third to one fifteenth of the total ketone bodies in the circulation during DKA.[2] Thus, the usual bedside tests for ketones provide a gross underestimation of the total ketone body concentration. This laboratory artifact has important implications for the management of patients with DKA: First, the absence of a positive nitroprusside reaction does not necessarily imply absence of ketoacidosis. Conversely, the persistence or even an increase in the color reaction of the nitroprusside test should not be assumed to be due to a deteriorating metabolic response to treatment. This is because with improvement in the metabolic status of the patient the concomitant increase in the cellular redox state results in the conversion of the "unmeasured" beta-hydroxybutyric acid to "measured" acetoacetate and an apparent worsening of the ketonemic state. False-positive reactions for ketones with the nitroprusside reaction, although rare, can occur due to the presence in the urine of drugs such as captopril.[2,3]

Lactic acidosis

Lactate is formed primarily as the end-product of anaerobic metabolism of glucose.[10] Lactate can be synthesized by virtually every tissue in the body, although under basal conditions the daily lactate generation of 15 to 20 mmol/kg is predominantly derived from muscle, skin, erythrocytes, brain, and the gastrointestinal tract.[10] Under basal conditions, the daily rate of lactate production is balanced by a matching degree of utilization. Lactate can be converted back to glucose by the gluconeogenic enzymes pyruvate carboxykinase and phosphoenolpyruvate carboxykinase (Fig. 3). Under basal conditions, liver accounts for approximately two-thirds, and the kidneys one-third, of lactate consumption. Lactic acidosis caused by hypoxia results from an overproduction of lactate by skeletal muscle and the gastrointestinal tract, with a concomitant reduction in the capacity for lactate utilization by the liver and kidney. Although DKA *per se* does not result in an increase in blood lactic acid concentrations, severe DKA may be complicated by tissue hypoxia, which results in lactic acidosis.

Fluid and electrolyte losses

Fluid and electrolyte abnormalities are virtually universal in patients with DKA, and, if unrecognized or mismanaged, can contribute significantly to the morbidity and mortality of DKA.[1-6] Fluid and electrolyte losses in DKA vary so that the extent of these losses is unpredictable in any given patient. However, estimates of losses that form the basis of the initial management of DKA have been formulated (Table 2). It is emphasized that these recommendations are only guidelines, that each patient should be closely monitored, and that the response to the initial therapy dictates any subsequent changes.

Water and electrolyte losses from the extracellular compartment occur via osmotic diuresis brought about by hyperglycemia, via the respiratory tract because of hyperventilation as a result of metabolic acidosis, and via the gastrointestinal tract because of vomiting. In DKA there is an osmotically driven shift of water from the intracellular to the extracellular compartment. This phenomenon results in clinical underestimation of the extent of dehydration and is responsible for the unusual laboratory finding of hyponatremia despite dehydration and hyperosmolarity. It is estimated that for every 3 mM increase in glucose there will be a 1 mM fall in plasma sodium concentration. Spurious hyponatremia may also result from lipemic plasma because sodium is distributed only in water, but the volume of the sample taken into account for calculation of sodium concentration includes the space occupied by lipids and other solids. This artifact can be avoided if special electrodes are used for the estimation of serum or plasma sodium concentration.

Serum potassium levels in DKA are variable but tend to be at the upper limits of normal in the majority of patients at initial presentation. However, even when serum potassium is normal, there is almost always depletion of total body potassium stores. Several factors contribute to these alterations of potassium balance. Serum potassium tends to be elevated because insulin deficiency, per se, will reduce the Na^+/K^+ ATPase activity with a decrease in sodium-potassium exchange across the cell membrane. In addition, acidosis will cause a movement of intracellular potassium to the extracellular-intravascular compartment in exchange for hydrogen ions moving into the cell along a concentration gradient. Hyperglycemia *per se* and impairment of renal function also tend to keep the serum potassium levels elevated. The potassium entering the intravascular compartment is then lost in part via osmotic diuresis and vomiting and, in part, via the actions of aldosterone, elevated in response to volume depletion.

Initiation of therapy may result in a rapid decrease in serum potassium levels with disastrous consequences if adequate potassium supplementation is not instituted, making hypokalemia one of the avoidable causes of fatality in DKA. Correction of acidosis, restoration of intravascular volume, administration of insulin, and improvement in renal function all tend to decrease extracellular concentration of potassium. In addition, if bicarbonate therapy is instituted, the hypokalemic effects of the above mentioned factors are compounded. [12]It is estimated that about one quarter to one half of the potassium administered during fluid replacement therapy is lost in the urine. Patients with urinary losses greatly exceeding these estimates (potassium sink) have been described; such patients are at a serious risk of hypokalemia. Hence, potassium supplements should be provided early in the course of therapy; contrary to the usual practice of avoiding potassium infusion in patients with renal failure, patients with DKA and compromised renal function may need careful potassium supplementation because insulin therapy will promote cellular uptake of extracellular potassium and favor the development of hypokalemia. These considerations about potassium balance in DKA emphasize the need for frequent and meticulous monitoring of serum potassium concentrations, with adjustments in the therapeutic regimen tailored to each individual patient's response rather than reliance on a "standard" protocol.[1-6,12,13]

Disturbances in phosphorus homeostasis must also be considered during management of patients with DKA. Because DKA is a catabolic state, it is accompanied by a shift of intracellular phosphate into the extracellular compartment, with subsequent urinary losses resulting in depletion of total body phosphorus. As in the case of potassium, serum phosphate concentrations do not provide an accurate estimate of the total body phosphate stores. Also, as with potassium, institution of insulin and fluid replacement therapy results in a shift of extracellular phosphate into the intracellular compartment and therefore frequently leads to a hypophosphatemic state.[1-4,13,14] Hypophosphatemia impairs insulin action and will result in a decrease in synthesis of ATP and other energy intermediates. Phosphate deficiency will also result in a depletion of 2,3-diphosphoglycerate (2,3-DPG). Depletion of 2,3-DPG leads to a shift in the oxygen-hemoglobin dissociation curve to the left; i.e., it increases the affinity of hemoglobin for oxygen and hence decreases the amount of oxygen released to the tissues. Concurrent acidosis shifts the oxygen-hemoglobin dissociation curve to the right (Bohr effect) so that the effect of 2,3-DPG deficiency is offset by DKA. However, after institution of treatment, the amelioration of the acidotic state may unmask the deleterious effect of hypophosphatemia on tissue oxygen supply. Inclusion of phosphate in the therapeutic regimen is therefore recommended and has been shown to lead to the normalization of 2,3-DPG levels within 24 hours, whereas without phosphate supplementation this process may take 3 to 4 days.[13] Phosphate is recommended and usually provided as potassium phosphate. This form of replacement confers an additional advantage in that it facilitates a reduction in the amount of chloride administered as potassium chloride to replace potassium losses and thus helps to avoid the development of hyperchloremic acidosis. Despite these theoretical reasons for phosphate supplementation, clinical studies have by and large failed to substantiate an unequivocal advantage of phosphate therapy in terms of either decreased morbidity and mortality or shortened recovery time.[14] Hence, the decision to administer phosphate must be made on an individual basis and not as a routine measure, especially as there exists a danger of precipitating hyperphosphatemia and hypocalcemia.[14,15]

Precipitating factors

The cardinal feature of DKA is a deficiency of insulin action brought about by an absolute or relative lack of insulin.[1,7,16] In newly-diagnosed patients, or when insulin therapy has been omitted, an absolute lack of insulin is responsible for the development of DKA.[7,16] By contrast, during acute illness, stress, most commonly due to an infection, causes DKA to result from a relative deficiency of insulin, with insulin's action opposed by the surge in the counter-regulatory hormones, glucagon, catecholamines, cortisol, and growth hormone.[1-4] Acute and severe emotional stress may be an important precipitating factor for DKA in children.[6,11] In most instances, emotional factors such as parental discord, peer pressure at school, and adolescent adjustment problems may serve to worsen an already disturbed metabolic state.[6,7] In rare instances these factors may appear to be the sole precipitating cause for DKA. However, the most common precipitating change in patients with established diabetes is deliberate or inadvertent omission of insulin.[7] Deliberate omission of insulin resulting in recurrent episodes of ketoacidosis may be pathognomonic for an intolerable home environment and may signal the patient's plea to be removed from this situation. The use of steroids or other drugs that antagonize insulin action may also precipitate DKA in a patient taking insulin. Examples include "bursts" of steroids in patients with asthma, with cystic fibrosis-related diabetes and post solid organ transplantation, where imminent rejection is treated by a combination of agents that inhibit insulin secretion such as cyclosporin or tacrolimus along with steroids that, together, can bring about diabetes and DKA.[2]

Clinical features

The classical patient with DKA is characterized by dehydration, acidosis with hyperventilation, with varying degrees of cerebral obtundation, and with peripheral circulatory compromise. Polyuria, polydipsia, and weight loss are nearly always present historically in a patient with DKA. Metabolic acidosis initiates hyperventilation to compensate for acidosis by respiratory alkalosis. This is the typical Kussmaul respiration: deep, sighing, and rapid.

However, in severe acidemia, respiration may be depressed, with an absence of Kussmaul breathing. In very young children, especially those below the age of 1 year, the rapidity of development of DKA may blur these symptoms, and the patient may present in coma without the parents noticing the classical triad of symptoms. The degree of cerebral obtundation is related to the degree of hyperosmolarity and may vary from drowsiness to deep coma.[3-6]

Vomiting is both a precipitating factor and a symptom of DKA. Acute abdominal pain is not uncommon in DKA and may simulate acute appendicitis or pancreatitis. Elevation in nonspecific serum amylase can occur in DKA, but without pancreatitis serum lipase is normal.[17] In most cases the abdominal pain, if not surgical in origin, resolves within a few hours of fluid and insulin treatment. Hence, it is recommended that a decision to intervene surgically be made only after an adequate trial of fluid and insulin therapy for DKA. However, appendicitis and other causes of a surgical abdomen must be carefully evaluated, including the possibility of bowel infarction from vascular obstruction in long-standing diabetes. Although, infection is a precipitating factor for DKA, the presence of an elevated white cell count with polymorphonuclear leukocytosis need not necessarily indicate acute infection; these findings may exist in DKA *per se* as part of an acute stress response. The presence of fever should be taken as an indicator of infection and excluded by clinical examination and appropriate laboratory tests.

Laboratory findings

Laboratory investigations in the management of DKA are required for three purposes: (a) diagnosis of DKA, to include blood glucose, blood acid-base status, and documentation of ketonemia; (b) identification of precipitating and complicating factors, to include complete blood count, serum electrolytes, renal function, chest x-ray, ECG, urine culture, and blood culture, if necessary; (c) monitoring the effect of the therapeutic regimen, to include serum electrolytes, glucose, phosphate, magnesium, calcium, ECG, acid-base status, and serum and urine ketones. Other investigations such as a cranial CT scan or abdominal ultrasound may be indicated, depending on whether the evolution of cerebral edema or an acute surgical abdomen is being considered.[18]

Treatment

The goals of treatment are: (1) correction of the metabolic disturbances, particularly hyperglycemia, ketonemia, and acidosis; (2) treatment of precipitating factors; (3) prevention and early identification of complications resulting from the therapy for DKA; and, (4) prevention of recurrence.

Although there are broad guidelines and principles that should be adhered to in managing DKA, it cannot be overemphasized that the management must be individualized, depending on the patient's initial condition and response to therapy. Children younger than 2 years of age or those with an arterial pH of less than 7.0, blood glucose greater than 1000 mg/dl, or altered mentation are best managed in an intensive care unit or an equivalent setting, where close monitoring of metabolic changes and meticulous supervision of therapy can be provided by experienced personnel. A flow sheet detailing the composition of intravenously administered fluid, oral fluid intake, fluid output, timing and dose of insulin administered, electrolyte and acid-base status, and clinical parameters (pulse, respiration, blood pressure, and conscious state) should be maintained; such a flow sheet is essential in monitoring the patient's progress. Bladder catheterization may be needed; urine bag collection or condom drainage usually provide an adequately accurate estimate of urine output in children. Repeated measurements of glucose, acid-base status, and serum electrolytes are obtained at 2-hour intervals for the initial 8 hours, at 4-hour intervals for the next 16 hours, and then every 6 to 12 hours until acidosis is completely resolved and the patient is fully conscious and able to tolerate an adequate oral fluid intake without vomiting.

The varying requirements with age and the relatively small volumes involved in the computation of fluid and electrolyte requirements of a child with DKA dictate that these be more carefully calculated than those of a typical adult. The maintenance fluid requirement of a child changes as the child grows but is constant when expressed per unit of surface area; it is not constant when expressed per unit of body weight. In general, 1500 ml per m^2 is accepted as maintenance fluid requirement. By contrast, dehydration is expressed as a percentage of body weight; i.e., 10% dehydration implies a loss of 10% of the body weight as water (Table 3). Because different patients have different body weights, it is imperative to relate dehydration to an individual's weight. At presentation, clinical assessment usually underestimates the degree of dehydration. For practical purposes, it can generally be assumed that patients in DKA are initially at least 10% dehydrated. The total fluid to be administered is the sum of maintenance and estimated deficit, plus ongoing losses. Table 4 outlines an example of a replacement procedure in a child of 30 kg and 1.0 M^2 in surface area. Clearly, this example can be modified to suit the weight and surface area of any individual patient in DKA but must take into consideration associated conditions such as cardiac or renal impairment. Replacement is extended over 36 to 48 hours in order to reduce the likelihood of too rapid a drop in plasma osmolality, a factor implicated by some as predisposing to cerebral edema.[19-25] However, it is not proven that medical treatment cause or can prevent cerebral edema in children with

DKA.[26-28] To reduce the potential for developing cerebral edema, the initial replacement fluid is generally recommended to consist of normal saline (0.9%) so that a gradual decrease in plasma osmolality is achieved. Potassium therapy is initiated in the second hour. Some of the potassium is given as the phosphate in order to provide phosphate repletion and to reduce the provision of excess chloride.

Fluid and electrolyte therapy alone often result in significant clinical and biochemical improvement.[13] Hydration alone benefits patients by restoring intravascular volume, decreasing blood concentrations of counter-regulatory hormones, and improving insulin-sensitivity of the tissues. It is recommended that insulin therapy be deferred until the second hour of fluid therapy, especially in established diabetics who may have received their dose of insulin within hours of presenting in ketoacidosis. However, insulin is absolutely essential to restore acid-base balance and resolve ketoacidosis.[2,3,7] The preferred method of insulin delivery is the continuous low-dose intravenous infusion as outlined in Table 5. Glucose concentrations often reach levels of 200 to 300 mg/dl before acidosis is completely resolved. Therefore, it is important to continue insulin administration at the standard rate of 0.1 unit/kg/hr, (or occasionally 0.05 unit/kg/hr,) while adding 5% or even 10% glucose to the infusate in order to maintain glucose concentrations between 200 and 300 mg/dl until bicarbonate levels exceed 15 mEq/L. Glucose contributes substantially to plasma osmolality, so the reason for maintaining glucose concentration in the range of 200 to 300 mg/dl is to prevent too rapid a fall in plasma osmolality, a factor implicated by some as predisposing to cerebral edema.[20-26]

The decision to switch from intravenous insulin therapy to subcutaneous administration of insulin is based on a stable cardiopulmonary status with normal peripheral perfusion and a blood glucose concentration near 300 mg/dl. Intravenous fluids and intravenous or subcutaneous insulin should be continued until the metabolic acidosis is corrected and the patient is able to tolerate food intake. Subcutaneous insulin therapy is initiated with regular (short-acting) insulin given in a dose 0.2 to 0.4 U/kg, with the subsequent dose being adjusted every 4 to 6 hours, depending on the response as judged by the blood glucose levels and ketonuria.

Bicarbonate administration is not routinely recommended.[2,12] The role of bicarbonate therapy in the management of DKA remains unclear. Severe acidemia (pH <less than>7) is considered detrimental because of its negative inotropic effect, direct peripheral vasodilatory effect resulting in hypotension, depression of cerebral function, and antagonism of insulin's action. However, the provision of insulin and fluids generally corrects ketoacidosis and elevates the blood pH so that in most patients with DKA a satisfactory outcome is achieved without the use of bicarbonate. We do not support the use of bicarbonate in patients with arterial pH greater than 7.0, because of the potential of drawbacks to the use of bicarbonate for DKA.[2,6] Among these drawbacks is hypokalemia, an effect caused by alkalosis shifting potassium intracellularly so that potassium replacement should be carefully adjusted to meet this additional requirement. Other established side effects of bicarbonate therapy include impaired tissue oxygenation with leftward shift of the oxyhemoglobin dissociation curve, rebound alkalosis, sodium overload, and a paradoxical fall in cerebrospinal fluid pH while systemic acidosis is being corrected. This occurs because HCO_3 associates with H^+ to form H_2CO_3 and this dissociates to H_2O and CO_2. Whereas, CO_2 diffuses freely across the blood brain barrier, HCO_3 diffuses poorly. Although there is no definite evidence for its efficacy even when the arterial pH is 7.0 or less, some authorities recommend that when the pH is 7.0 or below, 40 to 80 mEq per m^2 (1 to 2 mEq/kg of sodium bicarbonate) be infused over 2 hours, followed by reassessment of the clinical status of the patient. Bicarbonate should never be given as a bolus except during cardiopulmonary resuscitation.

Complications

With appropriate therapy, complications of DKA itself are uncommon, but the overriding concern is the precipitating event itself. Precipitating or associated factors for DKA such as myocardial infarction, adult respiratory distress syndrome, mucormycosis, rhabdomyolysis, emphysematous cholecystitis, or malignant otitis externa should be considered in adults but are not usually a consideration in childhood.[1,29] Iatrogenic management complications include hypoglycemia, hypocalcemia from too vigorous a use of phosphate, and hypokalemia from inadequate potassium replacement.[1,4,6,15]

In children, the major complication of concern during treatment for DKA is cerebral edema and related intracerebral complications.[20-28,30-32] This complication of DKA remains a serious problem in children, who are at a disproportionately higher risk for developing clinical cerebral edema as compared to adults with DKA. Clinically relevant cerebral edema is estimated to occur in 0.7%-1.0% of episodes of diabetic ketoacidosis in children.[26-28] The etiology of this potentially devastating sequence of events remains incompletely understood.[26-28] It is both practically and ethically difficult to conduct well-designed prospective studies because of the relatively small number of patients with this complication seen by any given physician or center. Thus, most of the data collated to date regarding this problem have been derived from retrospective studies amalgamating the experience of different physicians and treatment centers, the most recent of which identified approximately 60 episodes of cerebral edema over a 15 year period from a multi-center survey.[27]

Clinically, cerebral edema develops in patients, usually with new-onset diabetes, several hours after the institution of therapy when clinical and biochemical indices suggest improvement. Manifestations of cerebral edema include symptoms and signs of raised intracranial pressure such as headache, deterioration in consciousness, bradycardia, papilledema, development of fixed dilated pupils, and occasionally polyuria (secondary to diabetes insipidus), which may be misdiagnosed as osmotic diuresis due to hyperglycemia. Computerized tomography (CT) scanning has revealed that subclinical cerebral edema is common in children being treated for DKA.[18]

Magnetic resonance imaging and CT scanning have additionally indicated that at least some of these children have cerebral thrombosis and infarction in addition to cerebral edema.[26,31] In adults, monitoring by indwelling intrathecal catheters indicates that there is a rise in cerebrospinal fluid pressure in all patients during fluid and insulin therapy for DKA.[26] In children, subclinical cerebral edema may be present in the majority, as suggested by narrowing of the cerebral ventricles detected by CT scanning during treatment, and restoration to normal ventricular size after recovery.[18] The cause of this syndrome is believed by some to be a rapid correction of osmotic disequilibrium between brain cells and extracellular fluid brought about by hypotonic fluids and by a precipitous lowering of the blood glucose concentration.[29,20-28] This hypothesis is based on the tenet that in response to the hyperosmolar state of hyperglycemia, brain cells generate "idiogenic osmoles" which increase the intracellular osmotic pressure, thereby maintaining the intracellular water content of these cells.[19] With institution of treatment, there is a decrease in the plasma osmolality as a result of hydration and lowering of the plasma glucose concentration. In this milieu, if idiogenic moles dissipate at a rate slower than the rate at which the plasma osmolality is being lowered, then cerebral edema may be precipitated because the brain cells are hyperosmolar with respect to the extracellular compartment.[20-28] Experiments in animals, such as the rat, have suggested taurine as one of the idiogenic osmoles that accumulates in diabetic ketoacidosis.[19,23] Other mechanisms and factors implicated in the pathogenesis of cerebral edema in DKA include a direct effect of insulin on the influx of Na^+, K^+, and water into brain cells, activation of the plasma membrane Na^+, H^+ exchanger because of acidosis with movement of Na^+ into the cells,[32] inappropriate secretion of antidiuretic hormone, administration of bicarbonate, and cerebral hypoxia resulting in toxic activation of the N-methyl-D-aspartate (NMDA) receptor.[28] Proof for a dominant role for any single one of these factors is tenuous since none of these mechanisms provides a satisfactory explanation for all of the salient epidemiological features of this complication. In the recent comprehensive survey of cerebral edema in children,[27,28] the factors that conferred increased risk were low partial pressure of arterial carbon dioxide and high serum urea nitrogen at presentation, and treatment with bicarbonate.[27,33] All of these risk factors may reflect more severe metabolic decompensation and longer antecedent duration of metabolic disturbance before intervention. Thus, at the present time there is no clear explanation for the unique susceptibility of infants and children and the relative lack of this complication in adults with DKA. Also, this complication is rare in the syndrome of non-ketotic hyperosmolar coma where the initial hyperosmolarity is considerably greater than that usually encountered in DKA.[1] The observation that there is a preponderance of children with new onset IDDM with this complication compared to children with established IDDM may, again, reflect severity and duration, because the diagnosis of diabetes mellitus has not been considered or recognized until DKA supervenes.[27,28] Thus, the only way to avoid cerebral edema is to avoid DKA. One reason why a majority have subclinical brain swelling, whereas only a few (approximately 1%) manifest clinically apparent cerebral edema, may relate to the intracranial pressure-volume curve, which demonstrates a steep, exponential rise in intracranial pressure beyond a critical volume of cerebral mass.[34] For these reasons it is prudent to anticipate the possibility of clinical cerebral edema in all children treated for DKA, and to avoid DKA by heightening awareness of diabetes as a potential diagnosis in unexplained weight loss or other vague symptoms.[2,27,28] Some authorities believe that the risks can be reduced by limiting the rate of fluid administration to 4.0 L/m^2/day or less and avoiding the excessive use of bicarbonate.[20-25] It has also been suggested that fluid resuscitation in DKA should extend over 48 hours and that crystalloid solutions with an average Na^+ concentration of 125 mEq/L be utilized so that serum Na^+ levels increase as serum glucose levels decreases; hence, serum osmolality will remain relatively constant, and fluid shifts across the blood-brain barrier will be minimized.[25] We consider that in the absence of evidence to the contrary, it is advisable to moderate the rate of fluid administration and restrict the amount of free water provided during the initial phases of the rehydration protocol. As soon as intracranial hypertension is clinically suspected, measures should be taken to reduce brain swelling by the use of mannitol at 10 to 20 g/m^2/IV (0.25 to 1.0 g/kg IV) repeated at 2- to 4-hour intervals if necessary, reducing the rate of fluid administration, and instituting hyperventilation therapy. Retrospective studies suggest that these measures, instituted promptly, are lifesaving and may avoid neurological sequelae.[30-31] Heroic measures such as cerebral decompression via craniotomy are usually desperate measures. Once clinically obvious, cerebral edema is associated with a mortality of about 70% and only 7%-14% of these patients escape permanent impairment of neurological function.[31]

In summary, DKA is a medical emergency that dictates prompt and careful management, including close clinical and laboratory monitoring. Complications of DKA are uncommon in patients diagnosed promptly and managed appropriately. In children, prudent and prompt management usually results in excellent outcome and prognosis. Recurrent DKA reflects mostly deliberate omission of insulin, especially in adolescents and may be a plea for psychosocial intervention.

REFERENCES

1. Delaney MF, Zisman A and Kettyle WM. Diabetic ketoacidosis and hypergycemic hyperosmolar nonketotic syndrome. Endocrinol Metab Clin North Am 2000; 29:683-705.
2. Sperling MA: Diabetes mellitus. In Sperling, MA, editor. Pediatric Endocrinology, 2nd Edition, Philadelphia 2002, W.B. Saunders.
3. Foster DW and McGarry JD: The metabolic derangements and treatment of diabetic ketoacidosis, N Engl J Med 1983; 309:159-169.
4. Kitabchi AE and Wall BM: Diabetic ketoacidosis, Med Clin North Am 1995; 79: 9-37.
5. Lebovitz HE: Diabetic ketoacidosis, Lancet 1995; 345:767-772.
6. Sperling MA: Diabetic ketoacidosis, Pediatr Clin North Am 1984; 31:591-610.
7. Morris AD, Boyle DIR, McMahon AD, et al. Adherence to insulin treatment, glycaemic control, and ketoacidosis in insulin-dependent diabetes mellitus. Lancet 1997;350:1505-1510.
8. Munro JF, Campbell IW, McCuish AC, et al: Euglycaemic diabetic ketoacidosis, Br Med J 1973; 2:578-580.
9. Adrogue HJ, Wilson H, Boyd AE, et al: Plasma acid-base patterns in diabetic ketoacidosis, N Engl J Med 1982; 307:1603-1610.
10. Arieff AI: Pathogenesis of lactic acidosis, Diabetes Metab Rev 1989; 5:637-649.
11. Winter RJ, Harris CJ, Phillips LS, et al: Diabetic ketoacidosis: induction of hypocalcemia and hypomagnesemia by phosphate therapy, Am J Med 1979; 67:897-900.
12. Riley LJ, Cooper M, and Narins RG: Alkali therapy of diabetic ketoacidosis: biochemical, physiologic, and clinical perspectives, Diabetes Metab Rev 1989; 5:627-636.
13. Waldhausl W, Kleinberger G, Korn A, et al: Severe hyperglycemia:effects of rehydration on endocrine derangements and blood glucose concentrations, Diabetes 1979; 28:577-584.
14. Fisher JN and Kitabchi AE: A randomized study of phosphate therapy in

the treatment of diabetic ketoacidosis, J Clin Endocrinol Metab 1983; 57:177-180.
16. Menon RK and Sperling MA: Childhood diabetes. Med Clin North Am 1988; 72:15651576.
17. Moller-Petersen J, Andersen PT, Hjorne N, et al: Hyperamylasemia, specific pancreatic enzymes, and hypoxanthine during recovery from diabetic ketoacidosis, Clin Chem 1985; 31(12):2001-2004.
18. Krane EJ, Rockoff, MA, Wallman JK, et al: Subclinical brain swelling in children during treatment of diabetic ketoacidosis, N Engl J Med 1985; 312(18):1147-1151.
19. Arieff AI and Kleeman CR: Studies on mechanisms of cerebral edema in diabetic comas. Effects of hyperglycemia and rapid lowering of plasma glucose in normal rabbits. J Clin Invest 1973; 52:571-583.
20. Duck SC, Weldon VV, Pagliara AS, et al: Cerebral edema complicating therapy for diabetic ketoacidosis, Diabetes 1976; 25(2):111-115.
21. Duck SC and Wyatt DT: Factors associated with brain herniation in the treatment of diabetic ketoacidosis, J Pediatr 1988; 113:10-14.
21. Harris GD, Fiordalisi I, Harris W, et al: Minimizing the risk of brain herniation during treatment of diabetic ketoacidemia: a retrospective and prospective study, J Pediatr 1990; 117:22-31.
22. Hammond P and Wallis S: Cerebral oedema in diabetic ketoacidosis, Br Med J 1992; 305:203-204.
23. Harris GD, Lohr JW, Fiordalisi I, Acara M. Brain osmoregulation during extreme and moderate dehydration in a rat model of severe DKA, Life Sciences 1993; 53: 185-191.
24. Harris GD, Fiordalisi I, Finberg L, et al: Safe management of diabetic ketoacidemia, J Pediatr 1988; 113(1):65-68.
26. Muir A. Do doctors cause or prevent cerebral edema in children with diabetic ketoacidosis? Pediatr Diabetes 2000; 1:209-216.
27. Glaser N, Barnett P, McCaslin I, et al. Risk factors for cerebral edema in children with diabetic ketoacidosis. N Engl J Med 2001;344:264-269.
28. Dunger DB and Edge JA. Predicting cerebral edema during diabetic ketoacidosis. N Engl J Med 2001;344:302-303.
29. Carroll P and Matz R: Adult respiratory distress syndrome complicating severely uncontrolled diabetes mellitus: report of nine cases and a review of the literature, Diabetes Care 1982; 5:574-580.
30. Bello FA and Sotos JF: Cerebral oedema in diabetic ketoacidosis in children. Lancet 1990; 336:64.
31. Rosenbloom AL: Intracerebral crisis during treatment of diabetic ketoacidosis, Diabetes Care 1990; 13:22-33.
32. Van der Meulen JA, Klip A, and Grinstein S: Possible mechanism for

cerebral edema in diabetic edema in ketacidosis, Lancet 1987; 2:306-308.
33. Assadi FK, John EG, Fornell MT, et al: Falsely elevated serum creatinine concentration in ketoacidosis, J Pediatr 1985; 107:562-564.
34. Marmarou A, Shulman K, Rosende R. A nonlinear analysis of the cerebrospinal fluid system and intracranial pressure dynamic. J Neurosurg 1978; 38:332-344.

Chapter 11
INSULIN THERAPY AND OUTPATIENT DIABETES MANAGEMENT

Francine Ratner Kaufman, M.D.
Childrens Hospital Los Angeles, The Keck School of Medicine of University of Southern California, Los Angeles, CA

INTRODUCTION

Over the years since the completion of the Diabetes Control and Complications Trial (DCCT)[1,2,3] the benefits for infants, children and youth with type 1 diabetes of following a system of diabetes management that allows for optimal glycemia has become increasingly apparent. Not only is there reduction in long-term diabetes complications, but there is normalization of growth and pubertal development and improvement in physical and psychosocial well-being. Unfortunately, coupled with these benefits is the risk of increased episodes of hypoglycemia that might have neurocognitive consequences, particularly for young children. Therefore, the systems of diabetes management that improve glycemic control must be well-defined and carefully taught to patients and families. Certain aspects of diabetes care must also be conveyed to school personnel and other caregivers if pediatric subjects with type 1 diabetes are to maximally benefit from an intensive management approach. To accomplish this, the family must work in concert with a multidisciplinary diabetes team as well as their primary care provider.

While the goals of diabetes management are clear, to achieve the desired outcomes patients and families must integrate a comprehensive, rigorous diabetes regimen into their daily lives. The components of these regimens include measuring the blood glucose level at least 4 or more times per day. Insulin is administered according to what is best for the individual patient and his or her family so that glycemic targets can be met. These targets are set with pre-meal, post-meal, bedtime and night values so that defined actions are taken if glucose levels are outside the target ranges. Supplemental doses of insulin per an algorithm are given to correct an abnormally elevated glucose level and additional carbohydrate is administered to ameliorate hypoglycemia. Patients and families learn the effects of food and food types, activity and illness and how to dose insulin for alterations in the daily schedule. As such, comprehensive, intensive diabetes management can come to dominate daily life and complicate the fact that these children still need to reach the normal developmental milestones of infancy, childhood and adolescence, strive to succeed in school and in extracurricular activities, and develop independence and autonomy.

This chapter will review the multiple components of diabetes management focusing on the insulin regimens that can be used for pediatric subjects. The pharmacokinetics of the different insulin preparations will be addressed, as will the available methodologies for insulin administration. The emphasis will be on achieving the most intensive outpatient regimen that is possible for each new onset and established patient.

Table 1. The Onset of Action, Peak Action and Duration of Action of the Four Types of Insulin

Insulin Preparation	Onset of Action - hours	Peak Action - hours	Duration of action – hours	Maximal duration - hours
Rapid-acting				
Lispro (Humalog)	¼ - ½	1 - 2	3 – 5	4 – 6
Aspart (Novolog)	¼ - ½	1 - 2	3 - 6	5 – 8
Short-acting Regular	½ - 1	2 – 4	3 – 6	6 – 8
Intermediate-acting				
NPH (isophane)	2 – 4	8 – 10	10 – 18	14 - 20
Lente (Zinc suspension)	2 – 4	8 - 12	12 - 20	14 – 22
Long-acting				
Ultralente (Extended zinc suspension)	6 – 10	10 – 16	18 – 20	20 – 24
Glargine (Lantus)	1-2	none	(19) -24	24

Insulin Pharmacokinetics

Insulin can be obtained from pork pancreas or, it can be made identical to human insulin through recombinant DNA technology or chemical manipulation of pork insulin. Virtually all insulin treated patients should use human insulin preparations because human insulin has a more predictable time course, reduced antigenicity as evidenced by lower anti-insulin antibody titers and decreased immunogenicity compared to animal insulin. The 4 categories of available human insulin preparations are given in Table 1.

These four general categories of insulin preparations are determined by the time course of action. In general, insulin preparations with a longer onset of action and longer time to peak action have a longer duration of action. In addition, the greater the insulin dose, the wider the peak and the greater the duration of action. To assure that insulin has full potency, the individual manufacturer's storage recommendations and expiration dates must be followed. In general, insulin must not be frozen or exposed to direct sunlight or heated. Unused insulin should be stored in a refrigerator at 2-8 degrees C. After opening, insulin kept in the refrigerator should be discarded after 3 months and insulin kept at room temperature should be discarded after 1 month.

Rapid-acting Insulin

Rapid-acting insulin preparations have been genetically engineered to have a more rapid onset of action and a shorter duration of action when compared to short-acting regular insulin. This has been accomplished by manipulating the insulin molecule so that insulin molecules do not autoaggregate but rather remain monomeric or rapidly become monomeric. Insulin lispro (Lys(B28), Pro(B29)) has been prepared by switching the amino acid sequence at positions 28 and 29 of the B-chain. Insulin aspart is an analogue of human insulin in which the amino acid proline at the B28 position is replaced by aspartic acid. When given subcutaneously, these rapid-acting insulin preparations have an onset of action within 15-30 minutes, a peak action at 1-2 hours and duration of action of 3-5 hours. This allows for rapid-acting insulin to be given either immediately before the meal, within 10-15 minutes, or just after the meal. Immediate post-meal administration of rapid-acting insulin has been shown to be effective[4,5] particularly in young children in whom food intake may not be reliable. Rapid-acting insulin has been shown to lead to less hyperglycemia after eating and less hypoglycemia in the late postprandial period and at nighttime. Although there is this reduction in glycemic excursion, for the most part rapid-acting insulin has been shown to only minimally decrease or not change HbA1c in clinical trials. While the onset of action and duration of action of insulin lispro and insulin aspart are near identical, there may be a slightly longer duration of action of aspart compared to lispro. The clinical significance of this is likely to be negligible[6].

Short-acting Insulin

Short-acting regular or soluble insulin has a short duration of action and can be administered subcutaneously, intravenously, or intramuscularly. It is the insulin of choice for intravenous use. After intravenous injection, regular insulin has an immediate onset of action, a short half-life of 5-6 minutes, a peak glucose lowering effect in 20-30 minutes and duration of effect of 2-3 hours. After intramuscular injection, regular insulin has a peak effect in 1-1 ½ hours and duration of action of 3-4 hours. When given as a subcutaneous injection, the onset of action is1/2 to 1 hour, the peak effect is 2-4 hours and the duration of effect is 3-6 hours. Regular insulin can be given as a continuous intravenous infusion for the treatment of diabetic ketoacidosis, during the perioperative period, during childbirth, in combination with intravenous hyperalimentation and for acute illness. By supplying it in this way, rapid adjustments can be made to normalize glycemia.

Intermediate-acting Insulin

The intermediate-acting insulin preparations were designed so that insulin absorption would be delayed and insulin action prolonged. Insulin complexes with protamine (NPH) or zinc (lente) were made to have these properties. NPH insulin has an onset of action at 2-4 hours, a peak at 8-10 hours and duration of action of 10-18 hours. Lente has an onset of action at 2-4 hours, a peak at 8-12 hours and duration of action of 12-20 hours. Since the 1950's, these intermediate-acting insulin preparations have been used in combination with short-acting insulin, and now rapid-acting insulin, to allow patients to manage diabetes with 1, 2 or 3 insulin injections per day.

Long-acting Insulin

The first long-acting insulin in the clinical arena was ultralente insulin. This was prepared by forming an insoluble zinc-insulin complex that had an onset of action of 3-6 hours, a peak at 10-16 hours and duration of action of 18-24 hours. Insulin glargine was developed as a long-acting insulin preparation that is essentially peakless[7]. Insulin glargine has two molecules of arginine added to the B-chain and asparagine in position 21 of the A-chain is substituted with glycine. This results in a shift of the isoelectric point so that there is an onset of action in 1 hour and a duration of action of 24 hours[8]. Because of its pH, insulin glargine cannot be mixed with other insulin preparations. Initial studies in children have shown that it appears to be an effective insulin and that there are lower free insulin levels with its use when compared to NPH insulin[9, 10]. Although insulin glargine has been shown to result in less hypoglycemia in adults[11], due to little available clinical data as of this writing, statements about the ability to decrease hypoglycemic episodes or improve glycemic control in children with insulin glargine must be deferred. Other long-acting insulin preparations are under development. One such preparation, insulin detimer, is produced by adding fatty acid to regular insulin and maintaining a soluble form of insulin at a neutral pH[12]. A threonine at B30 is removed and the lysine at B29 is acylated with a C14 fatty acid. Insulin detimer is currently being studied to assess its usefulness as a basal insulin.

Pre-Mixed Insulin Preparations

Pre-mixed insulin has a fixed ratio of short or rapid-acting insulin to intermediate-acting insulin. Used in pen injector devices, pre-mixed insulin is available in a number of different combinations [such as 70/30 – 70% NPH/30% regular, 50:50 – 50% NPH/50% regular, 75/25 – 75% NPL (neutral protamine lispro)/25% insulin lispro] depending on the manufacturer. While pre-mixed insulin appears to have a role in improving adherence with the medical regimen in adults with type 2 diabetes, there is little evidence that it has benefit in children with diabetes and there is some provisional evidence that adolescents with diabetes have poorer metabolic control when they use pre-mixed insulin. By using pre-mixed insulin, adjustments for blood glucose levels and carbohydrate intake cannot be done without also changing the intermediate-acting insulin dose. Therefore, the role of pre-mixed insulin in pediatrics appears to be minimal[13].

Inhaled Insulin

Inhaled insulin (Exubera, Pfizer, Groton, CT) has recently been tested in wide-scale clinical trials[14]. The pharmacodynamic profile of this inhaled insulin is similar to that of short-acting regular insulin. Inhaled fast-acting insulin has a peak action at .25-.5 hours and a duration of action of 3 hours. Inhaled insulin has been shown in preliminary studies to be effective for the meal bolus in combination with basal insulin by injection. Children as young as 6 years have been enrolled in clinical trials and to date there has been good efficacy and little toxicity. Higher titers of insulin antibodies have been recognized in those receiving inhaled insulin. The significance of these antibodies is presently unknown.

Insulin Injection Devices

There are a number of devices that can be used to administer insulin[15]. These are listed in Table 2.

Table 2. Insulin Injection Devices

Insulin Syringes
Indwelling Catheters
Pen Devices
Automatic Injection Devices
Jet Injectors
Insulin Pumps

The traditional method for administering insulin is with a plastic fixed-needle syringe. These syringes are designed for single use and should be discarded with care to avoid transmitting blood-borne infections. Insulin syringes come in 1, 0.5 and 0.3 ml sizes with a standard or short 30 gauge (12.7mm) needle. Insulin can also be administered through subcutaneous indwelling catheters. These catheters are inserted usually after topical local anesthetic treatment of the skin and can be used multiple times for up to 3 days. Insulin pen injector devices obviate the need for accurately drawing insulin from a vial. The dosage is dialed up on a digital scale and pens facilitate giving insulin away from home and in school. The pen contains a prefilled insulin cartridge that is either a single type of insulin or a premixed insulin preparation; they are either disposable or the cartridge can be replaced; and they can be dialed to give full or half unit increments of insulin. Pens are particularly useful for patients routinely taking multiple injections or for patients who need a correction dose of insulin before meals or snacks on an intermittent basis. School personnel are particularly interested in giving insulin injections to young school-aged children with pen devices. Automatic injection devices used to hide the needle of the insulin syringe and jet injectors can be used by children who have needle phobia. Finally, insulin can be given by an insulin pump, which is an open-loop system that is worn externally.

Insulin Injection Sites and Reactions

Subcutaneous insulin can be given in a number of sites. Insulin can be injected in the front of the thigh, lateral thigh, abdomen, buttocks and lateral aspect of the arm. Disinfection of the skin at the injection site is not necessary since infection is uncommon, however, good hygiene is required. Children and youth should be encouraged to rotate injection sites, but to use the same part of the body at a particular time of the day, such as the arms for breakfast or abdomen for bedtime. They should be encouraged not to inject into the exact same location and the skin and subcutaneous area should be inspected for local reactions. Young children often will agree to be injected in only one body area for months or years. As long as there is no local effect, it may have psychological benefit to give young children some control over the diabetes regimen.

There are many factors that influence insulin absorption. Depending on where it is given and how the sites are rotated, the rate of absorption may be affected. In general, insulin absorption is faster in children who are younger and thinner, and who take a small dose of insulin. Absorption is also affected by site, the abdomen is faster than the buttock, the buttock faster then the leg; depth of injection, the deeper the faster; exercise; and ambient and body temperature.

Undesired reactions can occur as the result of insulin administration[16]. With purified, human insulin preparations, insulin allergy is rare. Local reactions, such as lipohypertrophy and lipoatrophy, are more common. Lipoatrophy, or the loss of localized subcutaneous fat in injection areas, is more common in young children and is due to a local immunologic reaction to impurities rather than true insulin allergy. It is a cosmetic problem and is usually ameliorated by injecting around the periphery of the lesions. Lipohypertrophy is due to an increase in subcutaneous fat deposition in the areas of chronic insulin injections or at the sites of pump catheter insertion. This problem is common in young children because there is less pain sensation in the hypertrophic areas. This makes them popular sites for repeated injection. The use of insulin can be associated with the development of edema. This edema is usually pedal and periorbital, and is self-limited in children. It is due to sodium and fluid retention, as well as an increase in vascular permeability. It occurs after administration of large doses of insulin, such as that which occurs during the treatment of ketoacidosis.

Initiation of Insulin Therapy

At the time of the diagnosis of type 1 diabetes, and after the resolution of diabetic ketoacidosis in those in whom it was present, daily subcutaneous insulin injections are begun. Most children and youth are started on 2 or 3 insulin injections per day. The total amount of insulin initially given is variable. For those subjects recovering from ketoacidosis, up to 1-2 U/kg/day of insulin may be required. Younger children and those who are not ill at presentation may be treated with ½-1 U/kg/day. The distribution of insulin is given in the Table 3. As shown, the total insulin dosage is initially split 2/3 in the morning, 1/3 in the evening. For 2 injections, the morning dose is split 1/3 short- or rapid-acting insulin and 2/3 intermediate-acting. The dinner dose is divided equally between short- or rapid-acting and intermediate-acting insulin. For 3 injections, the morning is the same as above and the evening dose is split before dinner of short- or rapid-acting insulin and before bed as intermediate-acting insulin. Thereafter, dosage adjustment becomes individualized according to blood glucose levels, carbohydrate intake and specific glycemic patterns. For example, if pre-breakfast glucose levels are below the target range, the evening intermediate-acting insulin is adjusted until fasting levels improve. Or if pre-lunch glucose levels are above the target range, the morning short- or rapid-acting insulin is increased. To optimize glucose control, most new-onset patients and families need to have almost daily contact with the health care team to learn how to alter the insulin regimen.

Table 3: Distribution of Insulin at Diabetes Diagnosis

	Morning	Dinner	Bedtime
2 injections	<u>2/3 total dose</u> 1/3 rapid or short 2/3 intermediate	<u>1/3 total dose</u> ½ rapid or short ½ intermediate	
3 injections	<u>2/3 total dose</u> 1/3 rapid or short 2/3 intermediate	<u>1/6 total dose</u> rapid or short	<u>1/6 total dose</u> intermediate or long

Most pediatric type 1 patients enter a remission or honeymoon phase of diabetes within 1 month of diagnosis. At this point, subjects are on a decreased dosage of insulin, often <1/3 U/kg/day. While in the past, patients would be weaned off insulin injections, this is no longer recommended. It appears advantageous to continue with the initially prescribed number of injections so that subjects remain accustomed to multiple injection therapy. During the remission phase, there is minimal glycemic fluctuation due to the endogenous production of insulin and negligible severe hypoglycemia due to the reduction in the dosage of exogenous insulin. The duration of the remission is variable, but it rarely persists more than 3-6 months. The end of the remission phase is characterized by increased variability of blood glucose concentrations, high HbA1c levels, increased insulin requirements and greater need to attend to diabetes management.

Over the long-term, many patients do extremely well on 2 or 3 insulin injections per day, however, others experience difficulty with wide fluctuations of blood glucose concentrations and unacceptably high HbA1c levels. This has led to more and more children eventually being placed on intensive regimens that utilize basal-bolus therapy. Basal-bolus therapy can be achieved with multiple daily insulin injections (MDI) combining an intermediate- or long-acting insulin (basal), with a rapid-acting insulin (bolus) given before meals. Basal-bolus can also be achieved with continuous subcutaneous insulin infusion with an insulin pump. These treatment regimens require that specific glycemic targets be set and success is measured by reduction in episodes of severe hypoglycemia, ketoacidosis and HbA1c concentrations.

While many pediatric patients are still hospitalized at the time of diabetes diagnosis, there has been a trend over the last decade to initiate insulin therapy as an outpatient. To be able to do this with success, a multidisciplinary team must teach the patient and family how to safely use insulin at home and be available to answer phone calls to trouble shoot if problems arise. This initial instruction is followed by a more comprehensive diabetes education program that is delivered over a number of days to weeks enabling the patient and family to learn as much about diabetes management as is possible. Many families will become virtually independent in the task of balancing insulin, food and activity, while other families will be incapable of adjusting an insulin dosage without interacting with the health care team. The challenge for the diabetes education team is to enable each child and family to be as successful in independent diabetes management as is possible.

Insulin Regimens

The basic concept of insulin therapy is to attempt to mimic normal physiology[17]. To do this, there must be sufficient insulin throughout the 24 hour period to cover basal insulin requirements and boluses of insulin to match carbohydrate and food intake. Changes in insulin levels need to coincide with alterations in activity. With this in mind, physiologic insulin replacement cannot be accomplished with two or three insulin injections per day, or conventional insulin therapy. For the most part, two injections of a mixture of rapid- or short-acting and intermediate-acting insulin normalize glycemia only in patients in the remission phase of diabetes. Three injections of a similar mixture before breakfast and a split of the rapid or short-acting insulin before dinner and the intermediate-acting insulin (or occasionally long-acting insulin) before bed is also unlikely to be physiologic. Despite this, the 3-injection regimen is widely used and may be the most common regimen for pediatric type 1 patients. This remains true because many patients/families and health care providers are reluctant to give more insulin injections, intensified regimens may be more difficult to teach and manage, and insulin delivery at school is often discouraged by school personnel. In addition, in the past the American Diabetes Association Standards of Care[8] asserted that intensive diabetes management was contraindicated in children younger than 2 years of age and that it should be instituted with extreme caution in children 2 to 7 years of age. However, it has become clearly evident that children and youth, including young children, can use intensive insulin regimens involving multiple injection therapy when coupled with education, support, dosage adjustment algorithms and close monitoring of the blood glucose level[19].

Multiple daily injection therapy (MDI) (intensive insulin therapy) is a more physiologic way to deliver insulin. When the emphasis is placed on the need to separate basal from bolus insulin, which allows for more liberal food choices with regard to content, amount and timing, this is referred to as flexible insulin therapy. Doses of basal insulin are given as intermediate- or long-acting insulin either two times a day before breakfast and bedtime or once every 24 hours (usually before bedtime). Bolus doses are given as either rapid-acting insulin immediately before the meal or short-acting insulin 20-30 minutes before the meal. The amount of the bolus dosage is determined by how much insulin is needed to be taken for the carbohydrate content of the meal (and protein content, if indicated) and for the premeal glucose level. For the most part, the basal insulin doses account for 50% of the total daily insulin requirement and the bolus doses the other 50%. Finally, insulin pump therapy (or continuous subcutaneous insulin infusion) may be the most effective way to achieve flexible insulin therapy and the optimal regimen for children of any age. Insulin pump therapy has been shown to be ideal for patients wishing to optimize glycemia, improve life style, reduce hypoglycemia, and prevent recurrent ketoacidosis or progression of diabetes complications[20-23].

Blood Glucose And Ketone Monitoring

It is critical to measure the blood glucose level multiple times during the day and intermittently during the night if glycemic targets are to be met. In a number of studies, it has been shown that frequency of blood glucose monitoring is highly associated with glycemic control[24-28]. In a large cohort of youth 7 to 16 years of age, it was the sole modifiable predictor of HbA1c levels[29]. At least 4 values per day need to be obtained on a routine basis before meals and bedtime. Additional tests are required at other times to determine if patterns of glycemic fluctuation are occurring. Occasionally, testing of the glucose level at midnight or 0200-0300 should be recommended to determine if there is nocturnal hypo or hyperglycemia. Blood glucose testing should be recommended after strenuous exercise, during illness or at other times, such as during traveling, when the usual routine is altered. Intermittently, the blood glucose level should be measured before the mid-morning or afternoon snack. Recently, there has been an emphasis on the postprandial period[30]. Since it is unknown how important peak glucose levels after meals are to adding to the glycemic burden of diabetes, it might be of value to obtain some 1-2 hour post meal glucose levels. These glucose levels are of particular relevance to those on basal-bolus regimens since postmeal levels will help determine how to dose bolus insulin.

There have been many advances that have facilitated making home glucose monitoring easier, faster, less painful and more relevant. Glucose measurements can be done on very small blood samples. Pre-prandial samples can be taken from the forearms. Forearm sampling, in addition to sampling areas other than the finger tips, are not valid in the non-steady, post meal state or in times of hypoglycemia. Results are available in 5 to 45 seconds from glucose meters small enough to fit in a pocket. Glucose meters store glucose values that can be displayed in a variety of forms and graphs either directly on the meter or on a home computer. This enables patients and their families to better identify undesired patterns and trends so that the diabetes regimen can be appropriately altered.

Recently, semi-invasive, continuous or frequent glucose monitoring devices have been developed. In the research setting, these glucose monitoring systems, such as the MiniMed CGMS ® (Medtronic, Inc, Northridge, CA) and the Cygnus GlucoWatch ® Automatic Glucose Biographer (Cygnus, Inc, Redwood City, CA), have been shown to facilitate identification of glycemic patterns and trends and lead to improvement in glycemic control[31-35]. The MiniMed system uses a glucose oxidase sensor that can measure subcutaneous glucose levels every 5 minutes. This can be worn presently for up to 3 days and the glucose results can be analyzed retrospectively. The Gluco Watch ®, recently approved for use in children, measures the glucose content of interstitial fluid through iontophoresis every 20 minutes for up to 12 hours. It contains alarms to detect hyper and hypoglycemia and when an abnormal value is displayed, confirmation with a standard home glucose monitoring device is required. The Gluco Watch ® has been associated with minor skin irritation in some individuals. When continuous systems can be used in the clinical arena to give patients and families real-time continuous glucose levels, it is likely that a marked improvement in short and long-term diabetes outcome will be appreciated. Eventually, it is anticipated that these will be linked to insulin infusion devices creating a near-artificial pancreas.

It remains important that patients measure urine or blood ketones during times of severe or sustained hyperglycemia, stress, fever or intercurrent illness. Blood ketones can now be measured with a home device that has a combined glucose and ketone sensor (Medisense/abbott Laboratories, Abington, U.K.)[36]. Any child who has vomiting or evidence of dehydration should determine if ketonuria or ketonemia is present. Urine ketone tests measure acetoacetate, while blood ketone tests assess for the presence of beta-hydroxybutyrate. Since beta-hydroxybutyrate is the predominant ketone body in diabetic ketoacidosis, urine measurement may give false negative results[37]. Patients on insulin pump therapy need to be able to assess for the presence of ketonuria or ketonemia since ketoacidosis can develop with failure of insulin delivery. The presence of ketones should lead to immediate evaluation and intervention since diabetic ketoacidosis requiring hospitalization can be avoided if recognized early and treated appropriately.

Glycemic Targets

In the DCCT, the intensification of diabetes management resulted in an increase in severe hypoglycemia in patients with type 1 diabetes. As a result, hypoglycemia has been labeled the rate-limiting step in placing patients on intensive management protocols[38]. Since it appears that young children are more susceptible to severe hypoglycemia, the target range for blood glucose levels and for HbA1c values are generally higher in young pediatric subjects. However, the fear that reducing HbA1c levels will lead to an unacceptable rate of severe hypoglycemia is generally unfounded. In a recent study, with an overall hypoglycemia event rate of 62 events per 100 person years, there was a high incidence of hypoglycemia even in those with poor metabolic control[29]. Despite the fact that the DCCT showed a 3-fold increase in severe hypoglycemia in those in the intensively managed group, this has not been borne out in other studies. Cox et al[39] showed no association between glycated hemoglobin levels and severe hypoglycemia in the 78 pediatric subjects in their study. In addition, other studies[40-43] have shown high rates of hypoglycemia in subjects with elevated HbA1c levels and no increase in hypoglycemia in those with low HbA1c values under intensive diabetes management.

Table 4. HbA1c Levels by Age

Infants	<7.5 – 8.0 %
Preschool	<7.5 – 8.0 %
School-aged	<7.0 – 8.0 %
Teens	<6.5 – 7.5 %

While there is much debate as to what target HbA1c levels should be[19], the most accepted goal for infants is to have an HbA1c level <7.5-8.0%; for pre-school children, <7.5-8.0% range; for school-aged children, <7.0-8.0% range, and for teens, <6.5-7.5%. Therefore, as the child becomes older, the primary concern shifts from avoidance of excessive hypoglycemia to avoidance of hyperglycemia as a means to decrease long-term diabetes complications. The DCCT showed it is difficult to achieve optimal glycemic control in adolescents[1, 2]. The 13-17 year subjects in the intensive arm of the DCCT only achieved a mean A1c of 8.06%, compared with 7.12% in the intensively treated adult group. Large multinational data collection has also shown that it is difficult to achieve optimal glycemic outcome in children and adolescents with type 1 diabetes[44] and studies from academic centers in the U.S. also show HbA1c levels that are generally unacceptably high[29].

The individual glycemic target of a patient must be determined understanding the developmental, cognitive and communicative capabilities of that individual. Table 5 shows the glycemic targets suggested by a number of reviews[45, 46]. Very young children with diabetes do not have the same glycemic targets as older children and teens. Infant and toddlers with diabetes should have a preprandial glucose target of 100-180 mg/dL and postprandial of <200 mg/dL. Preschool children should aim to have blood glucose levels between 70 or 80-150 mg/dL and <200 mg/dL during the pre and post-meal times, respectively. School-aged children and teens should use 70-140 or 150 mg/dL and <180 mg/dL for the pre and postprandial periods. Bedtime values should be at least within the target range to 20-30 mg/dl higher. For children who are susceptible to nocturnal or early morning hypoglycemia, bedtime values may need to be individually determined after repeated testing and correlation, as best as possible, between bedtime, middle of the night and morning readings. The goals for the middle of the night levels may also need to be individualized to help prevent aberrations of glycemia. Presently this can be accomplished by intermittent nocturnal testing or by the use of continuous glucose monitoring which has recently become available.

Table 5: Target Glucose Range for Different Age Groups

	0-2 years	3-6 years	7-12 years	>13 years
Premeal glucose mg/dl	100-180	70-150	70-150	70-150
2-3 hour post prandial mg/dl	<200	<200	<180	<180
Before Bed mg/dl	100-200	100-180	90-160	80-150
2-4 AM mg/dl	>100	>100	>90	>80

The point of the target range is that if the blood glucose levels are not within the target range action should be taken. If glucose levels are below target, glucose-containing substances should be ingested. If glucose levels are above target, this can be corrected with a supplemental dosage of insulin, increased activity or less carbohydrate-containing food with the scheduled meal. For an elevated blood glucose level, action should be taken immediately and although multiple parameters can be altered, administration of supplemental rapid-acting or short-acting insulin per an insulin correction algorithm is the most effective way to bring the glucose level back into the target range.

Insulin Dosage Adjustment

Insulin doses need to be adjusted to correct for an abnormal blood glucose level (correction algorithm), to account for exercise and activity, to match carbohydrate intake (insulin:carbohydrate ratio or carb supplement), to anticipate a change in the usual regimen (anticipatory supplement), and to correct an abnormal pattern in the basic or set dose of insulin. The amount of insulin given per the correction algorithm can be determined by taking into account age, overall insulin dosage and insulin sensitivity. Table 6 gives examples of typical algorithms that can be used by health care providers (and parents/patients) to determine how much extra rapid- or short-acting insulin their patients should be taking for every 50 mg/dl the blood glucose is above the upper limit of the target range to correct blood glucose levels. The dosage of insulin can also be determined by the 1800 or 1500 Rule. The 1800 Rule is used for rapid-acting insulin and the 1500 Rule for short-acting insulin. Insulin sensitivity is determined by dividing 1800 or 1500 by the total daily dose of insulin to determine how many mg/dl 1 unit of insulin decreases the blood glucose level[47].

Table 6: Examples of How to Determine the Amount of Insulin to be Given to Correct an Abnormal Blood Glucose Level, by Total Insulin Dosage or by Age

Insulin Dosage	Age	Amount/ 50 mg/dl that blood glucose is elevated
< 5 Units	< 5 years	¼ Unit
5-10 Units	6-9 years	½ Unit
10-20 Units	10-12 years	1 Unit
> 20 Units	Teens	2 Unit

For Immediate Correction of An Abnormal Blood Glucose Level: Add Insulin According to the Algorithm below if Blood Glucose is Above the Target Range.
Add Insulin Before Meals, Snacks, and at Bedtime (at Bedtime, give 50% of the Dosage and Check Blood Glucose in 2-3 Hours)

These insulin dosage algorithms can be taught to the patient and family by one or another methods. The algorithm can be written on a piece of paper, algorithms are available on plastic cards or they can be found in computerized devices such as an inexpensive hand-held plastic Insulin Dosage Guide that was developed in the author's center[47]. This Insulin Dosage Guide has resulted in a decrease in mean HbA1c values and mean blood glucose levels in a cohort of children and youth.

Patients/families can also learn how to give insulin supplements in anticipation of need (anticipatory supplements). Insulin doses can be either increased or decreased depending on anticipated food intake and activity level.

This requires that the patient/family understand the carbohydrate:insulin ratio. One way to determine this ratio is the following equation: divide 450 by the total units of insulin used per day to determine the number of grams of carbohydrate that requires 1 unit of insulin[20]. Adjustments for physical activity must also be done to avoid aberrations of glycemia. Increases in activity not only cause fluctuations at the time, but can result in delayed or nocturnal hypoglycemia. In general, for an isolated period of activity lasting ½ to 2 hours, a child will likely need to take 10-15 grams of carbohydrate for every ½ to 1 hour. This will depend on the starting blood glucose concentration, the level of activity and prior experience with similar exercise. Occasionally, activity can cause elevation of blood glucose levels. This usually occurs in the afternoon for children taking 2 or 3 insulin injections per day or if CSII is disconnected for greater than 1 ½- 2 hours. With repeated strenuous physical activity, the total daily insulin dose may need to be decreased by 10-20%. Finally, adjustments in the basic or set dose of insulin can be made in response to a pattern of glycemia that has been determined over a number of days[48]. Table 7 below gives guidelines used in the author's center as to how to made adjustments in the base or set dose of insulin.

Table 7. Principles used for Adjustments in Basic or Set Insulin Dose

Rapid-, Short-, Intermediate- or Long-acting insulin is adjusted after a pattern has been identified over 3-7 days	
Increase or decrease by 0.5, 1.0, 1.5 or 2.0 U (10% of the dose)	
Two or Three Insulin Injections	
Time of abnormal test	*Change this Insulin*
Before Breakfast	Evening intermediate- or long-acting
Before Lunch	Morning Rapid- or short-acting
Before Dinner	Morning intermediate- or long-acting
Before Bedtime	Evening rapid- or short-acting
In the night	Evening intermediate- or long-acting
Multiple Insulin Injections	The same as above except
Before dinner	Lunch rapid- or short-acting
Insulin Pump	
Change bolus dose if BG abnormal	<2-3 hours after the meal
Change basal dose if BG abnormal	>3 hours after the meal
Recheck to be sure the changes made return BG levels to the target range	

Sick Day Management

It is imperative that patients and families understand the importance of altering the diabetes regimen during intercurrent illness. Although children with diabetes are generally not more susceptible to illness or infection, once contracted, such processes can markedly deteriorate glycemic control. Illnesses associated with vomiting and diarrhea, particularly in young children, can lead to hypoglycemia. On the other hand, febrile illnesses can cause hyperglycemia as the result of elevation of the counterregulatory hormones leading to insulin resistance and gluconeogenesis. Either may lead to ketogenesis. In addition to teaching patients and families about sick day management, the diabetes health care team must be available 24 hours a day to provide guidance in managing intercurrent illness so that dehydration, ketoacidosis and hypoglycemia can be avoided.

Table 8. Patient Guidelines for Sick Day

Important Phone Numbers
Pediatrician:
Endocrinologist/diabetes team:
Emergency numbers:
Call diabetes team/physician for the following
Vomiting for more than 3-4 hours
Five or more diarrheal stools
Change in mental status, alertness
High fever (greater than 101F or 38.5 C)
Blood glucose > 300 mg/dl two times
Ketones
Evidence of bacterial infection, dehydration, trouble breathing
If You Are Concerned About Your Child
Begin a log sheet
Test blood glucose every 30-60 minutes, urine for ketones every void
Record results of test, temperature, number of voids, vomiting episodes, stools
Assess fluid intake (food is not important, only fluids)
Prevent Hypoglycemia
Reduce the dose of insulin for vomiting and poor oral intake
Give small dose of rapid-acting or short-acting insulin every 2-4hours according to blood glucose levels
Suggested dose for your child:
Prevent Diabetic Ketoacidosis
If blood glucose is elevated, give extra rapid-acting insulin every 2-3 hours
Suggested dose for you child:
Maintain Hydration
Give electrolyte- and glucose-containing solutions
For blood glucose < 250 mg/dl, give carbohydrate containing fluid
For blood glucose > 250 mg/dl , give noncarbohydate containing fluid
Attempt to get intake to exceed output

During acute illness, there should be heightened monitoring of blood glucose and ketones levels and modifications made to the routine diabetes regimen[49]. Blood glucose may need to be measured as frequently as every 30-60 minutes at the onset of symptoms. Insulin administration should not be stopped, but rather the dosage of insulin altered. Replacement of fluids should take precedent over trying to give food. If blood glucose levels are lower than target, glucose-containing fluids should be given in small quantities to normalize blood glucose levels. Insulin should be decreased by 20-50%. If persistent hypoglycemia occurs and patients are not able to retain glucose-containing solutions, the administration of a mini-dose of glucagon (for children $\leq$ 2 years, 20 μg or two "units" on the insulin syringe; for children > 2 years, 150 μg or 15 "units") has been shown to be of benefit[50] in acutely ameliorating hypoglycemia and allowing for subsequent retention of oral glucose-containing fluids. Although some centers advocate the use of anti-emetic suppositories, these agents must be given with extreme caution so as to not mask an acute abdomen or worsening ketosis. If there is associated hyperglycemia, supplemental insulin should be given dependent on the age of the child, blood glucose level, duration of hyperglycemia, severity of ketosis and comfort level of the family and health care provider. Usually 10-20% of the total daily insulin dose or 0.1 U/kg of rapid or short-acting insulin can be given every 2-4 hours until the blood glucose level falls to the <250 mg/dl. After that, continued supplemental rapid or short-acting insulin can then be given as 5-10% of the total daily dose or the usual dose can be increased by 10-20% so that intermediate or long-acting insulin is also administered. Non-glucose containing fluids should be given until the blood glucose level reaches 250 mg/dl. It is important to ingest fluids containing sodium and potassium if there has been excessive fluid loss with polyuria or vomiting. A sample of patient guidelines for sick day management are given in Table 8[49].

Components of the Outpatient Visit

Pediatric patients with diabetes should have comprehensive, multidisciplinary outpatient visits at regular intervals. The purpose of these visits is to assess health status, adjust the diabetes regimen as indicated, promote diabetes knowledge and competency, and motivate patients and families to improve short and long-term outcome. While there is conflicting data as to what the frequency of these visits should be[51], it has been shown that when outpatient follow-up is irregular and interrupted there is an increase in ketoacidosis, poor glycemic control and incidence of long-term complications. Our center[52] showed that visits as infrequent as one to two times per year were associated with significantly higher HbA1c levels than when visits were three to four times per year.

During outpatient visits, it is important to obtain a comprehensive interval history. As outlined in the American Diabetes Association Clinical Practice Recommendations for 2001,[15] and modified for pediatric patients, the following should be determined:

1. Frequency, causes and severity of hypoglycemia or hyperglycemia;
2. Results of home glucose monitoring from logbooks and blood glucose meter downloads,
3. Self-adjustments to the diabetes regimen,
4. Integration of home care management behavior, understanding of the diabetes management plan and goals,
5. Education assessment and needs,
6. Review of systems for intercurrent problems or diabetes complications,
7. Current medications,
8. Psychosocial issues,
9. Changes in life situations,
10. School performance, afterschool, weekend, and sports activities,
11. Risk-taking behavior, particularly for adolescence.

Diabetes health care providers should insure that the patient has routine pediatric care for well-child visits, to diagnose and treat other medical/psychosocial problems, and to administer immunizations and anticipatory guidance.

A comprehensive physical examination should be done and height, weight and pubertal development should be closely monitored. Head circumference should be plotted until age 3 years. Normalization of growth parameters and normal pubertal entrance and development are important goals of diabetes management. Chronic hyperglycemia and poor glycemic control can result in growth failure and delayed skeletal maturation and sexual maturity. Insulin overtreatment and recurrent hypoglycemia can lead to excessive weight gain. In addition, children and youth with type 1 diabetes are at increased risk for other autoimmune processes such as thyroid autoimmunity, collagen-vascular disease and celiac disease which can adversely affect growth and development. Eating disorders are common in adolescent girls with diabetes[53]. Therefore, deviations from normal growth velocities should be noted and lead to investigation as to the etiology. Blood pressure should be assessed at each visit. Elevation of the blood pressure may be the first sign of diabetic nephropathy and hypertension can accelerate diabetes complications. Blood pressure should be done with an appropriate cuff for the patient's size and results compared to age-specific norms. Blood pressure should be $< 85^{th}$ percentile for age.

In addition to what is done during a routine physical examination, specific emphasis should be placed on the ophthalmoscopic examination. After 5 years of diabetes, children and youth should have a yearly dilated eye exam, obtaining retinal photos if possible. The thyroid gland should be examined to determine size and consistency since 10-20% of subjects will have a palpable goiter. Thyroid enlargement may indicate authoimmune thyroid disease. The abdomen should be evaluated for the presence of fullness, which can be a sign of chronic constipation, inflammatory bowel disease, celiac disease or delayed gastric emptying. Assessment of liver size should be done to rule out the presence of hepatomegaly, which can be a sign of poor diabetes control. The feet should be examined and peripheral pulses palpated. The skin and joints should be evaluated for thickening and limitation of joint mobility, which in children can be signs of chronic poor glycemic control[54]. The finger-tips and forearms should be looked at for evidence that routine blood glucose monitoring is occurring, and insulin injection and pump catheter insertion sites should be evaluated for local reactions. Skin rashes and lesions, such as necrobiosis lipoidica diabeticorum and acanthosis nigricans, should be noted. A thorough neurologic examination should be performed to determine if there are any signs of neuropathy. Table 9 gives what should be monitored during follow-up visits with the health care team.

Table 9. Ongoing Monitoring: Physical Examination

	Frequency/ Recommendations
Weight, Height, BMI	Every 3 mo/ assess changes in percentile
Tanner stage	Every 3 mo/ note pubertal progression
Blood Pressure	Every 3 mo/ target < 90th % for age
Eye	Dilated fundoscopic exam every 12 mo after 5 years of diabetes
Thyroid	Every 3 mo/presence of goiter, signs of thyroid dysfunction
Abdomen	Every 3 mo/presence of hepatomegaly, fullness, signs of malabsorption, inflammation
Foot, Peripheral Pulses	Every 3 mo inspection/after age 12 years, thorough exam for sensation, pulses, vibration yearly
Skin, Joints, Injections Sites	Every 3 mo/injection sites, joint mobility, lesions associated with diabetes
Neurologic	Every 12 mo/signs of autonomic changes, pain, neuropathy

Ongoing Monitoring: Laboratory Examination

Test	Frequency
HbA1c	Every 3 mo
Microalbuminuria	Every 12 mo after puberty or after 5 years with diabetes
U/A, creatinine	At presentation and with signs or renal problems
Lipid profile	At diagnosis and every 12 mo
Thyroid function tests	Every 12 mo
Celiac screen	At time of diagnosis, if symptoms, at puberty
Islet antibodies	At diagnosis

At quarterly visits, HbA1c levels should be obtained. This measurement evaluates overall glycemic control by determining the amount of heme protein to which glucose has been nonenzymatically linked. This reflects the average blood glucose concentration over the preceding two to three month time period. For this reason, HbA1c has been referred to as the "diabetes report card." Preferably HbA1c values will be available at the time of the clinic visit so it can be determined if glycemic targets are being met. If HbA1c is elevated, it is best to have an in depth, face-to-face discussion at the time of the visit, rather than at a later date or over the phone. If the level is within the desired range, the patient, family and diabetes team can congratulate each other. For patients with higher than desired levels despite having put forth a maximal effort to manage diabetes, more radical modifications of the diabetes regimen can be considered.

Yearly thyroid function tests should be obtained. Thyroid autoantibodies are present in 20-30% of pediatric type 1 subjects, however, overt hypothyroidism occurs in 1- 5% and compensated hypothyroidism in 5-10%. A fasting lipid profile that includes total cholesterol, HDL cholesterol, LDL cholesterol and triglycerides should be obtained in children and adolescents after glucose control has been established. If values fall within age-adjusted norms, they should be repeated at yearly intervals. Urine microalbumin should be obtained beginning at puberty or after 5 years of diagnosis and then yearly. Microalbumin levels can be measured using a random microalbumin-to-creatinine ratio, timed overnight microalbumin assay-to-albumin excretion rate assessment, or 24 hour timed urinary microalbumin-to-albumin excretion rate measurement. Celiac disease has been reported to occur 10-50 times more often in children with diabetes when compared to the general population. Depending on the study, celiac disease may be present in 1-10% of children and adolescents with type 1 diabetes. Celiac disease should be considered in children and youth with gastrointestinal symptoms such as diarrhea, pain, flatulence, dyspepsia or aphthous ulcers. Unexplained hypoglycemia, dermatitis herpetiformis, and delayed growth or pubertal development can also be associated with celiac disease. A celiac screen, including antiendomysial IgA antibody quantitation, should be obtained[55]. At the time of diagnosis, patients should have liver function tests and a creatinine and urinalysis. Assessment of islet autoimmunity should be made by obtaining specific antibodies to islet antigens. This may help exclude the diagnosis of type 2 diabetes, particularly in adolescents.

Table 10. Check List That Can Be Used During The Health Care Visit

What to Ask and Assess During a Diabetes-Related Health Care Visit
History since last visit
Review of systems
Physical examination and laboratory
Adverse events since last visit
Intercurrent illness
Severe hypoglycemia
Ketosis/diabetic ketoacidosis
Emergency room visit or hospitalization
Paramedics
Contact with team since last visit - phone, fax, email
Down-load of blood glucose meter data
Mean blood glucose $\pm$ SD
Premeal blood glucose levels
Postmeal blood glucose levels
Insulin dose
Type of insulin, number of injections, timing
Correction algorithm
Dose for carbohydrate
Nutrition Plan – carbohydrate portions
Patient/family competence and education needs
Psychosocial issues
School and recreational activities
Number of days missed
Grades
Activities
Day care, other care providers
Complications – any detected by history, physical, laboratory
Evaluation and Plan

The Collaborative System of Care

The multidisciplinary diabetes care team consists of the following members:

Essential Members

1. Pediatrician specializing in diabetes/endocrinology (or a physician with special interest in childhood and adolescent diabetes),
2. Diabetes specialist nurse and/or diabetes educator
3. Dietitian

Health Care Professional who should be part of the multidisciplinary team, or who should be accessible

1. Psychologist/psychiatrist/counselor knowledgeable about diabetes and children
2. Social worker

These individuals will work together to provide expert practical guidance and skill training, educations advice and support for the psychological needs of the patient and family[13].

Active collaboration between the diabetes team and the primary care provider is essential for optimal outcome. The primary care provider must be kept informed and provide the medical home. He or she should know the patient's diabetes regimen, findings on quarterly evaluations, HbA1c results, the plan for managing intercurrent illness, issues surrounding the family, psychosocial adaptation of the patient and family, problems with school or during other activities, and adverse events and diabetes-related complications. The primary care provider in turn gives routine pediatric care, sees that developmental and behavioral issues are addressed, ensures that the family and child are adjusting to chronic illness and offers age and gender-appropriate anticipatory guidance.

The pediatrician or family practitioner can also help the patient obtain diabetes supplies, arrange subspecialty care visits and consult with the patient and family about whether the patient should intensify the diabetes regimen. As more clinical research becomes available to children and their family members, the pediatrician can help determine what experimental protocols might be most appropriate. Most importantly the pediatrician should serve as the patient's advocate with the parents, other caregivers, school personnel, coaches and the diabetes team.

Diabetes Care in School and Day Care Setting

The majority of individuals $\leq$ 19 years of age with diabetes in the U.S. attend school[56, 15]. It is imperative that parents and the health care team provide school personnel with the necessary information and training to deal with diabetes management. This should be in the form of as individualized Diabetes Health Care Plan. In addition, parents should be aware that federal laws protect children with diabetes. These laws include the Rehabilitation Act of 1973, Section 504, the Individuals with Disabilities Education Act of 1991 and the American with Disabilities Act of 1992. Under these laws, it is illegal to discriminate against children with diabetes. Families can ask to develop a formal 504 Plan, in addition to the Diabetes Health Care Plan, to obtain the necessary accommodations so that diabetes care is given with as little disruption to the school's and the child's routine.

The Diabetes Health Care Plan needs to include specific information about the following:

1. Blood glucose monitoring, including when and where testing should be done,
2. Insulin administration, if necessary, including doses and who can administer injections,
3. Meals and snacks, including amounts and timing,
4. Symptoms and treatment of hypoglycemia, including the use of glucagon,
5. Symptoms and treatment of hyperglycemia,
6. Ketone testing if indicated,
7. Management tasks the child can perform, those requiring supervision.

The school/day care center must allow the management of diabetes to proceed as outlined in the Diabetes Health Care Plan during school hours, after school and on field-trips. In addition, the school must guarantee privacy, training of backup personnel, access to the restroom and fluids, and permission to miss school without consequences for medical reasons and appointments. The specific responsibilities of the parents/guardians, the child and the health care team should also be outlined in the Diabetes Health Care Plan and supporting materials. Parents/guardians need to give the school/day care center all diabetes supplies and emergency information. The child must participate in diabetes-related tasks as allowed by his/her developmental stage and the health care team must be available for questions and emergency situations. In this way, children and youth can participate in day care, school and after school activities while they optimize diabetes outcome.

CONCLUSIONS

Many advances have been made in diabetes management over the last 1-2 decades. Further advances are anticipated over the next years while research progresses towards the cure of this devastating disorder. In the interim, the importance of effectively managing diabetes on a day-to-day basis cannot be underemphasized. Patients and families must be given effective tools to intensify management and meet glycemic goals. Follow-up visits must occur to insure optimal physical and psychosocial outcome. Partnerships must be developed between the patient, parents, family members, school and day care personnel, the diabetes team and the primary care provider. All must remain committed to a multi-component diabetes regimen that is as intensive and safe as possible.

REFERENCES

1. Diabetes Control and Complications Trial Research Group. The effect of intensive treatment of diabetes on the long-term development and progression of long-term complications in insulin-dependent diabetes mellitus. N Engl J Med 1993; 329, 977-986.
2. Diabetes Control and Complications Trial Research Group. Effect of intensive diabetes treatment on the development of long-term complications in adolescents with insulin-dependent diabetes mellitus: Diabetes Control and Complications Trial. J Pediatr 1994; 125, 177-188.
3. Diabetes Control and Complications Trial Research Group. Implementation of treatment protocols in the diabetes control and complications trial. Diabetes Care 1995 18, 361-376.
4. Chase HP, Lockspeiser T, Perry B, Shepherd M, MacKenzie T, Anderson J, Garg SK. The impact of the diabetes control and complications trial and humalog insulin on glycohemoglobin levels and severe hypoglycemia in type 1 diabetes. Diabetes Care 2001; 24, 430-434.
5. Brunner GA, Hirschberger S, Sendhofer G, et al. Post-prandial administration of the insulin analogue insulin aspart in patients with type 1 diabetes mellitus. Diabetic Medicine 2000; 17, 371-375.
6. Hedman CA, Lindstrom T, Arnqvist HJ. Direct comparison of insulin lispro and aspart shows small differences in plasma insulin profiles after subcutaneous injection in type 1 diabetes. Diabetes Care 2001; 24, 1120-1121.
7. Owens DR, Coates PA, Luzio SD, Tingergen JP, Kurzhals R. Pharmacokinetics of 125I-labeled insulin glargine (HOE 901) in

healthy men: Comparison with NPH insulin and the influence on different subcutaneous injection sites. Diabetes Care 2000; 23, 813-819.
8. Rosskamp R, Park G. Long-acting insulin analogs. Diabetes Care 1999; 22 (Suppl. 2):B109-B113.
9. Rosenstock J, Park G, Zimmerman J; U.S. Insulin Glargine (HOE 901) Diabetes Investigator Group. Basal insulin glargine (HOE 901) versus NPH insulin in patients with type 1 diabetes on multiple daily insulin regimens. Diabetes Care 2000; 23, 1137-1142.
10. Mohn A, Strang S, Lang AM, Edge JA, Dunger DB. Nocturnal glucose control and free insulin levels in children with type 1 diabetes by use of the long-acting insulin HOE 901 as part of a three-injection regimen. Diabetes Care 2000; 23, 557-559.
11. Ratner RE, Hirsch IB, Neifing JL, Garg SK, Mecca TE, Wilson CA. Less hypoglycemia with insulin glargine in intensive insulin therapy for type 1 diabetes. U.S. Study Group of Insulin Glargine in Type 1 Diabetes. Diabetes Care 2000; 23, 639-643.
12. Brunner GA, Sendlhofer G, Wutte A, et al. Pharmacokinetic and pharmcodynamic properties of long-acting insulin analogue NN304 in comparison to NPH insulin in humans. Exp Clin Endocrinol Diabetes 2000; 108, 100-105.
13. ISPAD. Consensus Guidelines 2000, ed, International Society for Pediatric and Adolescent Diabetes, Medical Forum International, Zeist, Netherlands.
14. Skyler J Lancet 2001; 357:331.
15. American Diabetes Association. Clincial Practice Recommendation 2001. Diabetes Care 2001; 24 (Suppl. 1), S1-S126.
16. White JA, Hirsch IB. Acute complications of diabetes. Endocrinol Metab 2000.
17. American Diabetes Association. Medical management of type 1 diabetes, 3rd edition. American Diabetes Association, Alexandria, VA, 1998.
18. American Diabetes Association. Standards of medical care for patients with diabetes mellitus. Diabetes Care 1997; 20(Suppl 1): S5-S13.
19. Kaufman FR. Diabetes in children and adolescents: Areas of controversy. Med Clin North Am 1998; 82, 721-737.
20. Kaufman FR, Halvorson M, Miller D, MacKenzie M, Fisher LK, Pitukcheewanont P. Insulin pump therapy in type 1 pediatric

patients: Now and into the year 2000. Diabetes Metab Res Rev 1999; 15, 338-352.

21. Kaufman FR, Halvorson M, Fisher LK, Pitukcheewanont P. Insulin pump therapy in type 1 pediatric patients. J Pediatr Endocrinol Metab 1999; 12, 759-764.
22. Steindel BS, Roe TF, Costin G, Carlson M, Kaufman FR. Continuous subcutaneous insulin infusion (CSII) in children and adolescents with chronic poorly controlled type 1 diabetes mellitus. Diabetes Res Clin Pract 1995; 27, 199-204.
23. Boland EA, Grey M, Oesterle A, Fredrickson L, Tamborlane WV. Continuous subcutaneous insulin infusion. Diabetes Care 1999; 22, 1779-1784.
24. Mortensen HB, Hartling SG, Petersen KE, the Danish Study Group of Diabetes in Childhood. A nation-wide cross-sectional study of glycosylated hemoglobin in Danish children with type 1 diabetes. Diabet Med 1998; 5, 871-876.
25. Mortensen HB, Villumsen J, Volund A, Petersen KE, Nerup J, the Danish Study Group of Diabetes in Childhood. Relationship between insulin injection regimen and metabolic control in young Danish type 1 diabetic patients. Diabet Med 1992; 9, 834-839.
26. Mortensen HB, Hougaard P. Comparison of metabolic control in a cross-sectional study of 1,873 children and adolescents with IDDM from 18 countries. Diabetes Care 1997; 20, 714-720.
27. Anderson B, Ho J, Brackett J, Finkelstein D, Laffel L. Parental involvement in diabetes management tasks: Relationships to blood glucose monitoring adherence and metabolic control in young adolescents with insulin-dependent diabetes mellitus. J Pediatr 1997; 130, 257-265.
28. Nathan DM, McKitrick C, Larkin M, Schaffran R, Singer DE. Glycemic control in diabetes mellitus: Have changes in therapy made a difference? 1996; 100, 157-163.
29. Levine B-S, Anderson BJ, Butler DA, Antisdel JE, Brackett J, Laffel LMB. Predictors of glycemic control and short-term adverse outcomes in youth with type 1 diabetes. J Pediatr 2001; 139, 197-203.
30. American Diabetes Association. Postprandial blood glucose. Diabetes Care 2001; 24, 775-778.
31. Bode BW, Gross TM, Thornton KR, Mastrototoro JM. Continuous glucose monitoring used to adjust diabetes therapy improves

glycosylated hemoglobin: A pilot study. Diabetes Research and Clinical Practice 1999; 46, 183-190.
32. Chase HP, Kim LM, Owen SL, et al. Continuous subcutaneous glucose monitoring in children with type 1 diabetes. Pediatrics 2001; 107, 222-226.
33. Garg SK, Potts RO, Ackerman NR, Fermi SI, Tamada JA, Chase HP. Correlation of finger stick blood glucose measurements with glucowatch biographer glucose results in young subjects with type 1 diabetes. Diabetes Care 1999; 22, 1708-1714.
34. Pitzer KR, Desai S, Dunn T, Edelman S, Jayalakshmi Y, Kennedy J, Tamada JA, Potts RO. Detection of hypoglycemia with the GlucoWatch Biographer. Diabetes Care 2001; 24, 881-886.
35. Lawlor MT, Laffel LMB. New technologies and therapeutic approaches for the management of pediatric diabetes. Current Diabetes Reports 2001; 1, 56-66.
36. Byrne HA, Tieszen KL, Hollis S, Dornan TL, New JP. Evaluation of an electrochemical sensor for measuring blood ketones. Diabetes Care 2000; 23, 500-503.
37. Fulop M, Murphy V, Michilli A, et al. Serum B-hydroxybutyrate measurement in patients with uncontrolled diabetes mellitus. Arch Intern Med 1999; 159, 381-384.
38. Cryer PE. Hypoglycemia: The limiting factor in the management of IDDM. Diabetes 1994; 43, 1378-1389.
39. Cox DJ, Kovatchev BP, Julian DM, et al. Frequency of severe hypoglycemia in insulin-dependent diabetes mellitus can be predicted from self-monitoring of blood glucose data. J Clin Endocrinol Metab 1994; 79,1659-1662.
40. Bhatia V, Wolfsdorf JI. Severe hypoglycemia in youth with insulin-dependent diabetes mellitus: frequency and causative factors. Pediatrics 1991; 88,1187-1193.
41. Nordfeldt S, Ludvigsson J. Severe hypoglycemia in children with IDDM: a prospective population study,1992 – 1994. Diabetes Care 1997; 20,487-503.
42. Beregszaszi M, Tubiana-Rufi N, Benali K, Noel M, Bloch J, Czernichow P. Nocturnal hypoglycemia in children and adolescents with insulin-dependent diabetes mellitus. Prevalence and risk factors. J Pediatr 1997; 131,27-33.
43. Kaufman FR. Searching for glycemic control in pediatric type 1 diabetes: A long way to go. J Pediatr 2001; 139, 174-176.

44. Danne T, Mortensen HB, Hougaard P, et al. Persistent differences among centers over 3 years in glycemic control and hypoglycemia in a study of 3,805 children and adolescents with type 1 diabetes from the Hvidore study group. Diabetes Care 2001; 24, 1342-1347.
45. Kaufman FR. (1997). Diabetes mellitus. Pediatr Res 1997; 18, 383-392.
46. Buckingham BA, Bluck B, Wilson DM. Intensive diabetes management in pediatric patients. Current Diabetes Reports 2001; 1, 11-18.
47. Kaufman FR, Halvorson M, Carpenter S. Use of a plastic insulin dosage guide to correct blood glucose levels of the target range and for carbohydrate counting in subjects with type 1 diabetes. Diabetes Care 1999; 22, 1252-1257.
48. Skyler JS, Skyler DL, Seigler DE. Algorithms for adjustment of insulin dosage by patients who monitor blood glucose. Diabetes Care 1981; 4, 311-318.
49. Kaufman FR, Halvorson M. New trends in managing type 1 diabetes. Contemporary Pediatrics 1999; 16, 112-123.
50. Haymond MW, Schreiner B. Mini-dose glucagons rescue for hypoglycemia in children with type 1 diabetes. Diabetes Care 2001; 24, 643-645.
51. Jacobson AM, Hauser ST, Willett J, Wolfsdorf JI, Herman L. Consequences of irregular versus continuous medical follow-up in children and adolescents with insulin-dependent diabetes mellitus. J Pediatr 1997; 131, 727-733.
52. Kaufman FR, Halvorson M, Carpenter S. Association between diabetes control and visits to a multidisciplinary pediatric diabetes clinic. Pediatrics 1999; 103, 948-951.
53. Meltzer LJ, Bennett Johnson S, Prine JM, Banks RA, Desrosiers PM, Silverstein JH. Disordered eating, body mass, and glycemic control in adolescents with type 1 diabetes. Diabetes Care 2001; 24, 678-682.
54. Rosenbloom AL. Skeletal and joint manifestations of childhood diabetes. Pediatr Clin North Am 1984; 31, 569-589.
55. Carlsson A, Axelsson IE, Borulf SK, et al. Prevalence of IgA-antiendomysium and IgA-antigliadin autoantibodies at diagnosis of insulin-dependent diabetes mellitus in Swedish children and adolescents. Pediatrics 1999; 103, 1248-1252.

56. American Diabetes Association. Care of children with diabetes in the school and day care setting. Diabetes Care 2000; 23 (Suppl 1), S100-103.

CHAPTER 12
INSULIN PUMP THERAPY

Jo Ann H. Ahern, APRN, MSN, CDE, Elizabeth A. Boland, APRN, MSN, CDE and William V. Tamborlane, MD
From the Yale-New Haven Children's Hospital/The Children's Clinical Research Center and the Yale University School of Medicine Department of Pediatrics, New Haven, CT

BACKGROUND

Continuous subcutaneous insulin infusion (CSII) pump therapy was introduced to treat patients with type 1 diabetes (T1DM) more than 20 years ago[1,2]. At that time, most children and adolescents were being treated with one or two daily injections of mixtures of NPH and regular insulin of animal origin and treatment was adjusted based on urinary glucose excretion. With these inadequate methods, it's not surprising that glucose levels often averaged over 300 mg/dl and that the children were at high risk for the later development of the devastating complications of diabetes. CSII offered the opportunity to more closely simulate the patterns of plasma insulin levels seen in normal children. The more predictable pharmacokinetics of fast-acting versus intermediate-acting insulin[3] and the administration of bolus doses immediately prior to each meal were two obvious advantages of this approach to insulin replacement. The development of newer, smaller pumps with variable basal rate profiles allowed for a closer match in insulin needs, particularly overnight, leading to a reduction in nocturnal hypoglycemia.

The development of pump therapy in the late '70's coincided with the introduction of self monitoring of blood glucose (SMBG), HbA1c assays, and more aggressive approaches to conventional insulin therapy, using multiple daily insulin injections (MDI). It was suggested that these new technologies might finally provide the means to achieve glucose levels closer to normal. The achievement of this improved level of control would allow the diabetes community to determine if microvascular complications of diabetes could be prevented or delayed[1]. This issue was finally resolved in 1993 with publication of the results of the Diabetes Control and Complications Trial[4]. Even in the relatively small subset of adolescents who were 13-17 years of age on entry in the DCCT, intensive treatment significantly reduced the risk of onset and progression of retinopathy and microalbuminuria[5]. Subsequent follow-up of adolescents in the DCCT has shown that the risk of these complications remained reduced four years after completion of the DCCT, even though HbA1c levels no longer differed between former intensive and former conventional treatment group patients [6]. Thus, it has been recommended that the goals of treatment in children with diabetes should be to achieve glucose and HbA1c levels as close to normal as possible beginning at diagnosis.

Despite the pharmacokinetic and other recognized advantages of CSII over conventional insulin injection regimens and the requirement for fewer shots than MDI therapy, CSII was used in very small numbers of children until recently. Factors that limited more widespread use of this method of insulin delivery in children were the large size and difficulties in use of early pumps, psychological issues about wearing an external device, the extra costs of pump therapy[7], and the introduction of insulin pens for more convenient MDI therapy. The most important obstacle to use of these devices, however, was uncertainty regarding the long-term benefits of intensive treatment itself.

Over the past decade there has been a number of important improvements in pump technology that have made the devices easier for children with diabetes to use. They are smaller, programming is simpler, they have more alarms, spring-loaded devices are available to inject the catheters under the skin, and the quick release mechanism in the infusion set allows the pump to be disconnected while leaving the catheter or needle in place under the skin. The results of the DCCT removed the most important obstacle to use of pumps in children; namely, the uncertainty regarding the benefits of intensive treatment itself. The demonstration that glycemic control has a preeminent role in the pathogenesis of microvascular complications has been accompanied by a dramatic increase in the use of insulin pumps in children in the United States and elsewhere. As pediatric treatment teams have been challenged to find more effective methods to achieve intensive treatment goals, the newer, smaller, safer, and easier to use insulin pumps have been rediscovered. Over the past four years there has been a more than 20-fold increase in the number of patients under 20 years of age starting on insulin pumps annually in the U.S. Despite the newly found popularity of CSII in children, some pediatric endocrinologists continue to question the justification for its use. This is due, in part, to the lack of published data regarding this "new" approach to treatment of childhood diabetes.

While there have been no randomized comparisons of CSII and MDI in youth with well established diabetes, the DCCT results provide a gold standard by which to judge the usefulness of CSII in non-randomized studies and descriptive reports of clinical outcomes. During the course of the DCCT, intensively treated adolescents were able to achieve and maintain HbA1c levels at a mean of 8.1% (normal ≤ 6.0 %)[5]. However, improved diabetes control was achieved at the cost of a 3-fold increase in the risk of hypoglycemia compared to conventional treatment. During the first 12 months of study, the frequency of severe hypoglycemic events requiring the assistance of another person in intensively treated adolescents was approximately 1 event per patient per year and 40% of these episodes resulted in seizure or coma.

EFFICACY OF CSII IN YOUTH: YALE EXPERIENCE

Enthusiasm for the use of CSII in our patients was renewed as a result of our experience in the DCCT. We were anxious to apply the pump technology to our clinic population to achieve improved levels of diabetes control. Furthermore, we decided to test this formally in the adolescent population in a study we called the ABC's (Adolescents Benefit from Control) of Diabetes Study. One of the aims of this study was to determine whether DCCT recommendations regarding intensive therapy could be achieved in a large group of adolescents in a single center. The study also addressed the question of whether the increased burdens of intensive therapy had adverse psychosocial effects in teenagers[8]. As in the DCCT, the 75 patients enrolled in our study were allowed to select their method of insulin administration; 25 selected CSII and 50 patients selected MDI.

Both MDI- and CSII-treated patients initially exhibited improved metabolic control during the first six months of study. However, this level of control was more difficult to sustain with MDI treatment, so that $HbA1_c$ levels were higher in MDI vs CSII patients after 12 months (8.3 vs 7.5%, Figure 1). Most impressive, the rate of severe hypoglycemia was 50% lower with CSII versus MDI, even in the face of lower HbA_{1C} levels in the CSII group[8]. In general, psychosocial well-being improved in both groups of adolescents. However, CSII-treated patients felt that it was easier to cope with diabetes. We concluded from these results that in comparison to MDI, CSII provided a safer and easier means to achieve intensive treatment goals in adolescents.

Figure 1

Yale Adolescent Study
Metabolic control: 12 months of treatment

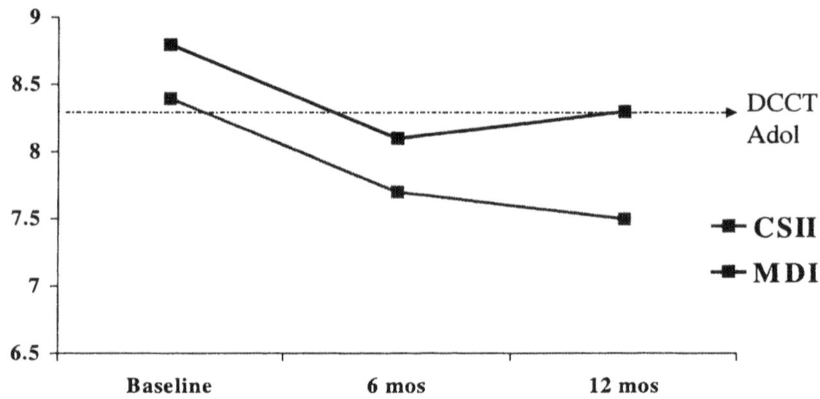

Boland et al: Diabetes Care 1999;22:1779-1784

Interpretation of how our ABC's of Diabetes Study results translate to the diabetes clinic setting was limited because of the small sample size, failure to include children less than 12 years of age, and the research environment in which the study was performed. It should also be noted that all of the teenagers in our adolescent study were using regular insulin[7], whereas most CSII-treated patients are currently using lispro or aspart insulin. In CSII-treated adults, lispro insulin has been shown to lower HbA1c levels and reduces the risk of hypoglycemia compared to regular insulin[9], presumably due to the more rapid onset and shorter duration of premeal bolus doses[10].

Following the success of the ABC's Study, our multidisciplinary treatment team has made much more extensive use of CSII in the Pediatric Diabetes Clinic. Consequently, the number of children using CSII has grown dramatically and almost all are using rapid acting insulin analogs. In a recent report, we described clinical outcomes in the first 161 patients (aged 18 months to 18 years) who were started on CSII in our Pediatric Diabetes Clinic since 1997[11]. Only patients with T1DM who had been followed in our

Children's Diabetes Clinic for at least one year prior to the start of pump therapy were included in the study and clinical data were collected prospectively before and during pump treatment using standardized report forms. Of the 161 children who were studied, 26 were preschoolers (< 7 yrs), 76 were school-aged (7-11 yrs) and 59 were adolescents (12-18 yrs). In the three age groups, mean $HbA1_c$ levels were 7.1% in the preschoolers, 7.8% in the school-aged and 8.1% in the adolescents prior to the start of CSII. There was a significant and consistent reduction in mean $HbA1_c$ levels by 0.6-0.7% after 12 months of CSII in all three groups that was maintained at the most recent visit, 26±9 months after the start of CSII (Figure 2). Improved diabetes control was achieved with CSII without increasing daily insulin doses and in association with a 32 % decrease in the frequency of severe hypoglycemic events (Table 1). The greatest decrease in the frequency of severe hypoglycemia was in the pre-school patients. From these data, we concluded that CSII is an effective alternative to injection therapy in a large Pediatric Diabetes Clinic setting and that even very young patients can utilize CSII to safely lower $HbA1_c$ levels[11].

Table 1. Frequency of severe hypoglycemia during 12 months before and after CSII in the first 161 children started on pump therapy in the Yale Diabetes Clinic between 1997 and 2000. Data are shown as the number of events, and in parenthesis, event rate (number/patient/year)

	Prepump	Postpump
Preschool	11 (0.42)	5 (0.19)
School age	25 (0.33)	17 (0.22)
Adolescents	20 (0.33)	16 (0.27)
Total	56 (0.35)	38 (0.24)*

*p<0.05 vs prepump

Figure 2

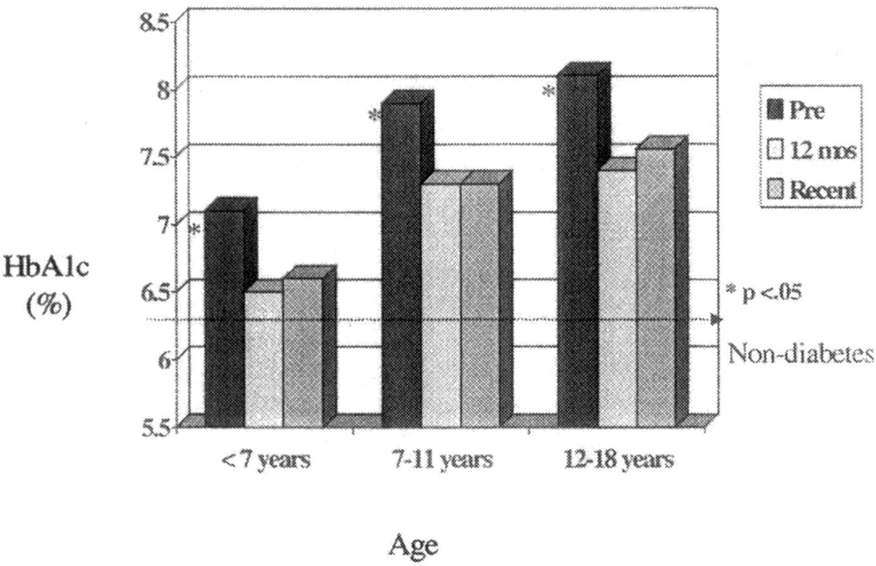

The number of youngsters utilizing CSII in our Diabetes Clinic has continued to grow. Nearly half of the patients (i.e., 300 out of 630 children <18 years) are currently using CSII and the results to date have been excellent. The most recent $HbA1_c$ level in our pump patients was 7.3±1.2% (mean ± SD); whereas HbA1c levels averaged 8.0±1.6% in those using injection therapy. Moreover, more than 95% of children who have started pump treatment have remained on this therapy, as of their last clinic visit.

EFFICACY OF CSII IN YOUTH: RESULTS AT OTHER CENTERS

In view of the relatively recent increase in use of CSII in children, it is not surprising that published data regarding the efficacy of this approach to therapy is relatively sparse. There has been only one randomized, prospective study comparing CSII and MDI in youth with diabetes and that study compared the two therapies in newly diagnosed patients[12]. Although HbA1c levels were lower in the CSII group, beta cell function was not prolonged[12]. Tubiana-Rufi et al. were the first to demonstrate the usefulness of pump therapy in very young patients[13]. They studied infants and toddlers who were experiencing recurrent episodes of hypoglycemia while on injection therapy. After switching to pump treatment, the frequency of severe hypoglycemic events was sharply reduced without sacrificing overall diabetes control.

In a preliminary report, Buckingham and colleagues noted improved diabetes control and greater parent satisfaction with treatment in their infants and toddlers who switched from injection to pump therapy[14].

Maniatis and colleagues at the Barbara Davis Center in Denver have reported their clinic experience in applying CSII in children and adolescents with T1DM[15]. Data from 56 patients (7-23 years old) were collected during regularly scheduled visits at a frequency similar to non-CSII patients. Compared to pre-pump values, there was only a modest decrease in HbA1c levels from 8.5% to 8.3%. However, the rate of severe hypoglycemia before and on CSII therapy also decreased from 12.3 to 9.5 events per 100 patient years and a statistically significant proportion of patients reported a decrease in seizure frequency. There was no clinically significant increase in BMI, even in the patients with improved metabolic control. They concluded that CSII is an appropriate option for some children in routine pediatric diabetes care. It can effectively decrease the HbA1c and reduce hypoglycemic episodes, without producing an abnormal increase in BMI. In preliminary communications, White, et al.[16] and Celona-Jacobs, et al.[17] have also reported a reduction in the frequency of severe hypoglycemia in children with CSII, even though HbA1c levels did not change appreciably. Children who started on CSII at the Joslin Clinic experienced only at transient lowering of HbA1c levels that was difficult to sustain[18].

Kaufman et al. have examined whether insulin pump treatment when used only at night could improve fasting and nighttime blood glucose levels in children less than 10 years of age without having adverse effects[19]. The rationale for the study was that there may be a group of 7-10 year olds who would not be able to use the pump when at school due to lack of school nurses but could use it at home under the supervision of their parents. Ten children with T1DM were studied using a randomized, crossover design with 6 weeks of treatment with each form of therapy (CSII just at night, with injections during the day vs. only injections). Compared to baseline and injection therapy periods, improved control was observed with CSII. They concluded that use of the CSII at night alone should be considered in young children who are incapable of independently managing an insulin pump. Of course an alternative approach is to organize and educate school personnel and other caregivers regarding the use of CSII when a parent or guardian is not present.

PRACTICAL ASPECTS OF CSII IN YOUTH

The approach utilized at our center to initiate and manage pump therapy in children and adolescents will be briefly summarized in this section. The reader is also referred to other useful reviews and monographs that discuss special considerations in using CSII in youth with T1DM[20,21].

Multidisciplinary Team Management

As with MDI, successful use of CSII depends in part on the skill and enthusiasm of the multidisciplinary team of clinicians who are dedicated to the treatment of childhood diabetes. At our center, the diabetes nurse specialists (all advanced practice nurses) are the key members of the team who interact most frequently with the patients and parents[22]. These primary nurse managers remain in close contact with the families between office visits by telephone, email, and fax to adjust the treatment regimen and to maintain their commitment to treatment goals. Other members of the team, including the dietitian, social worker, and pediatric endocrinologist, support the patients whenever their particular expertise is required or desired.

Patient Selection

Family is a key component in making the decision for the best method to achieve glucose goals as close to normal as possible. Even in adolescents, successful management of diabetes depends on an effective partnership between the parent and child[23]. In order to be considered for CSII, the child or parent must be performing at least 4 blood glucose tests per day, be committed to the goals of intensive treatment, have demonstrated consistent follow-up of regularly scheduled clinic appointments and be knowledgeable regarding general principles of diabetes management (Table 2). Knowledge of carbohydrate counting and use of carbohydrate to insulin ratios and correction boluses is preferred. Adolescents must want to try CSII themselves. Many of our patients are exposed to other children using insulin pumps at diabetes camp and at school and request this form of treatment for themselves. We introduce the idea of switching from injections to an insulin pump in patients who are having wide swings in blood glucose, are having frequent episodes of hypoglycemia, are very active in sports, or have irregular meal schedules. Patients and parents are given videos and printed materials that describe further what this therapy entails.

Table 2: Getting CSII started

Indications
- An infant /toddler
- Older children themselves want to try CSII
- Wide and unpredictable swings in blood glucose
- Hypoglycemia
- Need increased flexibility for sports and irregular meal schedules

Eligibility Criteria
- 4 blood glucose tests per day
- Committed to intensive treatment goals
- Supportive and knowledgeable family
- Consistent follow-up of schedules visits

Starting Treatment

The first step in switching from injection therapy to CSII is to secure insurance coverage for the costs of the device and disposable supplies. In most cases, this is an easier task than in the past. We do not admit the children to the hospital or require adherence tests like wearing a saline pump or doing multiple daily injection prior to the start of pump therapy. Instead, initiation of pump therapy is accomplished in two, 60-90 minute outpatient sessions. During the first session, they are instructed on basic pump features including setting basal rates and giving bolus doses, as well as filling the reservoir, priming the tubing and injecting the catheter. Initial basal rates and bolus doses are determined at this time.

We start most children on a basal rate that is equal to 50% of the TDD of insulin that the patient is presently taking by injections. Children require an increased basal rate from 9PM to 3AM and decreased one from 3AM to 6AM. They are then given a chart with their insulin/carbohydrate ratio and correction boluses (Table 3). Thus, the initial basal rate in a child who is receiving a total dose of 30 units of insulin per day would be 15 units divided by 24 hours or 12AM 0.7, 3AM0.5, 7AM-9PM 0.6 and 9PM 0.7 units/hour. All patients use rapid acting insulin analogs unless they have had some unusual reaction to these insulins[24] or for special sports.

Table 3_ Sample worksheet for patient/parent/school/sitters for pre-meal bolus doses and correction doses

Insulin Pump Doses

0.3 units/carb

Patient Name

MEALS		CORRECTION	
Carbs (G)	INSULIN	BG	Insulin to add
5	0.1	150-180	0.1
10	0.2	181-210	0.2
15	0.3	211-240	0.3
20	0.4	241-270	0.4
25	0.5	271-300	0.5
30	0.6	301-330	0.6
35	0.7	331-360	0.7
40	0.8	361-390	0.8
45	0.9	391-420	0.9
50	1	421-450	1
55	1.1	451-480	1.1
60	1.2	481-510	1.2
65	1.3	511-540	1.3
70	1.4	541-570	1.4
75	1.5	571-600	1.5

Several approaches can be taken for the selection of the initial insulin to carbohydrate ratios used for bolus doses with CSII. If the patients are already using carbohydrate to insulin ratios with injection therapy, these ratios can be used for CSII as well. However, this approach may underestimate meal requirements with CSII, if they are using pre-meal mixtures that include intermediate acting insulin. We usually start with insulin to carbohydrate ratios that are based on age. For each 15-gram serving of carbohydrate, we start with 0.3units for children <5 years, 0.5 units for 5-7 year olds, 0.7 units for 8-11 year olds, 1.0 units for 12-14 year olds and 1.5 units or more in 15-18 year olds. Initial correction doses, are usually based on the insulin to carbohydrate ratio -- the amount of insulin required for 15 grams of carbohydrate will also lower glucose levels by approximately about 100 mg/dl (Table 3).

After completion of the first visit, parents and the patients are asked to check blood glucose levels before meals, and at 12 AM and 3AM for the next 2-3 days. They call in blood glucose results the next day and come in for a second visit on the day after. The main purpose of the second visit is to have the patients demonstrate that they can refill the pump and change the catheter site and are also able to change basal rates based on our recommendations. They are scheduled for a regular follow-up visit in three months. Further adjustments in bolus and basal insulin doses are made over the telephone based on blood glucose results, as we would do with any other patient.

Site Selection and Care

There are several different infusion sets and these need to be evaluated for each patient based on size of the patient and preference. Some infusion sets disconnect right on the set, whereas others leave a three-inch segment of tubing connected to the infusion set. Some sets require additional tape to hold them in place, whereas others are self-sticking. For the very thin or young child, a catheter that goes in at an angle is the catheter of choice. Those who are older and have enough subcutaneous fat tissue can utilize catheters that go in at a 90-degree angle. Ninety degree angle sets come in shorter lengths for thin children. Most infusion sets are inserted with a spring-activated devise that makes insertion simpler and almost painless. The site should be cleansed with an IV Prep pad prior to inserting the set. Patients should not use alcohol pads, as they dry out the skin. Usually, the infusion set is placed in either the buttocks or abdomen. In children, the buttock is the preferred site because the catheter is less likely to come out. The site needs to be changed every 2-3 days. Use of a topical anesthetic cream is not usually necessary. If families request that such a cream be used, we usually recommend Ela-max® because of its quick action (15 minutes) and the fact that it does not cause vasoconstriction like other products such as Emla®.

DKA Prevention

All patients who use pump treatment must continue to test blood sugar levels at least four times/day. Since the pump contains only rapid acting insulin, patients can develop diabetic ketoacidosis rapidly if the pump malfunctions or the catheter dislodges[25]. The way to avoid this is to test frequently. If the pre-breakfast blood glucose level is greater than 250 mg/dl, the catheter should be changed, especially if the child will be going off to school. If any glucose level is greater than 250mg/dl at other times of the day, a correction bolus should be given, and the patient should recheck blood glucose level in one hour. If there is no reduction in the blood glucose, a correction dose should be given with an insulin syringe or pen and the site should be changed. Ketones should be checked if glucose is >250 two times in a row or patient feels nauseous. If ketonuria is present, a correction insulin dose should be given by injection, and the site should be changed immediately.

Hypoglycemia Treatment

Once patients begin pump therapy, they often need less carbohydrate for treating a low blood glucose level. This is may be due to the shorter duration of the insulin used with pump treatment. Since there is no large depot of insulin under the skin, hypoglycemia is more quickly reversed than on injection therapy. Parents and patients are often surprised by this and will need to relearn how much carbohydrate is needed to treat a low glucose level. We usually recommend either glucose tablets or juice for treatment, and that 8 gm of carbohydrate be taken if blood glucose is 51-70 mg/dl, 15 gm if it is 41-50 mg/dl and 30 gm if it is below 40 mg/dl.

Day Care and Nursery School Issues

Children in the day care setting may provide a challenge to insulin pump treatment. Most day care programs have cooperated with the parents and the diabetes treatment team. Young children are not able to check glucose levels or give bolus doses without assistance. In many instances, it has been helpful to incorporate the bolus dose for morning snack into the basal rate profile. For example, if the child is eating a morning snack of 15gms of carbohydrate at 10:30 AM and the insulin to carbohydrate ratio is 0.3 units/15 gm CHO, we increase the basal rate by 0.3 units between 10 to 11 AM. This approach causes less disruption of normal activities and allows the day care provider to give a snack without worrying about giving a bolus at this hectic time of day. At lunch, the day care provider/nursery school teacher checks the glucose level and gives a bolus based on the insulin to carbohydrate ratio and blood glucose level (Table 3). Day care providers must be able to check blood glucose and recognize the signs/symptoms of hypoglycemia in this young age group. They should also be given specific guidelines for treatment of hypoglycemia.

School Issues

School is one of the barriers that need to be overcome with pump treatment. Every school has its own policies to care for children with diabetes and children treated with the insulin pump. Most of the young children go to the nurse to check the blood sugar level before lunch and to receive their lunch bolus. The parent who packs a lunch for the child counts the carbohydrates and places a card with the amount in the child's lunch bag. The nurse has a written protocol with the insulin/carbohydrate ratio and the correction bolus doses. If the child has been giving the correct bolus doses on a regular basis, the parents and nurse may agree that the child can do this without supervision. If this results in doses being missed, then the child goes back to doing these tasks in the nurse's office. Older children are encouraged to check glucose levels and give bolus doses before lunch on their own and preferably in the classroom.

Sports and Exercise

Most children are involved in activities that involve exercise in one form or another. Many are involved in organized sports. Using the pump makes this easier but each sport requires doing something different with the pump.

Swimming

The pump is removed for this sport. Most swimmers don't want any "drag" so even if the pump is waterproof, it is removed. Since the patient is on rapid acting insulin, it cannot be off for more than 2 hours. We ask them to re-connect and give 1 hour's basal rate as a bolus and then remove it again for 2 more hours if necessary. Another option is to take some Regular insulin before removing the pump and that will allow 4-5 hours off of the pump. If families live at the beach in the summer, some choose to switch the insulin in the pump to Regular instead of Lispro or Aspart. This allows more time off of the pump. Most do not do this for only a day at the beach or pool.

Soccer, football, basketball, hockey, and tennis

These sports involve spurts of activity and are very aerobic. The pump is usually removed for these sports and the need for bolus doses before and after the pump is removed is determined by trial and error. Because children are more active during practices, blood glucose levels may drop. However, with competitive games, blood glucose levels can rise significantly because of the stress of the event, as well as the fact that the children may have less playing time. When starting a new sport, they should not take a bolus before disconnecting. Instead, they simply check blood glucose levels at half time and again at the end of the practice or game. If glucose levels rise dramatically during the game, then a bolus dose should be taken before removal and/or at the half time of the next game. If glucose levels fall during practices, a small snack without a bolus before or during the practice may be necessary.

Baseball

Most of our patients wear the pump during this sport since the activity is minimal most of the time. If the child is a catcher or pitcher, he/she may need to put a temporary basal rate in at ½ the usual basal rate. For those that slide, the pump could be removed when at bat. Again some choose to remove the pump and take regular insulin for the game.

Hiking, biking and skiing

For these activities that are usually prolonged, the pump should be set at a temporary basal rate of ½ of the usual basal for the duration of the activity. This works very well since the pump will automatically return to the normal basal rate at the end of the activity. If the activity is terminated early, the temporary basal rate can be cancelled manually by going into the program and adjusting the duration down to 0.

Gymnastics/Dance

These activities can be tricky. Most do not want to wear the pump during these activities. Many of the patients become hypoglycemic in the first hour and then hyperglycemic at the end of the activity. Some need to remove the pump ½ hour before the activity begins in order to remain normoglycemic for the first hour, but are then hyperglycemic at the end. Some choose to eat a snack and take a bolus before so that they have a little insulin "on board" during the activity. Some refuse to eat before. If glucose level is normal or high at the end of the activity, the patients are instructed to bolus 1 hour's basal rate plus the correction bolus if >140mg/dl.

There is no "right" way for all patients to accommodate these activities. Different methods may be utilized until satisfactory results are achieved. These are simply some examples of different methods that have worked for most pump patients.

THE FUTURE

Even with CSII, management of childhood diabetes is difficult and the risk of severe hypoglycemia remains unacceptably high. These problems are related, in part, to limitations in the ability of conventional pre-meal and bedtime self-monitoring of blood glucose (SMBG) to reflect overall glucose control. Results of studies with continuous glucose monitoring systems have shown that conventional SMBG often misses marked post-prandial hyperglycemia and asymptomatic nocturnal hypoglycemia in youth with T1DM[26,27]. By combining continuous glucose monitoring with CSII, clinicians may have a means to more fully utilize the variable basal and bolus dose capabilities of CSII leading to even safer and more effective treatment. Even more exciting, however, is the prospect of combining the capabilities of these technologies. We may finally be at the threshold of the development of a practically applicable artificial pancreas, a prospect that has been anticipated for more than 25 years[28].

ACKNOWLEDGEMENTS

This work was supported by grants from the National Institutes of Health (RR06022), the Juvenile Diabetes Research Foundation, and the Stephen I. Morse Pediatric Diabetes Research Fund.

REFERENCES

1. Tamborlane WV, Sherwin RS, Genel M, Felig P. Reduction to normal of plasma glucose in juvenile diabetics by subcutaneous administration of insulin with a portable infusion pump. N Engl J Med 1979; 300:578.
2. Pickup JC, Keen H, Parsons JA, Alberti KGMM. Continuous subcutaneous insulin infusion: an approach to achieving normoglycemia. Br Med J 1978; 1:204-207.
3. Lauritzen T, Pramming S, Deckert T, Binder C. Pharmacokinetics of continuous subcutaneous insulin infusion. Diabetologia 1983; 24:326-329.
4. DCCT Research Group. The effects of intensive diabetes treatment on the development and progression of long-term complications in insulin-dependent diabetes mellitus. The Diabetes Control and Complications Trial. N Engl J Med 1993; 329:977-986.
5. The DCCT Research Group. The effect of intensive diabetes treatment on the development and progression of long-term complications in

adolescents with insulin-dependent diabetes mellitus: the Diabetes Control and Complications Trial. J Pediatr 1994; 125:177-188.
6. DCCT/EDIC Research Group. Prolonged beneficial effects of intensive therapy of diabetes during adolescence: microvascular outcomes four years after conclusion of the Diabetes Control and Complications Trial. J Pediatr 2001; 139: 804-812
7. DCCT Research Group. Resource utilization and costs of care in the Diabetes Control and Complications Trial. Diabetes Care 1995; 18:1468-1478.
8. Boland EA, Grey M, Fredrickson L, Tamborlane WV. CSII: a "new" way to achieve strict metabolic control, decrease severe hypoglycemia and enhance coping in adolescents with type I diabetes. Diabetes Care 1999; 22:1779-1894.
9. Zinman B, Tildesley H, Chiasson TJ, Tsue E, Strack T. Insulin lispro in CSII: results of a double-blind crossover study. Diabetes 1997; 46:440-443.
10. Howey DC, Bowsher RR, Brunelle RL, Woodworth JR. [Lys(B28),Pro(B29)]-human insulin. A rapidly absorbed analogue of human insulin. Diabetes 1994; 43:396-402.
11. Ahern JH, Boland EA, Doane R, Vincent M, Tamborlane WV. Insulin pump therapy in pediatrics: a therapeutic alternative to safely lower therapy HbA1c levels across all age groups. Pediatric Diabetes, in press
12. de Beaufort CE, Houtzager CMGJ, Bruining GJ et al: Continuous Subcutaneous Insulin Infusion (CSII) Versus Conventional Injection Therapy in Newly Diagnosed Diabetic Children: Two-year Follow-up of a Randomized, Prospective Trial. *Diabetic Medicine*, 6:766-71, 1989
13. Tubiana-Rufi N, deLonlay P, Block J, Czernichow P. Remission of severe hypoglycemia incidents in young diabetic children treated with subcutaneous infusion. Arch Pediatr 1996; 3:969-976.
14. Buckingham BA, Paguntalan H, Fassl B, Wilson DM. Continuous subcutaneous infusio (CSII) in children under five years of age. Diabetes 2001; 50 (Suppl. 2): A107.
15. Maniatis AK, Klingensmith GJ, Slover RH, Mowry CJ, Chase HP. Continuous subcutaneous insulin infusion therapy for children and adolescents: an option for routine diabetes care. Pediatrics 2002; 107:351-356.
16. White NH, Hollander AS, Sadler M, Daniels L. Risks and benefits of continuous subcutaneous insulin infusion (CSII) therapy in children. Diabetes 2001; 50 (Suppl. 2):A66

17. Celona-Jacobs N, Weinzimer SA, Rearson M, Hartz D, Katz L, Murphy K. Insulin pump therapy in children: a cautionary tale. Diabetes 2001; 50 (Suppl. 2): A67.
18. Laffel L, Loughlin C, Ramchandani N, Butler D, Laffel N, Levine B-S, Anderson B. Glycemic challenges of pump therapy (CSII) in youth with type 1 diabetes (T1DM). Diabetes 2001; 50 (Suppl.2):A66.
19. Kaufman FR, Kim C, Halvorson M, Pitukcheewanont P. Use of insulin pump therapy at nighttime only for children 7-10 years of age with type 1 diabetes. Diabetes Care 2000; 23:579-582.
20. Boland EA. Teens Pumping it Up, 2nd Edition. Sylmar, CA:MiniMed, 1998.
21. Kaufman FR, Halvorson M, Miller D, Mackenzie M, Fisher, LK, Pitukcheewanont P. Insulin pump therapy in type 1 pediatric patients: now and into the year 2000. Diabetes Metab Res Rev 1999; 15:338-352.
22. Ahern JA, Ramchandani N, Cooper J, Himmel A, Silver D, Tamborlane WV. Using a primary nurse manager to implement DCCT recommendations in a large pediatric program. The Diabetes Educator 2000; 26:990-994.
23. Grey M, Boland EA, Davidson M, Li J, Tamborlane W. Coping skills training for youth on intensive therapy has long lasting effects on metabolic control and quality of life. J Pediatr 2000; 137:107-114.
24. Griffin ME, Feder A, Tamborlane WV. Lipoatrophy associated with lispro insulin in insulin pump therapy: an old complication, a new cause? *Diabetes Care* 24:174, 2001.
25. Attia N, Jones TW, Holcombe J, Tamborlane WV. Comparison of human regular insulin and lispro insulin after interruption of CSII and in the treatment of acutely decompensated IDDM. Diabetes Care 1998;21:817-821.
26. Boland EA, Monsod T, DeLucia M, Brandt C, Fernando S, Tamborlane WV. Limitations of conventional methods of self monitoring of blood glucose: lessons learned from three days of continuous glucose sensing in pediatric patients with type I diabetes. Diabetes Care 2001; 24:
27. Kaufman FR, Gibson LC, Halvorson J, Carpenter S, Fisher LK, Pitukcheewanont P. A pilot study of the continuous glucose monitoring system: clinical decisions and glycemic control after its use in pediatric type 1 diabetic subjects. Diabetes Care 2001; 24:2030-34.
28. Albisser M, Leibel BS, Ewart TG, *et al.* Clinical control of diabetes by the artificial pancreas. Diabetes 1974; 23:397-404.

Chapter 13

EDUCATION

Educating the child and family

Jean Betschart Roemer, MN, MSN, CPNP, CDE
Children's Hospital of Pittsburgh, Pittsburgh, PA

INTRODUCTION

It long has been recognized that education is a cornerstone of diabetes treatment. Daily decisions must be made based on understanding of the pathophysiology of diabetes regarding food, schedules, exercise, medication, and recognition and treatment of symptoms. Where poor knowledge or understanding of the principles of diabetes management and skills exist, self-care is likely to be poor with resulting poor glycemic control. Self-management skills are essential in order to manage diabetes effectively on a daily basis. However, even when knowledge and skills are present, without motivation to accurately perform necessary management tasks and make sound decisions, optimal glycemic control may not be achieved. Certainly this is true in both the adult population as well as pediatrics where a child or adolescent does not have the maturity and skills to consistently perform self-care, relying on parents and caregivers to do so. Diabetes education, therefore, is an essential and important component of diabetes care for children and teens with diabetes and their families.

There are inherent differences in the diabetes education and management of children and adolescents versus adults. These differences are primarily due to the dynamic nature of the developmental process and are integral to physical, cognitive, and emotional development. The health care team must understand and be sensitive to developmental issues as they foster the child and family finding a balance between self-care practices and the physical and social tasks of childhood and adolescence. Recent advances in research, technology and international efforts to promote diabetes education have improved awareness of the importance of educational support in managing children and teens and their families. Yet, these advances come with the price of a great burden of responsibility on families to do what is required of them in order to manage the diabetes.

Children and their parents must accurately measure and give injections, monitor blood glucose at least four times daily, follow a meal plan, monitor urine for ketones, be always prepared for hypoglycemia and keep records of it all. It is the child, parent and/or caregiver who must shoulder the tasks for self-management. Beyond the daily requirements, the child must be assessed by a healthcare provider at three month intervals for appropriate growth and weight gain, thyroid screening, general health, psychosocial issues, pubertal development, complications screening and diabetes control.

The treatment of diabetes in children and adolescents continues to be a challenge for health care providers. It is often difficult for children and families to be consistent about their diabetes regimen. Some do well in certain areas, such as taking medication or monitoring, yet struggle with other components such as food issues or keeping records. Patience, guidance and promoting as much flexibility in the plan as possible helps children and their families follow a specific treatment plan.

GENERAL GOALS OF DIABETES EDUCATION FOR CHILDREN, ADOLESCENTS AND THEIR FAMILIES

The nature of pediatric diabetes education is such that extensive time must be spent in the education, support and management of a child's insulin doses, food and exercise in order to achieve reasonable glycemic control. The current term for this is self-management education or self-management training[1].

The daily care and well being of children and teens depends in part on the quality and quantity of their educational experiences. However, even with quality experiences, other factors such as support and stability must also be present in order for knowledge to be able to be translated into daily practices. Therefore, the goal of education is not just to impart information, but to motivate patients and parents to use their knowledge to make well-informed decisions that will improve diabetes control on a daily basis. An informed and motivated person will have increased self-management skills, self-monitoring skills, adherence to overall management, and improved glycemia[1].

Data from the Diabetes Control and Complications Trial (DCCT) indicate that few people will maintain regimens that do not fit their lifestyle, culture and health care beliefs[2].Although the study has only been done in adults and adolescents, it can most likely be generalized to children as we consider their family characteristics. There has been little research on the optimal way to teach parents and children. However, a multidisciplinary team which includes physicians, nurse educators, dietitians, social service personnel, psychologists offers distinct advantages to meet the unique characteristics and individual needs of each child and family.

Pediatric diabetes education is unique in that it must be clearly targeted toward the developmental age of the child and also meet the needs of adult learners who are parents and caregivers. There has not been consensus regarding the best way and time to educate newly diagnosed children and their families. The benefits and outcomes of inpatient and outpatient education have not shown much difference regarding rates of readmission and/or emergency room visits, knowledge test scores, sharing of responsibilities, adherence to the diabetes regimen, family functioning scores, coping skills and perceptions of quality of life[3]. In an inpatient setting, the child and parents may be more available, but may also be in acute grief from the diagnosis itself, and the child may not feel well. Initial in-depth and ongoing education is crucial and can be the hospital, the outpatient setting or the home. Developmentally, different ages bring different diabetes-related concerns. Therefore, the multidisciplinary team of health professionals is important to education and follow-up in order that developmental issues are addressed completely at appropriate times.

The outpatient setting may be cost effective and have the advantage of keeping the child and parents in familiar surroundings, thus making the diagnosis less frightening. However, families may have reluctance or difficulty completing all of the outpatient education classes, or have a tendency not to take the education seriously. The best possible glycemic control can only be a result of diligence and commitment.

How much and when to teach must also tailored to the educational background, level of stress, wellness, and readiness to learn of each family. Ideally, the child should receive developmentally appropriate education and all family members and caregivers should also be educated when they are ready to learn. Initially, some people can only learn concrete skills and survival information whereas others may immediately be able to absorb more abstract information. Survival skills include those, which are essential to the immediate safety of the child. For some families, survival skills may be all they can ever learn. In any case, the chronicity of diabetes and the ongoing nature of the education process make follow-up evaluation essential and education on going.

Survival Skills: Minimum Skill Requirements for Caregivers of Children with Diabetes:

- monitor blood glucose
- test urine for ketones
- recognize signs of hypoglycemia
- treat hypoglycemia (includes glucagon)
- mix and inject insulin
- rotate injection sites
- understand basic meal plan
- know who and when to call for help

A Comprehensive Education Program would also Include Information Regarding:

- etiology and pathophysiology of diabetes
- signs, symptoms and treatment for hyper and hypoglycemia
- property of insulin
- insulin adjustment
- exercise and its implications for glycemic control
- daily balancing of insulin, food, exercise and scheduling
- sick day guidelines
- DKA prevention and treatment
- maintaining and using a daily log for pattern adjustments
- acute and chronic complications of diabetes and how to prevent them

The goals of diabetes education and treatment for children, adolescents and their families are to achieve normal growth and development, optimal glycemic control, positive psychosocial adjustment of diabetes and to prevent the acute and chronic complications of diabetes[4]. A team of professionals including physicians, nurse educators, dietitians and psychosocial experts best meets these goals[5].

An assessment of the level of understanding, knowledge and acceptance of diabetes is the first step in the education process. Prior experiences with other family members or friends who may have had diabetes can bring strong biases and misinformation. Assessment of the health beliefs, cultural impact, social situation, lifestyle and readiness to learn must be completed before an educational plan can be developed. Then a comprehensive, individualized teaching plan for a child or adolescent can be made that includes an assessment of the child's:

- personality characteristics
- maturity level
- developmental stage (pre-school, latency age, etc.)
- level of family support
- other supports
- eating patterns
- exercise and sports
- school considerations

The outcome of the assessment results in an individualized plan of education, which must of necessity be planned over time and dynamic, based on their situation, current needs and family lifestyle. The plan also accounts for the child and family's adaptation and acceptance of the diagnosis and how fully the child and family are able to follow their prescribed treatment plan. The child's participation in diabetes education with age-appropriate material suitable for the child's developmental level is essential. Assessment tools include a self-report, observation of the child's and parent's behaviors as related to the treatment plan, and physical examination.

BEHAVIORAL AND PSYCHOSOCIAL CONSIDERATIONS

People who cope well with diabetes seem to find a balance as they fit diabetes into their usual lifestyle. The demands of diabetes affect the lifestyle of the child and family, and visa versa. For the parent of a newly diagnosed child, there is a grief process, which follows the diagnosis. There is the perception of the loss of a healthy child, guilt, and uncertainty, which affects quality of life. Developing effective stress management and coping and problem solving skills is as important to successful therapy as insulin administration, meal planning, blood glucose monitoring and exercise[6].

Due to the chronic, unrelenting and persistent nature of caring for a child with diabetes, dealing with the daily regimen can become an overwhelming task. Well-adapted families function effectively with few limitations other than those imposed by the disease. However, few major chronic childhood diseases affect families and their social network as profoundly as diabetes[7].It is well established that children at greater risk for acute and chronic complications of diabetes may come from families in which there are few supports, lower socioeconomic status, or chaotic home environments. Family stresses can contribute to parental behaviors of abuse, or neglect, the degree of which may not be recognized by professionals involved in their care[8].

When episodes of severe hypoglycemia do occur, they can be frightening for caregivers who may then purposefully allow hyperglycemia. However, parents, adolescents and children who have adequate education with a problem-solving approach to their diabetes management, as well as psychosocial support can limit severe hypoglycemia, hyperglycemia and DKA. Active self-control and training are probably the most useful tools for prevention[9]. Therefore, on-going diabetes education and support are essential to the goal.

In a child with diabetes, the safety and predictability of normal life are replaced with a sense of vulnerability, need for control, and blame of self, parents and others[10]. Likewise, parents also express guilt and anxiety about the possibility of acute and chronic complications. When other medical and/or psychosocial problems exist, diabetes care must be integrated into sometimes already overly stressed situations, leading to compromised glycemic control.

It is incumbent upon the health care provider to take into account these dynamics in the support and education of the family.

DEVELOPMENTAL CONSIDERATIONS

The diagnosis of diabetes impacts the mental, emotional and overall well being of the child. Lifestyle and freedom are affected, and in some instances diabetes can contribute to emotional disturbance both in the child and family[11]. A child or adolescent also must cope with the normal developmental issues of growing up, and must somehow integrate diabetes management into them.

Educational Considerations for Infants and Toddlers

There are a number of developmental factors to be considered when teaching parents to manage a young child with diabetes. Parents and caregivers of young children must learn to plan tasks considering the normal developmental needs and personality of the child yet address the specific requirements of diabetes management. This involves a certain amount of organization, forethought and ability to prioritize. Safety issues are paramount to this age group who do not have verbal skills to express how they are feeling. Although hyperglycemia and ketoacidosis is always a concern, the educational focus for very young children is the prevention and treatment of hypoglycemia. Infants and young children cannot verbally communicate their feelings. Therefore it is incumbent on parents and caregivers to carefully observe behavior and provide protection from hypoglycemia.

Infants may require significant amounts of sleep and toddlers need daily naps, which must be considered when planning the daily diabetes regimen. Parents and caretakers can be shown how to fit naps into the child's schedule at times, which do not interfere with meals or snacks. Educational issues revolve around monitoring, recognizing hypoglycemia even during sleep, and finding a routine which generally allows the infant sufficient uninterrupted sleep while also preventing hypoglycemia.

Although infants usually eat predictably, regular scheduled nightly feedings are important for avoiding hypoglycemia in infants. A three to four hour flexible feeding schedule is effective for maintaining a steady blood glucose level. Breast milk, if possible, is preferable over formula for supplemental feedings so that there will not be caloric differences from one feeding to the next. In order to prevent hypoglycemia, infants older than 4 months of age may be given additional cereal by spoon along with their bottle at feedings prior to the peak effect of insulin[12].

Due to the spontaneous and sporadic nature of physical activity in infants, balancing food with insulin and activity in order to prevent hypoglycemia can be challenging. Eating habits that are normal for a toddler can be worrisome for the parent of a child with diabetes who must always be prepared to provide carbohydrates in the form of milk or juice if the child will not eat. From 5 to 30 g. of carbohydrate is recommended for treating hypoglycemia in infants taken in the form of Karo syrup, undiluted baby fruit juice, glucose water, Jello water or a small tube of commercially prepared gel cake decorator frosting. Honey should be avoided for treatment of hypoglycemia in infants due to an association with infantile botulism[10].In the case of severe hypoglycemia in a child less than 6 years, 0.5 mg glucagon must be administered subcutaneously.

Frequent monitoring also plays an important role for parents and caregivers who must always be on the lookout for hypoglycemia. Monitors which can test serum glucose from sites other than fingers, toes, and heels in young children are helpful in giving a wide range of sites. Considerations for meters in infants and toddlers are ease of use, blood sample size, and ability to test for ketones and accuracy.

All parents have difficulty with the concept of having to inject their young child repeatedly. The hesitancy is normal and natural, but health care professionals can assist parents to adopt a firm and no-nonsense approach to injections. It is important to teach parents how to hold their squirming child to minimize discomfort yet insure that the injection is given without difficulty and to hug or play with the child afterward. In the education process, it is useful for parents to inject themselves with the needle of an empty syringe to allow them to know what it feels like and to hopefully allay fears that injections are quite painful. Toddlers can benefit from the use of Band-Aids as minor choices to allow a feeling of control over the process.

One of the most important educational considerations for parents of a young child to learn is when to call for help. This concern prompts a plan of care with action guidelines so that parents, caregivers, day care settings, preschool's and others know parameters of safety. Guidelines should include who to call and phone numbers for signs of illness, vomiting, diarrhea, ketonuria, dehydration, hyperglycemia > 300 mg/dl, and severe hypoglycemia including the use of glucagon.

The health care provider can encourage expressive play so that children have an opportunity to work through diabetes related issues. The advantages of play therapy have been well recognized in young and school aged children. Guided play, puppet play and other forms of creative expression are useful educational strategies to assist young children in the expression of their concerns about diabetes and its impact on their life.

Educational Considerations for School Age Children

The challenge for parents of a school age child is to fit diabetes care into the child's normal activities in a way that provides optimum diabetes control, emotional adjustment and school performance. Children with diabetes can become worried about themselves because of the inordinate amount of attention focused on their blood glucose, food and health. Understandably, parents also might be overprotective and therefore the child may not be able to achieve a level of independence normal for his age[13]. One difficulty is that many of the demands of diabetes care do not necessarily fit into normal developmental tasks for a child. Although concerns about hypoglycemia and hyperglycemia are present, one of the primary issues of this age group is that of feeling different from peers [14].For a child, who must eat when friends don't eat, or who shouldn't eat when friends do eat, or who eats pretzels when others are eating cupcakes, feeling different due to diabetes can be a problem.

Therefore it is necessary to try to provide a flexible regimen to minimize differences. Of course, in providing the flexible regimen, the concept itself necessitates multiple daily injections (MDI) or an insulin pump, both of which can be done discreetly but might also promote feelings of difference. Parents, schoolteachers and others who are sensitive to the issues can help to minimize the problem.

Healthcare providers can suggest certain tasks that might help the caregiver and child be organized and prepared to treat hypoglyemia by:

- Keeping a steady supply of juice boxes and crackers to pack in backpacks, school nurses office, and on the soccer field, etc.;
- Asking the school for the lunch menu monthly. Decisions can be made whether to buy or pack lunch based on preferences and the diabetes regime.
- Arranging a plan of care with the school regarding monitoring blood and treating hypoglycemia. (See Section XX on Schools)
- Testing frequently before, during and after sports when exercising strenuously.
- Monitoring 4 a.m. blood glucose if the child has been hypoglycemic during the day or evening, hasn't eaten well, or has exercised strenuously.

Educational Considerations during Adolescence

The adolescent period is a time of rapid biologic change accompanied by increasing physical, cognitive and emotional maturity. Adolescents with diabetes display normal growth patterns and onset and progression of pubertal development[15]. However, metabolic control, indicated by rising HbA1c levels deteriorates during adolescence despite significantly higher insulin doses[16 17]. Poor control during the adolescent period is often blamed on nonadherence to the prescribed regimen and the spontaneity of adolescent life. Attitudes of experimentation, rebellion, risk taking and independence are characteristic of adolescence. In those with diabetes, diabetes management may become the issue around which independence struggles revolve. Thus, there are both biologic and developmental reasons for deteriorating metabolic control during the teen years.

The educational process must recognize and support these differences. Lack of knowledge in diabetes management is not always or often the problem when poor control exists, but rather is a symptom of chaotic home environment, parental over or under-involvement or concern, or even the frank omission of insulin. Adolescent females who develop ketoacidosis might do so because they fail to take their insulin for the purposes of weight control. The adolescent period is a challenging and frightening time for parents who have difficulty transferring responsibility of care to their teen who may or may not take on the responsibility. The task of the health professional educator is to engage the teen as an advocate for their health and well being.

The following educational strategies for health care providers who work with adolescents might help to establish a positive relationship:

- Convey enjoyment in working with adolescents.
- Develop a primary relationship with teens and a collaborative one with parents.
- Provide honest communication and don't minimize their feelings.
- Be willing to listen. Listen to what is being said as well as what is not being said.
- Promote feelings of normalcy.
- Discuss perceptions of barriers.
- Problem-solve diabetes issues together.
- Invite friends, and other supportive people to join in
- Address adolescent issues such as tobacco, drug, and alcohol use, driving issues, sexuality, and all night activities. The educator must be comfortable discussing these issues.
- All educational materials must be developmentally appropriate and adjusted to the age, ability and attention span of the individual.
- Foster association with others through support groups, diabetes camps, or diabetes fund-raising activities.

Adolescents can often manage their own diabetes regimen with guidance and supervision. Many teens are conscientious regarding their diabetes tasks. Others see diabetes as a nuisance and can be reluctant to perform their self-care activities. They can accurately measure and inject insulin or insulin pump, monitor blood and keep records. Adherence issues are not usually not ones of capability but in having the time and interest to care for diabetes. Diabetes is not the first priority in the life of a teen. Teens who do best often have parental involvement in their care[18].

Health care professionals must be aware that adolescents frequently falsify numbers in their records, or will transpose them. For example a 312 may be recorded as a 213 or a 432 may be recorded as a 132. When insulin doses are being adjusted based on false readings, the practice can indeed be dangerous. Verification of numbers in memory meters is a useful practice although many adolescents have several meters, which makes the detective work difficult. Those with parents who regularly double-check their meter memory and are involved in diabetes related decisions on a daily basis tend to be more accountable and diligent in their record keeping and self-management.

Educational Considerations in Children and Teens with Type 2 Diabetes

Children and adolescents with type 2 diabetes pose their own educational challenges. Due to the familial nature of type 2 diabetes and the propensity toward obesity, these children often live in an environment where parents have diabetes, are also overweight and are sedentary. They may not recognize the need to modify behavior and make lifestyle changes. Weight loss and weight control are the educational focus.

All children with type 2 diabetes and their families should receive comprehensive self-management education[19]. Self-management education should include teaching self-monitoring of blood glucose, medication, increasing exercise and developing healthy eating habits. Focus must be to encourage healthy eating habits for the entire family, including decreasing high-caloric high fat food choices. Obviously, the goal of education is not that the adolescent merely knows he is to do this, but to help the teen translate knowledge into practice. Helping the adolescent find a way to promote healthy lifestyle practices is important. This may involve limiting their television viewing or playing of computer games. One of the educational challenges is to motivate adolescents with type 2 to care for themselves. Educational Strategies for Adolescents with type 2 diabetes include:

- Engage the whole family in healthy lifestyle practices
- Encourage the teen to find a friend who enjoys exercise or weight control to stimulate his/her exercise program and dietary efforts
- Encourage the teen to find a sport or activity that is fun and that can be done regularly, such as dancing, tennis, golf aerobics, biking, etc
- Help the teen set limits for their own TV or computer time (e.g. 2 hours a day or less)

DIABETES IN THE SCHOOL AND DAY CARE SETTING

One of the hardest things for a parent to do under normal circumstances is to entrust a young child's care to someone else. Most parents are comfortable with a baby-sitter in the home for short periods of time, but when the child has diabetes there are even larger concerns. Parents must feel comfortable that those who are responsible for their child's safety are well informed, knowledgeable and committed to taking care of the child in the best possible way.

There are two pieces of legislation, which help to support the care of children with diabetes in school. The first is the American Disabilities Act, which is civil rights legislation designed to protect people with mental or physical disabilities from discrimination based on that disability. In addition, the Individuals with Disabilities Education Act of 1991 to guarantee free, appropriate public education for children with special needs[20].

Appropriate diabetes care in the school and day care setting is necessary for the child's immediate safety, long-term well being, and optimal academic performance. School personnel must have an understanding of diabetes and must be trained in its management and in the treatment of diabetes emergencies[21]. Children must be allowed to incorporate their diabetes care into the normal school setting and be encouraged to participate in all activities.

The parent and school personnel must create a plan of care for the child in school with input from the child and health care team. It must be reviewed and revised regularly. In order to facilitate the child's entrance into the school setting, a collaborative meeting should be set up prior to the start of school. The parent, child, and key school personnel should participate. (These may include the principal, teacher, nurse, cafeteria aid, playground aid, bus driver, gym teacher and/or coach.) This meeting should be a forum for determining the child's diabetes needs, individual preferences, and the school's policies. The plan should include:

- a routine plan of care
- designated responsibilities (who does what)
- designated persons responsible for emergencies.
- the place emergency supplies are kept
- phone list
- critical action plan (when to call parent or physician)
- plan for communication with parents or caregivers.

(See Plan of Care for schools: Figure 1 * Permission to publish sought from American Diabetes Association.)

There have been persistent difficulties for students with diabetes in the school especially in the area of monitoring blood glucose in the classroom as well as the use of glucagon to treat severe hypoglycmeia. The American Diabetes Association as well as the American Association of Diabetes Educators recommend that students be permitted to monitor in the classroom or anywhere, as well as treat severe hypoglycemia with glucagon[21,22].

The goal for all concerned is for the child to have a positive school experience. The ages at which children are able to perform self-care tasks are very individual and variable. Therefore, a child's capability and willingness to provide self-care in the school setting should be respected and may vary from one child to the next. The school personnel should feel comfortable in their role and be well educated by the parent, school nurse, or medical team. It is also important that they understand the rationale for the demands of diabetes so that they are not anxious about their duties, or take the diabetes casually. The parent should feel that even in the constraints of a busy school that their child will be well cared for and that they will be contacted for any problems arising. If there are concerns, the child's medical team can often provide assistance to smooth over difficulties. By working together as a team, which has a common goal, children can have a successful, happy and safe school experience.

SUMMARY

Pediatric diabetes education is unique in its differences and can be challenging. There must be consideration to and education of all family members and caregivers, the child or adolescent, and the school system. Children and teens must be regularly and carefully assessed for growth, development, and glycemic control which is accompanied by education and anticipatory guidance. There should be an ongoing educational plan for each child as well as an individualized care plan at school. Each should be regularly revisited and updated. Good communication between all members of the health care team is essential. It is critical that families feel secure in their ability to care for diabetes and have an honest and open working relationship with their health team.

REFERENCES

1 American Diabetes Association Clinical Practice Recommendations. Diabetes Care 24(1):33-43, 2001.

2 Brown S. Studies of educational interventions and outcomes in diabetic adults: A meta-analysis revisited. Patient Education Counseling 16:189-215, 1990.

3 Siminerio L. Comparing outpatient to inpatient diabetes education for newly diagnosed pediatric patients: an exploratory study. Doctoral thesis of Pennsylvania State University Graduate School Department of Health Education 1998.

4 Betschart J. Childhood and Adolescence. Core Curriculum on Diabetes Education 4th Ed. Franz, Ed, 2000.

5 Becker, D. Management of insulin dependent diabetes mellitus in children and adolescents. Current Opinion in Pediatrics 3:710-23, 1991.
6 Boland EA, Grey M. Coping strategies of school-age children with diabetes mellitus. Diabetes Educ 22:592-7, 1996.
7 Arslanian S, Becker D, Drash A. Diabetes in the child and adolescent. In Wilkins 4th ed. The diagnosis and treatment of endocrine disorders in childhood and adolescence. Springfield, IL: Chas. Thomas, 961-1027, 1994.
8 Horan P, Gwynn C, Renzi D. Insulin dependent diabetes mellitus and child abuse: Is their a relationship? Diabetes Care 9:302-7, 1986.
9 Norfeldt S, Ludvigsson J. Adverse events in intensively treated children and adolescents with type 1 diabetes. Acta Paediatr 88:1184-93, 1999.
10 Citrin W, Tapp J, Wine H. Diabetes counseling issues: The patient and family. In Pediatric and adolescent diabetes medicine Chicago: YearBook Publishing: 369-90, 1987.
11 Kovacs M, Feinberg T, Paulauskas S, et al: Initial coping responses and psychosocial characteristics of children with insulin dependent diabetes mellitus. J Pediatr 106:827-834, 1985.
12 Betschart J. Childhood and Adolescence. In: Core Curriculum for Diabetes Education. 4th Edition. Franz M. Ed. American Association of Diabetes Educators. Cpt 17, 2001.

13 Betschart J. Children and Adolescents with Diabetes. In: Nursing Clinics of North America: 28:1:35-43, 1991.
14 Puczynski S, Betschart J. Foundation for the future: understanding the child with diabetes in the classroom. American Association of Diabetes Educators, 1991.
15 Clarson C, Daneman D, Ehrlich R The relationship of metabolic control to growth and pubertal development in children with insulin dependent diabetes. Diabetes Research 2:237-41, 1985.
16 Amiel S, Sherwin R, Simonson D, et al. Impaired insulin action in puberty: A contributing factor to poor glycemic control in adolescents with diabetes. N Engl J Med 315:215-9, 1986.
17 Daneman D, Wolfson J, Becker D, et al. Factors affecting glycosylated hemoglobin values in children with insulin dependent diabetes. J Pediatr 99:847-53, 1981.
18 Follansbee D. Assuming responsibility for diabetes management: What age? What price? Diabetes Educ 15:347-53, 1989.

19 American Diabetes Association. Type 2 Diabetes in Children and Adolescents. Diabetes Care 23:3:381-9, 2000.
20 American Diabetes Association. Your School and your Rights. Discrimination against Children with Diabetes in the Public School System. Alexandria, VA: American Diabetes Association, 1996.
21 American Diabetes Association. Care of Children with diabetes in the school and day care setting. Diabetes Care 24(1l): S108-112, 2001.

22 American Association of Diabetes Educators Position Statement: Management of Children with Diabetes in the School Setting. AADE 200 Member Resource Guide, 1 xvii, 1999.

Chapter 14
NUTRITION

Lea Ann Holzmeister
Nutrition Consultant, Tempe, AZ

INTRODUCTION

Medical nutrition therapy (MNT) is an integral component of diabetes management[1]. MNT for children and adolescents with diabetes influenced by a number of advances that have allowed practitioners to adopt a more flexible approach to managing diabetes. Critical developments in pediatric diabetes nutrition management include revised nutrition recommendations[2], nutrition practice guidelines for type 1 and type 2 diabetes[3], results of the Diabetes Control and Complications Trial (DCCT) [4], and pharmacological advances.

The American Diabetes Association (ADA) evidence-based nutrition recommendations for children and adolescents attempt to translate research data and clinically applicable evidence into nutrition care. Nutrition recommendations for children with type 1 diabetes focus on achieving blood glucose goals without excessive hypoglycemia[5,6,7]. Nutrition recommendations for youth with type 2 diabetes focus on treatment goals to normalize glycemia and to facilitate a healthy lifestyle[8].

The Diabetes Care and Education Practice Group of the American Dietetic Association has developed a set of nutrition practice guidelines for type 1 diabetes that help to formulate a logical and sequential plan of nutrition care to improve metabolic control in patients with diabetes. Field-test results, which included pediatric patients, showed that nutrition practice guidelines can empower patients and their families and improve metabolic control by influencing eating and nutrition related behaviors. These guidelines were designed for use in children and adolescents with the assumption that each child's specific growth, learning, and social needs are addressed. Nutrition practice guidelines also outline the referral process for nutrition therapy as well as the level of nutrition care. This information helps primary care providers when referring patients to the registered dietitian for MNT. The levels of nutrition care indicate frequency and type of interventions.

Results of the Diabetes Control and Complications Trial (DCCT) and the United Kingdom Prospective Diabetes Trial (UKPDS) convincingly demonstrate the importance of prevention of diabetes-related complications [9,10]. In both trials, MNT was essential in achieving diabetes treatment goals [11,12]. The DCCT provided valuable information about the role of various flexible nutrition intervention strategies. Recent advances in the pharmacological treatment of diabetes, such as flexible insulin regimens and algorithms have also played a role in the formulation of the current recommendations and guidelines.

Goals of Medical Nutrition Therapy in Children and Adolescents

The goals for MNT provide a reference for nutrition care and are used when developing a nutrition care plan for children and adolescents with diabetes. Whereas these goals provide a reference point for care, the specific nutrition and health needs of the individual pediatric patient must be considered when formulating a nutrition care plan.

- Achieve blood glucose goals without excessive hypoglycemia
- Improve health and maintain normal growth, weight, and pubertal development with adequate nutrition
- Prevent/treat obesity and hyperlipidemia
- Prevention, delay, or treatment of nutrition-related risk factors and complications

Maintaining normal blood glucose control without excessive hypoglycemia is the primary treatment goal in children with diabetes. Care must be taken to prevent hypoglycemic events in young children, who are at risk of impaired brain development resulting from multiple hypoglycemic episodes[13,14].

Nutrient recommendations for children and adolescents with diabetes are based on requirements for all healthy children[2,15]. Healthful eating habits are important to ensure intakes of essential vitamins and minerals and to maintain normal growth and development. Energy requirements in children and adolescents vary considerably with age, weight, sex, height, stage of development, and level of physical activity. The ideal method for estimating calorie needs is a food/nutrition history of a typical daily intake as obtained from a 24-hour recall or 3-day food record, providing that growth and development are within normal limits. A typical daily intake of calories can be compared to reference intakes for normal growth and development[16]. Adequacy of caloric intake can be evaluated by monitoring weight gain and growth patterns using the pediatric growth charts from the Centers for Disease Control[17].

Achieving good metabolic control is essential to normal growth and development[18]. Five to ten percent of children with type 1 diabetes will experience growth abnormalities. Growth and weight-gain data should be recorded at diagnosis and every 3-4 months. Careful consideration of a child's appetite must be given when determining energy requirements. Withholding food or having a child overeat consistently without an appetite for food in an effort to control blood glucose must be discouraged[2].

Children with type 1 diabetes often present at diagnosis with weight loss that is restored with proper insulin treatment and adequate energy intake. When catch-up growth and weight are established, calorie intake should be adjusted. Children with intensively managed diabetes exhibit a tendency to gain more weight than children on conventional insulin regimens, possibly secondary to improved glycemic control and more efficient utilization of nutrients[19]. Therefore it is important to routinely monitor growth and weight gain.

One component of successful treatment of children and adolescents with type 2 diabetes can be defined as cessation of excessive weight gain with normal linear growth[20]. Slowed weight gain may be accomplished by calorie reduction may be accomplished by decreasing high-calorie high-fat food choices.

The macronutrient composition of the nutrition prescription is individualized according to blood glucose and plasma lipid goals and requirements for growth and development[2]. Protein and fiber requirements for children with diabetes are no different than for children without diabetes. Carbohydrate contributes over half of the calorie intake in healthy children. For children with diabetes taking insulin, the total carbohydrate content of meals and snacks is a primary determinant of postprandial glucose response and premeal insulin dose[21, 22]. Individuals receiving intensive insulin therapy should adjust premeal insulin based on carbohydrate content of meals and snacks. Children on fixed daily insulin doses should try to be consistent in day-to-day carbohydrate intake[2].

Evidence suggests that dietary sucrose does not increase glycemia more than isocaloric amounts of starch therefore it is no longer recommended that the intake of sucrose and sucrose containing food by people with diabetes be restricted because of concern about aggravating hyperglycemia[2]. However, limiting sucrose-containing food to proper serving sizes in children and adolescents is essential for a nutritionally balanced diet.

With diabetes as a major risk factor in the development of cardiovascular disease, maintaining normal blood lipid levels in children with diabetes is an important goal of MNT. Children and adolescents in groups at high risk of developing lipid abnormalities should be screened and monitored according to guidelines issues by the National Cholesterol Education Panel (NCEP) Report of the Expert Panel on Blood Cholesterol Levels in Children and Adolescents and the American Academy of Pediatrics[23,24].

Table 1. Classification of Total and LDL Cholesterol Levels in Children and Adolescents form Families with Hypercholesterolemia or Premature Cardiovascular Disease

Category	Total Cholesterol (mg/dL)	LDL-Cholesterol(mg/dL)
Acceptable	<170	<110
Borderline	170-199	110-129
High	≥200	≥130

An initial goal in lipid management is achievement of glycemic goals followed by a stepwise approach to the dietary management of lipid abnormalities suggested by the NCEP. This approach recommends a reduction in total fat, saturated fat, and cholesterol for children over the age of 2 years. The NCEP Step I diet consists of approximately 30% of total calories from fat, with less than 10% of calories from saturated fat and less than 300 milligrams of cholesterol per day. If, after at least 3 months on the Step-One Diet, the minimal goals of therapy are not achieved, a Step-Two Diet with a further reduction of saturated fat to less than 7 percent of total calories and cholesterol intake to less than 200 milligrams per day. A study of the dietary intake of children with type 1 diabetes, aged 4-9 years, found that saturated fat intake exceeded the NCEP recommendations[25]. Children with elevated blood lipids can benefit from reducing the amount of fat, saturated fat, and cholesterol in the diets without adversely affecting growth, nutritional status, or pubertal maturation[26].

Preventing, delaying, and treating nutrition-related risk factors and complications is an important goal of MNT. Proper treatment of hypoglycemia should be an integral component of the nutrition prescription. Proper management of diet, including consumption of regular, consistent meals and snacks with a balance of nutrients can reduce the incidence of hypoglycemia.

Nutrition Assessment

Effective MNT supports families in working within their lifestyle, abilities, and readiness to change[3]. A thorough nutrition assessment provides invaluable information for providing this support to patients. Components of the pediatric nutrition assessment include[27]:

- Pattern of growth and weight gain
- Food history and activity patterns
- Results of blood glucose monitoring, glycated hemoglobin, urine tests, and lipids
- Insulin regimen
- Support systems
- Socioeconomic factors
- Barriers to learning/readiness for change

The nutrition assessment includes an evaluation of usual food intake, eating habits, physical activity habits, and attitudes toward nutrition and health. This information is essential when developing individualized meal plans. The components of a nutrition and activity history for children and adolescents of varying ages have been delineated[27]. A pediatric diet history form can be used to save time while identifying important components necessary to formulate an individualized meal plan[28].

Nutrition Intervention and Treatment

Nutrition intervention regimens are based on self-management education in the context of approaches to meal planning, pharmacological interventions and physical activity patterns. Self-management education is based on a child's glycemic control goals, readiness to change, and current level of self-management. Effective nutrition intervention promotes normal growth, individualization, and consistent eating patterns[3].

Meal Planning Approaches

Individualized food plans utilizing nutrition assessment data are designed to meet basic nutrition guidelines and specific management goals. The basic concepts of meal planning are taught at initial diagnosis and flexibility within the meal plan is implemented during continuing education. Children and adolescents must be taught the basics of meal planning in a developmentally appropriate manner, with specific details provided to parents and other family members.

Adolescents in the DCCT used a wide variety of meal plan techniques, such as carbohydrate counting, exchange lists, calorie counting, and simplified meal planning guidelines[11]. Since dietary compliance is a particularly difficult part of the treatment regimen it is important to select an approach that will promote adherence, individual needs, and level of understanding. A meal plan self-efficacy index can be used to determine whether specific meal plan methods are challenging for an adolescent[29].

The meal plan system selected should consider the developmental age of the patient. Toddlers and young children have variable appetites due to rapid changes in growth and this results in variable intake. These children often prefer a "grazing" meal and snack schedule, consuming smaller amounts of food more frequently throughout the day. Older children and preadolescents tend to eat more consistent amounts at the same time each day because of school schedules and more predictable appetites. Older children typically eat three meals and at least two or three snacks each day. Adolescents often eat at inconsistent times with the amounts of carbohydrate being consumed being quite variable.

Carbohydrate counting is a meal planning approach that focuses on carbohydrate as the main macronutrient that affects post-prandial blood glucose levels. This system has been in use since the 1920's and was one of the primary approaches used in the DCCT by individuals taking multiple daily injections or using an insulin pump. In the DCCT, carbohydrate counting was found to be effective in allowing flexibility in food choices, promoting self-management of diabetes, and achieving the outcomes goals. Carbohydrate counting helps make a more concrete and immediate connection between blood glucose control, food, physical activity, and medication.

Carbohydrate counting can be used as a meal plan approach to set carbohydrate targets at each meal and snack or can be used to better manage the more variable eating habits of some children and adolescents by working with a carbohydrate-to-insulin ratio to cover carbohydrate intake. Carbohydrate counting principles are taught using carbohydrate grams and/or carbohydrate servings based on the exchange groups and food labels. Three levels of carbohydrate counting, basic, intermediate, and advanced are available to help ease patients and families into the system and assure both an understanding of basic concepts and sound application.

The carbohydrate counting meal plan is developed according to the usual amount of carbohydrate eaten at meals and snacks, which can vary according to age, level of activity, and usual eating patterns. Education is provided about the importance of selecting a variety of foods from all food groups to ensure a nutritionally adequate diet. Carbohydrate counting focuses only on the carbohydrate portion of the eating plan and this offers an easier and less structured approach for children and adolescents who often have vacillating appetites and food preferences. Parents and children are taught potential strategies for managing the variations in their blood glucose levels, such as changing insulin doses or the amount of timing of carbohydrate intake, or adjusting their physical activity.

Until recently, the *Exchange System for Meal Planning* was the most widely used meal plan approach in pediatrics. This approach provides a solid base of knowledge about food composition, portion sizes, and the effect of food on blood glucose. The exchange lists have been expanded and updated to reflect the trend of carbohydrate counting for blood glucose control. An important advantage of this system is the emphasis on obtaining an overall nutrition balance by selecting foods from all the major food groups.

Other meal planning systems such as USDA Food Guide Pyramid, nutrition guidelines, fat or calorie counting may be used, especially for children with type 2 diabetes. Intervention strategies should be culturally appropriate, sensitive to family resources, and provided to all caregivers[20].

Physical Activity

Physical activity promotes cardiovascular health, enhances social interaction and can help decrease the chances of obesity. Developing physical skills during childhood may also promote continued adherence to appropriate levels of physical activity during adulthood.

Usual levels of physical activity in children and adolescents should be taken into account when developing a food plan and food adjustments for additional activity is discussed at diagnosis and reviewed regularly. Toddlers and very young children have intermittent moderate activity throughout the day, usually in the form of unstructured play. Small frequent meals and snacks usually afford prevention of exercise related hypoglycemia. School-aged children and adolescents are more likely to participate in planned moderate to rigorous exercise in the form of physical education classes or organized sports. Additional carbohydrate prior to or during the activity can be offered.

Physical activity is an important treatment modality for type 2 diabetes in children and adolescents. Exercise can decrease insulin resistance and is an important component of weight management. Replacing sedentary activities such as television viewing and computer use have been shown to be an effective method to increase physical activity in children. Family involvement in physical activity can provide positive reinforcement. Children and adolescents with type 2 diabetes who participate in physical activity will increase calorie expenditure. Adjustments in the meal plan for physical activity will not be necessary unless oral hypoglycemic medications or insulin are used.

In general, physical activity reduces insulin requirements in children with type 1 diabetes. Hypoglycemia due to physical activity can be managed by an increase in carbohydrate consumption or a reduction in exogenous insulin. It is generally suggested that children increase intake carbohydrate for exercise instead of reducing insulin dose since children may need the additional calories for sustaining proper growth.

Hyperglycemia associated with insulin deficiency, resulting from an improper insulin regimen or a missed injection, may not require the addition of carbohydrate before exercise. Instead, additional postexercise carbohydrate, such ah as a larger supper or bedtime snack, to prevent delayed hypoglycemia may be needed.

Pharmacological Interventions

A variety of insulin regimens are utilized in pediatrics. At the time of diagnosis, a conventional insulin regimen may be used. However, many patients eventually transition to a more intensive therapy regimen such as multiple daily injections or continuous subcutaneous insulin infusion (CSII), depending on blood glucose values.

Short and rapid-acting insulin intake is matched to carbohydrate intake. Intensive diabetes management may include developing insulin-to-carbohydrate ratios for increased flexibility in meal planning. Typically, one unit of insulin per 15-20 grams of carbohydrate is used. However, in children and adolescents, this ratio often varies with age, pubertal maturation, and activity level as well as meal composition and timing. Frequently the insulin required in relation to the carbohydrate consumed is higher in the morning hours. Young children may require a smaller insulin-to-carbohydrate ratio while insulin-resistant teenagers may require as much as 2 units for every 15 grams of carbohydrate.

CSII offers another treatment option for intensive diabetes management in children and adolescents. CSII can allow for greater flexibility in food intake by offering the ability of the child to respond to a physiological hunger cues and food intake schedule rather than a predetermined insulin dose schedule. This may help children develop normal eating behaviors and prevent psychological consequences of food restriction sometimes present in rigidly structured meal plans. Advanced carbohydrate counting is often utilized with CSII. In advanced carbohydrate counting, carbohydrate-to-insulin ratios are determined by using a consistent meal plan while adjusting the premeal insulin dose. Premeal, bedtime blood glucose levels, insulin doses, carbohydrate intake, and physical activity records are used to calculate the carbohydrate-to-insulin ratio. Patients and parents must be able to acquire the meal plan skills to make daily adjustments in food and insulin doses.

For children and adolescents with type 2 diabetes, oral diabetes medicines and or insulin may be indicated if nutrition and exercise interventions are not effective in reaching blood glucose goals. Certain blood glucose lowering oral agents may cause hypoglycemia therefore patients may require planned snacks. Sulfonylureas promote insulin secretion therefore an afternoon or evening snack may be needed. Biguanides increase insulin sensitivity and therefore do not generally cause hypoglycemia.

REFERENCES

1. American Diabetes Association: Standards of medical care for patients with diabetes mellitus (Position Statement). Diabetes Care 24(Suppl 1): S33-S43, 2001.
2. Franz MJ, Bantle JP, Beebe CA, Brunzell JD, Chiasson J, Garg A, Holzmeister LA, Hoogwerf B, Mayer-Davis E, Mooradian A, Purnell JQ, Wheeler M: Evidence-based nutrition recommendations for diabetes and complications. Diabetes Care, (awaiting publication in 2001).
3. The American Dietetic Association: Nutrition Practice Guidelines for Type I and Type II Diabetes Mellitus. Chicago, The American Dietetic Association, 1996.
4. The DCCT Research Group: The effect of intensive treatment of diabetes on the development and progression of long-term complications in insulin-dependent diabetes mellitus. N Engl J Med 329:977-86, 1993.
5. Wise E, Kolb E, Sauder S: Effect of glycemic control on growth velocity in children with IDDM. Diabetes Care 15:826-830, 1992.
6. Danne T, Weber B, Hartman R, Enders I, Burger W, Hovener G: Long-term glycemic control has a nonlinear association to the frequency of background retinopathy in adolescents with diabetes. Diabetes Care 17:1390-1396, 1994
7. Donaghue KC, Fung A, Hing S, Fairchild J, King J, Chain A, Howard NJ, Silink M: The effect of pre-pubertal diabetes duration on diabetes. Diabetes Care 20:77-80, 1997.
8. American Diabetes Association: Type 2 diabetes in children and adolescents (Consensus Statement). Diabetes Care 23:381-389, 2000

9. Diabetes Control and Complications Trial Research Group: The effect of intensive treatment of diabetes on the development and progression of long-term complications in insulin-dependent diabetes mellitus. N Engl J Med 329:997-986, 1993.
10. UK Prospective Diabetes Study (UKPDS) Group: Intensive blood-glucose control with sulphonylureas or insulin compared with conventional treatment and risk of complications in patients with type 2 diabetes (UKPDS 33). Lancet 352:837-853, 1998.
11. Delahanty LM, Halford BH: The role of diet behaviors in achieving improved glycemic control in intensively treated patients in the Diabetes Control and Complications Trial. Diabetes Care 16:1453-1458, 1993.
12. UKPDS Group. UK Prospective Diabetes Study 7: Response of fasting plasma glucose to diet therapy in newly presenting type II diabetic patients.Metabolism39:905-12, 1990.
13. Ryan C, Vega A, Drash A: Cognitive deficits in adolescents who developed diabetes early in life. Pediatrics 75:921-927, 1985.
14. Rovet JF, Ehrlich RM, Hoppe M: Intellectual deficits associated with early onset of insulin-dependent diabetes mellitus in children. Diabetes Care 10:510-515, 1987.
15. Food and Nutrition Board, National Research Council: Recommended Dietary Allowances, 10th ed, Washington, D.C. National Academy Press, 1989, p.285.
16. Food and Nutrition Board, National Research Council: Recommended Dietary Allowances, 10th ed, Washington, D.C. National Academy Press, 1989, p.285.
17. http://www/cdc.gov/growthcharts
18. Wise E, Kolb E, Sauder S: Effect of glycemic control on growth velocity in children with IDDM. Diabetes Care 15:826-830, 1992.
19. The DCCT Research Group: The effect of intensive treatment of diabetes on the development and progression of long-term complications in insulin-dependent diabetes mellitus. N Engl J Med 329:977-986, 1993.
20. American Diabetes Association: Type 2 diabetes in children and adolescents (Consensus Statement). Diabetes Care 23:381-389, 2000.
21. Rabasa-Lhoret R, Garon J, Langelier H, Poisson D, Chiasson J-L: The effects of meal carbohydrate content on insulin requirements in type 1 diabetic patients treated intensively with basal bolus(ultalente-regular)insulin regimen.Diab Care 22:667-3,1999.
22. Slama G, Klein JC, Delage A, Ardila E, Lemaignen H, Papoz L, Tchobroutsky G. Correlation between the nature and amount of

carbohydrate in meal intake and insulin delivery by artificial pancreas in 24 insulin-dependent diabetics.Diabetes30:101-5, 1981.
23. Expert Panel on Blood Cholesterol Levels in Children and Adolescents: Treatment recommendations of the National Cholesterol Education Program report of the Expert Panel on Blood Cholesterol Levels in Children and Adolescents. Pediatrics 89(Suppl):525-584, 1992.
24. American Academy of Pediatrics Committee on Nutrition: Cholesterol in children. Pediatrics 101:141-147, 1998.
25. Randecker GA, Smiciklas-Wright H, McKenzie JM, Shannon BM, Mitchell DC, Becker DJ, Kieselhorst K:The dietary intake of children with IDDM. Diabetes Care 19:1370-1374, 1996.
26. Obarzanek E, Kimm SY, Barton BA, Van Horn L L, Kwiterovich PO Jr, Simons-Morton DG, Hunsberger SA, Lasser NL, Robson AM, Franklin FA Jr, Lauer RM, Stevens VJ, Friedman LA, Dorgan JF, Greenlick MR. Long-term safety and efficacy of a cholesterol-lowering diet in children with elevated low-density lipoprotein cholesterol: seven-year results of the Dietary Intervention Study in Children(DISC).Pediatrics. 107(2):256-64, 2001.
27. Holzmeister LA: Medical nutrition therapy for children and adolescents with diabetes. Diabetes Spectrum 10:268-274, 1997.
28. McLennan CL, Hartz DJ: Use of a pediatric diet history form to create individualized, consistent carbohydrate meal plans. Diabetes Spectrum 24:457-464, 1998.
29. Remley D, Cook-Newell M: Meal planning self-efficacy index for adolescents with diabetes. Diab Educator 25:883-890, 1999.

Chapter 15
ADOLESCENTS WITH DIABETES MELLITUS

Fergus Cameron MD FRACP and George Werther MD FRACP
Department of Endocrinology and Diabetes, Royal Children's Hospital, Australia

INTRODUCTION

Adolescence is a challenging and complex stage in human development, involving major physical, hormonal, emotional and psychological changes, which affect both the young person involved, and members of his or her family[1]. The burden of having to deal with a chronic disease such as diabetes at this time of life adds further to the potential for instability and turmoil. Diabetes is almost always insulin-dependent or type 1 at this age, although type 2 is now increasingly recognized in adolescence, particularly in African and Native American and similar ethnic groups[2].

Diabetes affects most aspects of adolescence, including the physiologic processes of growth and puberty, and the emotional and social transitions into adulthood. Conversely, the various physiologic, psychologic and behavioral changes of adolescence have significant impact on diabetes and its management. These include the effects of rapid growth and sexual development with their associated hormonal changes, the various behaviors associated with the growing independence from parents and associated potential conflicts, and experimentation with alcohol and drugs, and other rebellious behaviors. Diabetes in the adolescent also has a number of co-morbidities, both organic and psychosocial, some peculiar to this stage of development. It is also the period when the vascular complications of diabetes have their genesis and may first appear.

The management of diabetes in the adolescent is thus highly challenging, requiring awareness of, and attention to, all of these components of the adolescent and his or her diabetes. This requires a multi-disciplinary approach, involving pediatric diabetologist, nurse-educator, dietician, social worker, psychologist, youth workers, peer group support and others. In this chapter we will review current knowledge and understanding of diabetes in adolescence, dealing both with the underlying mechanisms and dynamics, as well as practical approaches to management.

GROWTH, PUBERTY AND DIABETES

If diabetes is diagnosed before puberty, linear growth prior to diagnosis has been variously described as being reduced, increased or unchanged[3-6]. Following diagnosis, linear growth prior to puberty may be impaired, especially if diabetic control is poor. This inverse relationship between growth and poor diabetic control is more marked during puberty, such that the pubertal growth spurt may be impaired, as well as the onset of puberty being delayed[7-13]. Following menarche, menstrual dysfunction is more common, including secondary amenorrhoea and irregular cycles, as well as polycystic ovary syndrome[11, 14]. Improved diabetic control, involving more adequate insulinisation, often leads to restoration of linear growth[15] and restoration of regular menstrual cycles[14].

The GH/IGF axis, which plays a central role in the growth acceleration of puberty, can be significantly disordered in the adolescent with poor diabetic control, contributing to both growth impairment and greater insulin resistance[16]. Circulating GH is significantly elevated in adolescents with diabetes, contributing to both increased insulin resistance and the “dawn phenomenon” of rising early morning blood glucose[16]. There is also a dissociation of GH and IGF-I levels, so that IGF-I levels are depressed in adolescents with poor control. Hepatic insensitivity to GH is thought to result from reduced expression of the GH receptor, which is regulated by insulin, so that adequate insulinisation reverses the apparent GH resistance and low IGF-I, providing a mechanism for restoration of linear growth[17, 18]. The other important components of the IGF system are the IGF binding proteins, which regulate IGF availability for its receptors. GH regulates the major carrier of circulating IGF-I, IGFBP-3; it may be suppressed in poorly controlled diabetic adolescents, further accounting for low circulating IGF-I[19]. In contrast, IGFBP-1, which shows diurnal variation, is negatively regulated by insulin, so that it is markedly elevated when diabetic control is poor at times of inadequate insulinisation, such as prior to the morning insulin injection[20, 21]. IGFBP-1 is thought to function as a “counter-regulatory” hormone, rapidly binding free IGF-I, which has insulin-like effects when it is in excess. Persistently elevated IGFBP-1 levels would therefore further reduce IGF-I availability, so contributing to growth failure.

METABOLIC CONTROL

Deteriorating metabolic control of diabetes during adolescence has been reported by several groups[22-25]. (Figure 1). Common reasons for

Figure 1: Data from Dabaghdao et al (4), showing longitudinal changes in BMI, insulin dosage and metabolic control (HbA1c) through puberty and adolescence. (Reproduced with permission of Blackwell Publishers, London, UK)

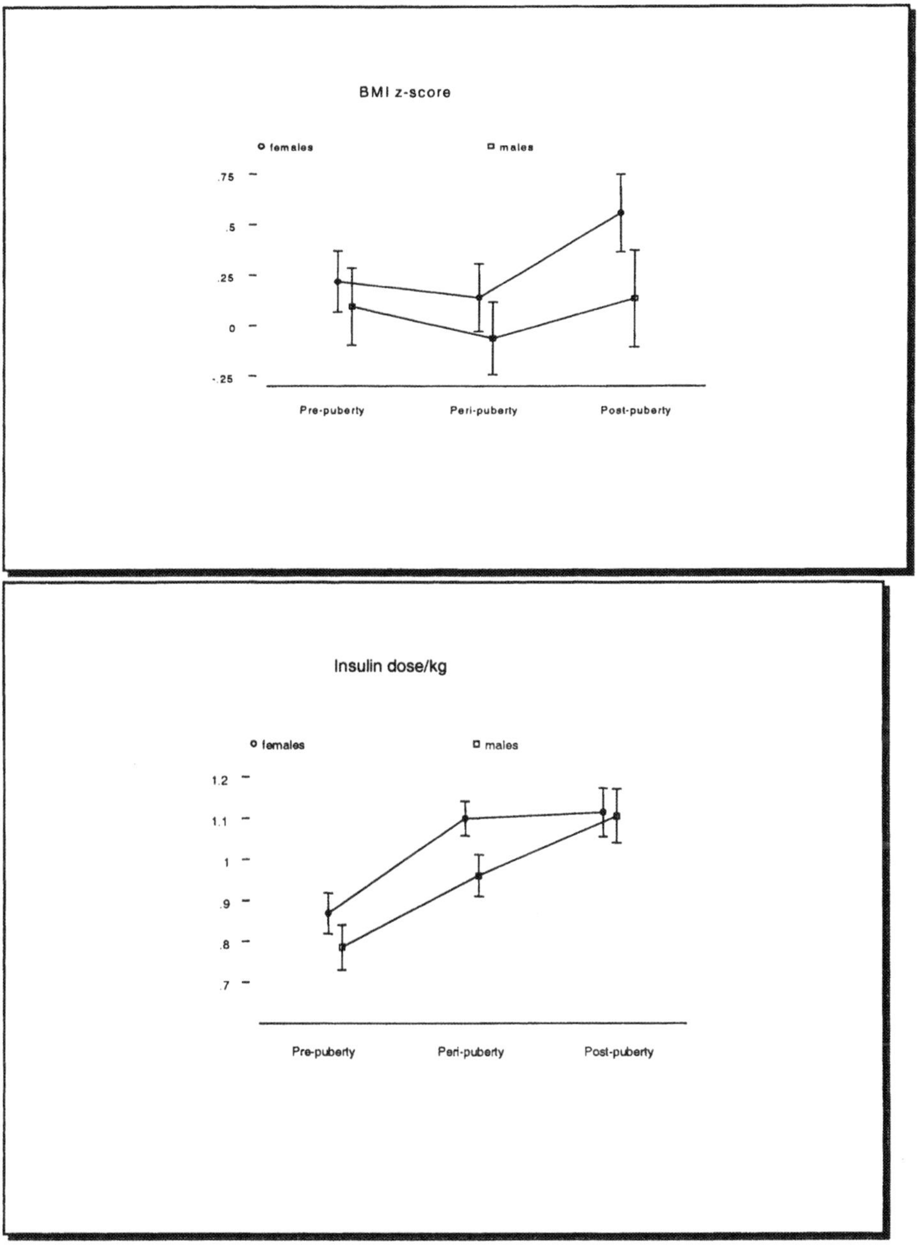

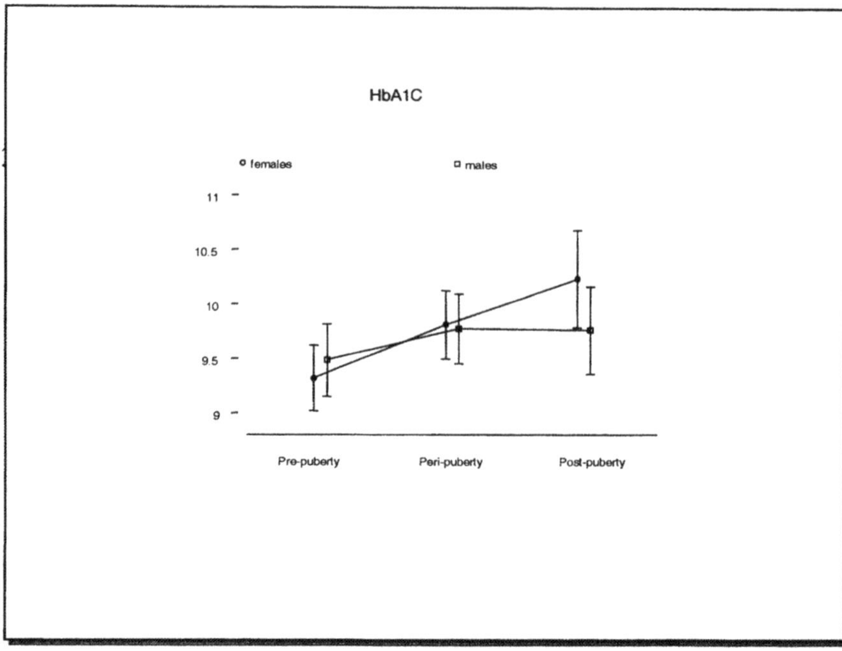

worsening metabolic control include erratic meal and exercise patterns[26,27], poor compliance[28], deliberate risk taking behaviour[29], eating disorders[30, 31, 32] and endocrine changes associated with puberty[33], leading to greater insulin resistance. Inadequate insulinisation in the face of increasing insulin requirements is thus a common cause of deteriorating control. Previous studies addressing the issue of deteriorating diabetic control in this age group have also highlighted maladaptive lifestyle practices acquired during adolescence, and the impact of these practices upon diabetic control[34-38]. Our studies (Figure 1)[25] and others[24] have shown that females were more likely to have deterioration in metabolic control. Our recently, published longitudinal data showed that diabetes control at the completion of childhood is to some extent predictive of diabetes control at the end of adolescence[25]. In the total study group, over half the study group completed adolescence with a mean HbA1C of $\pm$ 1 % to that with which they had in late childhood. The vast majority of patients (82%) had a mean post-adolescent HbA1C within 2% of their mean post-childhood value. Significantly, only 11% and 2% of patients had mean HbA1c values that decreased by greater than 1 and 2 percent respectively from pre- to post-puberty[25]. This data suggests that intervention programs designed to improve diabetes control through adolescence should also aim to optimize diabetes control in late childhood.

ADHERENCE

As adolescents adjust their priorities towards the competing demands of their social life and an erratic life-style, adherence with treatment regimens often falters[39-42]. Adolescents may increasingly resent the impositions placed on their lives by diabetes including parental and medical supervision of their diabetes care. The intrinsic nature of diabetes and factors such as chronicity, complex and invasive treatment procedures, and dietary restriction further mitigate against treatment adherence[43]. One study has reported rates of non-adherence with various aspects of diabetes treatment of up to 90%[39]. In addition to this La Greca et al[40] have shown that youth administer insulin incorrectly 40% of the time and frequently monitor blood glucose levels incorrectly. There are a number of risk factors associated with poor adherence, including emotional disturbance, family dysfunction, poor school performance and difficult peer relationships[44-47]. Poor adherence has been linked with "learned helplessness"[48], with the relationship between psychiatric illness and treatment adherence being unresolved[49]. The immediate consequences of poor adherence to either therapy or blood glucose monitoring include severe hypoglycemia and ketoacidosis. The medium to long term outcomes of poor adherence include the early appearance of diabetic retinopathy and nephropathy[50, 51]. Optimizing adherence to medical and lifestyle regimens is therefore critical when caring for adolescents and young adults. Guidelines aimed at fostering better adherence and adaptive lifestyle choices place much emphasis upon: negotiating therapy regimens with adolescent patients that are attainable and sustainable; focussing on the successful activities undertaken by the adolescent; building emotional strength; and allowing adolescents to express their feelings[52]. From a clinician's perspective the most helpful thing to do is to maintain a comfortable and mutually respectful relationship with an adolescent who is having trouble adhering to a diabetic regimen. Small gains should be emphasized and encouraged whilst maintaining ongoing family support.

IMPACT ON BODY HABITS AND IMAGE – EFFECTS ON INSULIN SENSITIVITY

As can be seen from Figure 1, increases in body mass index (BMI) frequently occur during adolescence, particularly in females[23, 25, 53, 54]. Holl et al reported increases in standardized BMI in both diabetic males and females thorough adolescence. Whilst this group found no association with total daily dose of insulin and weight gain there was a positive association between multiple daily injections (>3) and BMI[55]. Increases in BMI may result in insulin resistance and an increased insulin requirement for glycemic control. Increasing insulin resistance during adolescence is the norm for both sexes[56], accounting for the well-recognized increasing insulin requirement, particularly during the pubertal growth spurt, from less than 1unit/kg/day to as high as 2 units/kg/day[56, 57, 58]. Doses higher than this usually indicate dietary non-adherence or omission of insulin injections. Some authors have reported sexual dimorphism in insulin sensitivity during this period[56-58], with earlier rises in adrenal androgens, estrogen and growth hormone contributing to increased insulin resistance in females. We have found this to be a feature only in early adolescence, with both sexes having a reported mean total daily insulin dose proportionate to body weight (TDDI/W) of 1.1 unit/kg/day by the completion of puberty[25]. Further to this, in our experience TDDI/W increases in female adolescents prior to BMI, suggesting that in addition to diet and exercise, daily insulin dose may be contributory.

Notwithstanding the mechanism of increase in BMI, this event is frequently associated with marked distress by female adolescents and may be coincident with the appearance of an eating disorder[31,32, 59]. In one recent study, subthreshold eating disorders were found to be almost twice as common in adolescent females with type 1 diabetes as in their non-diabetic peers[60]. Many female adolescents with diabetes rapidly learn how to manipulate weight gains by altering insulin dosage[61-64]. The combination of either anorexia nervosa or bulimia and diabetes can result in multiple hospital re-admissions for poor glycemic control early appearance of diabetes-related complications and considerable familial disruption[62]. Such patients and their families require care from a large multidisciplinary team, often at considerable expense of time and resources.

IMPACT UPON EDUCATION AND LIFESTYLE – THE ROLE OF DRUGS AND OTHER RISK-TAKING BEHAVIOURS

Adolescent actions can also be impulsive and seemingly without regard to consequence. Physical risk-taking and recreational drug use, in particular, may result in significant injury or, more tragically, death[65, 66]. Physical morbidity, psychopathology and mortality may arise in this context through accidental overdose, ingestion of unknown and multiple agents, infection and the combination of an altered sensorium with risk-laden activity. Confusion between effects of drug or alcohol excess and hypoglycemia can have tragic results if hypoglycemia is overlooked. When emerging sexual interest is added to this mix, unwanted teen-age pregnancy and sexually transmitted disease often ensue. Diabetes significantly increases the risks associated with pregnancy in particular. Adolescents with diabetes therefore have to assume more responsibility than their non-diabetic peers. In particular they must assume responsibility for diabetes control and maintain control in the face of a changing hormonal environment and lifestyle. In addition to this increased burden of responsibility, diabetic adolescents also encounter the reality of the risks of diabetes-related complications with the clinical advent of regular complication screening.

In many respects diabetes can act as an obstruction to adolescent passage. Diabetes is a potent touchstone for areas of potential conflict with parents and care-givers (such as locus of control issues) [67, 68]. Ironically, diabetes may also increase the likelihood of risk-taking behaviours[29] and may interfere with conformity to a peer group[69]. Poorly controlled diabetes is associated with subtle neuropsychological deficits which can impact on academic achievement and ultimately reduce career options and life style choices[70, 71, 72]. There is evidence that the deterioration seen in both psychological well being and metabolic control during adolescence are linked, with non-adherence with the treatment regimen acting as a mediating variable[73, 74]. It is not surprising therefore that the convergence of diabetes and adolescence is frequently associated with conflict and a subsequent deterioration in diabetic control[22-24].

QUALITY OF LIFE/FUNCTIONAL HEALTH STATUS

While it is generally accepted that children and adolescents with diabetes suffer a greater burden of psychosocial ill-health and poor quality of life or functional health, simple assessment tools for these outcomes have until recently been lacking. Studies using two tools, the diabetes quality-of-life questionnaire (DQOL) and the Child Health Questionnaire (CHQ) have been published[75, 76]. The DQOL is a disease-specific tool designed specifically for use in the DCCT[77, 78]. It has been subsequently modified to deal with adolescents and children[79], to include a diabetes life satisfaction scale, a disease impact scale, and a disease-related worries scale. In the context of the DCCT, the DQOL found no adverse effects upon quality of life amongst adolescents during intensive treatment regimens[80]. Unlike the DQOL, the CHQ is a generic tool that allows comparison between children and adolescents with and without diabetes. The CHQ is a parent/self-report tool that quantifies disease impact upon general health, psychosocial health and family cohesion. In published data from our clinic[76], parents reported that for adolescents aged 12-18 years, general health was markedly lower, parental impact (in terms of time and emotion) was high and family activities mean scores were moderately lower (Figure 2).

Figure 2: Child Health Questionnaire data in children and adolescents with diabetes (76). (Reproduced with permission of Blackwell Publishers, London, UK)

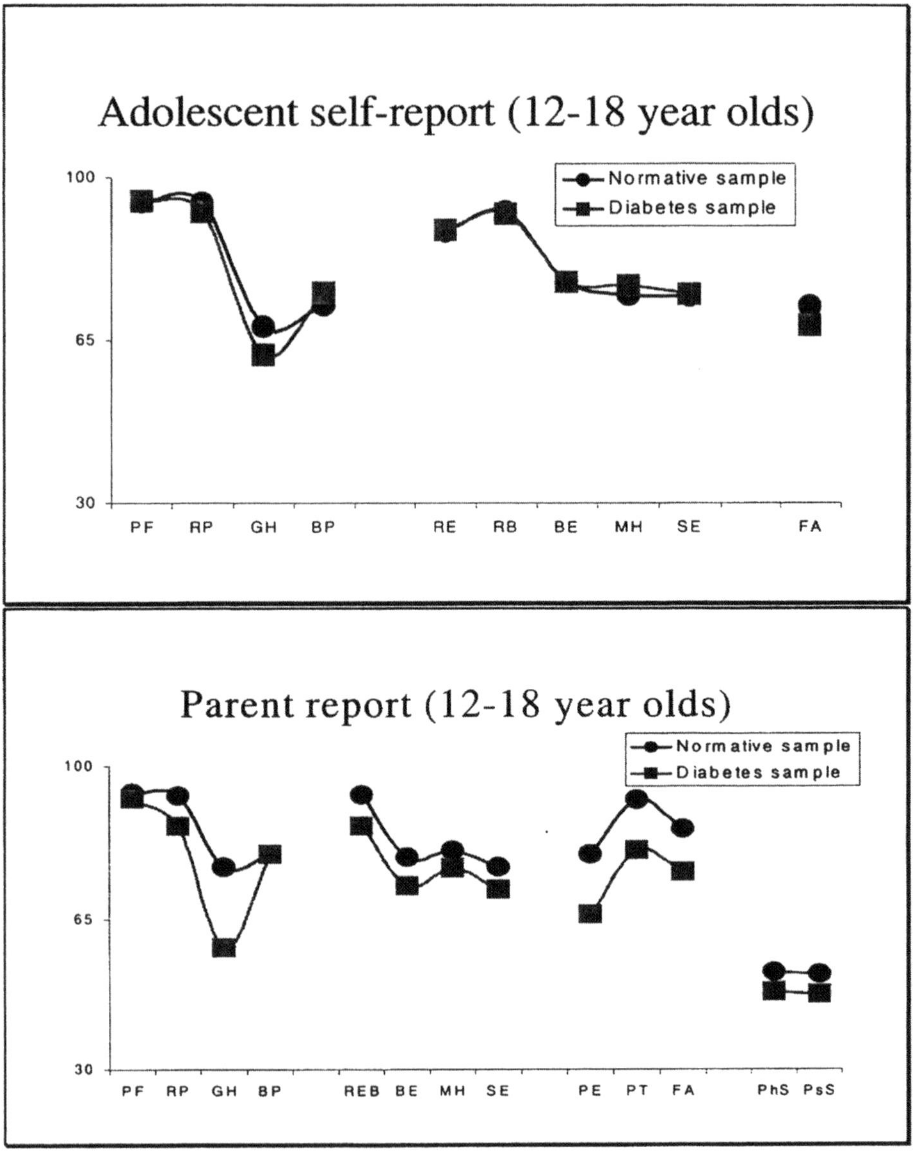

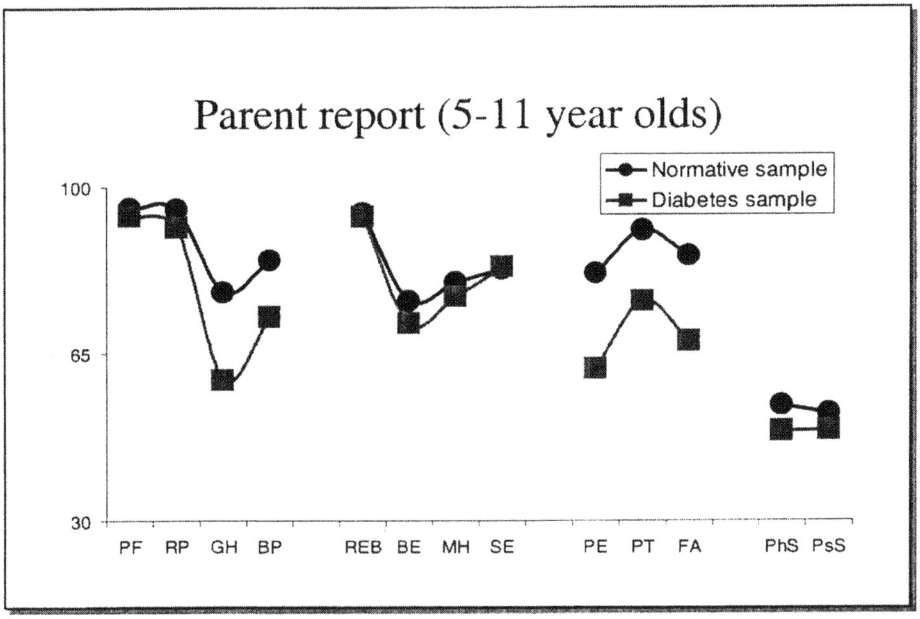

Adolescents with diabetes were reported by their parents as having poorer emotional and behavioral outcomes and poorer self-esteem outcomes than the non-diabetic adolescents. Interestingly, while parents reported a significantly lower quality of life for their adolescent offspring, the adolescents with diabetes rated themselves similarly to adolescents without diabetes. This may be due to the fact that adolescents with diabetes genuinely perceive their health to be similar to that of their peers. Alternatively, even when health concerns are present, this form of adolescent self-report may not be the ideal way of describing their impact. Finally, adolescents may not wish to report themselves to be different.

PEER SUPPORT AND EDUCATION

Effective strategies for education and support are orientated around peer-support models[81]. Positive role-modeling, diabetes camps, buddy-systems and peer counseling are approaches that are gaining increasing usage within diabetes clinics that deal with adolescents[81, 82]. Techniques that foster resiliency life skills are also garnering interest from clinicians who deal with adolescents and chronic disease, although specific diabetes research in this field is lacking. Apart from printed material directed at adolescents, newer approaches such as internet-based programs, multimedia and video packages such as our recently released "Keep Your Life On

Line"[83] attempt to deal holistically with a range of issues such as sex, drugs, alcohol, smoking and diabetic complications, all relevant to the life of an adolescent with diabetes.

TRANSITION

At the completion of adolescence and secondary education thought must be given toward transition of patients to adult diabetes care services. This should coincide with a major degree of autonomy in self-care by the young adult in question. Unfortunately it is during this period that the greatest risk for sudden death exists[84]. Pediatric diabetologists have a critical role to play in preparing their adolescent patients for this process. Frequently they have been involved in their patient's care for many years and the thought of transition may be greeted with trepidation by both adolescents and parents. In our clinics, adolescents themselves have reported that they think transition should occur after 17 years of age and that in such clinics they expect confidentiality and privacy and some degree of informality[85]. Unfortunately the issue of successful transition from a pediatric or adolescent clinic to an adult program remains problematic. Anecdotally we experience large drop-out rates during the process of transition despite transition workshops and active collaboration with other adult diabetes services in our region.

Adolescents should be made aware of the different adult clinics available and the different practice-style of those clinics. The adult diabetes clinic may be busier, less pastoral in their approach than pediatric diabetes clinics. Diabetologists treating adult patients assume that patients are wholly responsible for their own lifestyle decisions and actions and that the clinician's role is simply to provide advice and encouragement along the way. In some centers, specific young adults' clinics are provided. These clinics are often staffed by a combination of both pediatric and adult diabetologists. The purpose of such clinics is an attempt to ensure successful transition. Unfortunately, if transition is not made and patients are lost to ongoing specialist care, diabetes control usually deteriorates markedly, maladaptive lifestyle practices become entrenched and the early appearance of diabetes-related complications frequently results.

CONCLUSION

Diabetes in the adolescent is complex and challenging in the extent of physiological, psychological and sociological consequences and, conversely, in the impact of these on diabetes control. Adolescents with diabetes can neither be considered simply as young adults nor as large children. The satisfactory outcome of diabetes in young people emerging from adolescence must be judged primarily by the extent to which microvascular and related complications are avoided, for this is the time when they have their genesis. Of similar importance is the maintenance of overall physical and psychological health and continuing motivation to strive for optimal diabetic control into the future. The clinician supporting the adolescent with diabetes through these difficult years must have understanding and insights into the complex nature of the biology of adolescence and its interaction with diabetes.

REFERENCES

1. Thomas AM and Hauser ST. Psychosocial Challenges and Issues. In: Werther GA, Court JM: eds. *Diabetes and the adolescent.* Miranova Publishers, Melbourne 1998: 35-55
2. Dabelea D; Pettitt DJ; Jones KL; Arslanian SA. Type 2 diabetes mellitus in minority children and adolescents. An emerging problem. Endocrinol Metab Clin North Am, 1999; Dec, 28:4, 709-29, viii
3. Hoskins, P., Leslie, R., Pyke, D. Height at diagnosis of diabetes in children: a study in identical twins. Br Med J 1985; 290, 278-280
4. Leslie, R., Lo, S., Millward, A., Honour, J., Pyke, D. Decreased growth velocity before IDDM onset. Diabetes1991; 40, 211-16
5. Emmerson, A., Savage, D. Height at diagnosis in diabetes. Eur J Pediatr 1988; 147, 319-320
6. Brown, M., Ahmed, M., Clayton, K., Dunger, D. Growth during childhood and final height in Type I diabetes. Diabetic Med 1994; 11, 182-187
7. Herber, S., Dunsmore, I. Does control affect growth in diabetes mellitus? Acta Paediatr Scand 1988; 77, 303-305
8. Stewart-Brown, S., Lee, T., Savage, D. Pubertal growth in diabetics. Arch Dis Child1985; 60, 768-769
9. Rogers, D., Sherman, L., Gabbay, K. Effect of puberty on insulin-like growth factor I and HBA1 in type I diabetes. Diabetes Care 1991; 14, 1031-1035
10. Connors MH . Growth in the diabetic child. [Review] Pediatric Clinics of North America 1997; 44(2):301-6,
11. Kjaer, K., Hagen, C., Sando, S., Eshoj, O. Epidemiology of menarche and menstrual disturbances in an unselected group of women with insulin-dependent diabetes mellitus compared to controls. J Clin Endocrinol Metab 1992; 75, 524-29

12. Schriock, E., Winter, R., Trasiman H. Diabetes mellitus and its effects on menarche. J Adolesc Health Care 1984; 5, 101-104
13. Clarson, C., Daneman, D., Ehrlich, R. The Relationship of Metabolic Control to Growth and Pubertal Development in Children with Insulin-Dependent Diabetes. Diab Res 1985; 2, 237-241
14. Adcock, C., Perry, L., Lindsell, D. Menstrual irregularities are more common in adolescents with type I diabetes: association with poor glycemic control and weight gain. Diabetic Med 1994; 11, 465-470
15. Rudolf, M., Sherwin, R., Markowitz, R., et al. Effect of intensive insulin treatment on linear growth in the young diabetic adolescent. J Pediatr 1982; 101, 333-339
16. Dunger, D., Cheetham, T. (1996) Growth hormone insulin-like growth factor axis in insulin-dependent diabetes mellitus. Horm Res, 46, 2-6
17. Menon, R., Arslanian, S., May, B., Cutfield, W., Sperling, M. (1992) Diminished growth hormone-binding protein in children with insulin-dependent diabetes mellitus. J Clin Endocrinol Metab, 74, 934-938
18. Clayton, K., Holly, J., Carlsson, L., et al. (1994) Loss of the normal relationships between growth hormone, growth hormone-binding protein and insulin-like growth factor I in adolescents with insulin dependent diabetes mellitus. Clin Endocrinol, 41, 517-524
19. Batch, J., Baxter, R., Werther, G. (1991) Abnormal regulation of insulin-like growth factor binding proteins in adolescents with insulin-dependent diabetes mellitus. J Clin Endocrinol Metab, 73, 964-968
20. Batch, J., Baxter, R., Werther, G. (1991) Abnormal regulation of insulin-like growth factor binding proteins in adolescents with insulin-dependent diabetes mellitus. J Clin Endocrinol Metab, 73, 964-968
21. Holly, J., Dunger, D., Edge, J., Smith, C., Chard, T., Was, J. (1990) Insulin-like growth factor binding protein-1 levels in diabetic adolescents and their relationship to metabolic control. Diabetic Med, 7, 618-623
22. Anderson B, Ho J, Brackett J, Finkelstein D, Laffel L. Parental involvement in diabetes management tasks: relationships to blood glucose monitoring adherence and metabolic control in young adolescents with insulin-dependent diabetes mellitus. J Pediatr 1997; 130: 257-265.
23. Mortensen HB, Robertson KJ, Aanstoot HJ, Danne T, Holl RW, Hougaard P et al. Insulin management and metabolic control of type 1 diabetes mellitus in childhood and adolescence in 18 countries. Hvidore Study Group on Childhood Diabetes. Diabet Med 1998; 15: 752-9.

24. Vanelli M, Chiarelli F, Chiari G, Tumini S, Costi G, di Ricco L et al. Metabolic control in children and adolescents with diabetes: experience of two Italian Regional Centers. J Pediatr Endocrinol Metab 1999; 12: 403-9.
25. Dabaghdao P, Vidmar S and Cameron FJ. Deteriorating diabetic control through adolescence- do the origins lie in childhood? *Diabetic Medicine (in press)*
26. Loman DG, Galgani CA. Physical activity in adolescents with diabetes. Diabetes Educ 1996; 22: 121-5.
27. Webb KL, Dobson AJ, O'Connell DL, Tupling HE, Harris GW, Moxon JA et al. Dietary compliance among insulin-dependent diabetics. J Chronic Dis 1984; 37: 633-43.
28. Cerkoney KA, Hart LK. The relationship between the health belief model and compliance of persons with diabetes mellitus. Diabetes Care, 1980; 3: 594-598.
29. Patterson JM, Garwick AW. Coping with chronic illness; a family systems perspective on living with diabetes. In Werther GA, Court JM: eds. *Diabetes and the adolescent.* Miranova Publishers, Melbourne 1998: 3-34.
30. Peveler R, Fairburn C, Boller I, Dunger D. Eating disorders in adolescents with IDDM. Diabetes Care 1992; 15: 1356-1360.
31. Rodin G, Johnson L, Garfinkel P, Daneman D, Kenshole A. Eating disorders in female adolescents with insulin dependent diabetes mellitus. Int J Psychiatr Med 1986; 16: 49-57.
32. Rosmark B, Berne C, Holmgren S, Lago C, Renholm G, Sohlberg S. Eating disorders in patients with insulin-dependent diabetes mellitus. J Clin Psychiatry 1996; 47: 547-550.
33. Amiel SA, Sherwin RS, Simonson DC, Luritano AA, Tamborlane W. Impaired insulin action in puberty: a contributing factor to poor glycemic control in adolescents with diabetes. New Engl J Med 1986; 315: 1273-1280.
34. Boardway RH, Delamater AM, Tomakowsky J, Gutai JP. Stress management training for adolescents with diabetes. J Pediatr Psychol 1993; 18: 29-45.
35. Grey M, Boland EA, Davidson M, Li J, Tamborlane WV. Coping skills training for youth with diabetes mellitus has long-lasting effects on metabolic control and quality of life. J Pediatr 2000; 137: 107-113.
36. Nurick MA, Johnson SB. Enhancing blood glucose awareness in adolescents and young adults with IDDM. Diabetes Care 1991; 14: 1-7.

37. Peveler RC, Davies BA, Mayou RA, Fairburn CG, Mann JI. Self-care behaviour and blood glucose control in young adults with type 1 diabetes mellitus. Diabet Med 1993; 10: 74-80.
38. Wdowik MJ, Kendall PA, Harris MA, Keim KS. Development and evaluation of an intervention program: "Control on Campus". Diabetes Educ 2000; 26: 95-104
39. Cerkoney, K.A. and Hart, L.K. (1980) The relationship between the health belief model and compliance of persons with diabetes mellitus. *Diabetes Care*, 3, 594–598.
40. LaGreca, A., Auslander, W., Greco, P., Spetter, D., Fisher, E. and Santiago, J. (1995) I get by with a little help from my family and friends: Adolescents' support for diabetes care. J Pediatr Psych 1995; 20:449–476.
41. Bryden KS, Neil A, Mayou RA, Peveler RC, Fairburn CG, DungerDB. Eating habits, body weight, and insulin misuse. A longitudinal study of teenagers and young adults with type 1 diabetes.Diabetes Care 1999;22:1956-60.
42. Du Pasquier-Fediaevsky L, Tubiana-Rufi N. Discordance between physician and adolescent assessments of adherence to treatment: influence of HbA1c level. The PEDIAB Collaborative Group. Diabetes Care 1999;22:1445-9.
43. Charron-Prochownik D, Becker D Factors affecting adherence. In Werther GA, Court JM: eds. *Diabetes and the adolescent.* Miranova Publishers, Melbourne 1998:pp 57-67.
44. Hanson, C.L., Henggeler, S.W.and Burghen, G.A. (1987) Model associations between psychosocial variables and health-outcome measures of adolescents with IDDM. Diabetes Care, 10, 752–758.
45. Hanson, C.L., DeGuire, M.J., Schinkel, A.M., Henggler, S.W. and Burghen, G.A. (1992) Comparing social learning and family systems correlates of adaptation in youths with IDDM. J Ped Psych, 17, 555–572.
46. Hanson, C.L., DeGuire, M.J., Schinkel, A.M. and Kolterman, O. (1995) Empirical validation for a family-centered model of care. Diabetes Care, 18, 1347–1356.
47. Hauser, S.T., Jacobson, A.M., Lavori, P., et al. (1990) Adherence among children and adolescents with insulin-dependent diabetes mellitus over a four-year longitudinal follow-up. II. Immediate and long-term linkages with the family milieu. J Ped Psych, 15, 527–542.

48. Kuttner, M. J., Delameter, A. M. and Santiago, J. V. (1990) Learned helplessness in diabetic youths. Journal of Pediatric Psychology, 15, 581–594.
49. Blanz, B. J., Rensch-Riemann, B. S., Fritz-Sigmund, D. I. And Schmidt, M. H.(1993) IDDM is a risk factor for adolescent psychiatric disorders. Diabetes Care, 16, 1579–1587.
50. Cooper ME, Allen TJ, Couper J. Nephropathy and hypertension. In Werther GA, Court JM: eds. *Diabetes and the adolescent.* Miranova Publishers, Melbourne 1998:pp 139-156.
51. Donaghue K. Retinopathy. In Werther GA, Court JM: eds. *Diabetes and the adolescent.* Miranova Publishers, Melbourne 1998:pp 157-174.
52. Rubin R. Working with diabetic adolescents. In: Practical Psychology for Diabetes Clinicians: How to Deal with the Key Behavioral Issues Faced by patients & Health Care Teams. B Anderson and R Rubin (eds), pp 13-23. Alexandria, VA: American Diabetes Association.
53. Bognetti E, Macellaro P, Novelli D, Meschi F, Ciralli F, Chiumello G. Prevalence and correlates of obesity in insulin dependent diabetic patients. Arch Dis Child 1995; 73: 239-42.
54. Domargard A, Sarnblad S, Kroon M, Karlsson I, Skeppner G, Aman J. Increased prevalence of overweight in adolescent girls with type 1 diabetes mellitus. Acta Paediatr 1999; 88: 1223-8.
55. Holl RW, Grabert M, Sorgo W, Heinze E, Debatin KM. Contributions of age, gender and insulin administration to weight gain in subjects with IDDM. Diabetologia 1998; 41: 542-7.
56. Amiel, S., Sherwin, R., Simonson, D., Lauritano, A., Tamborlane, W. (1986) Impaired insulin action in puberty. A contributing factor to poor glycemic control in adolescents with diabetes. N Engl J Med, 315, 215-19
57. Arslanian SA, Heil BV, Becker DJ, Drash AL. Sexual dimorphism in insulin sensitivity in adolescents with insulin-dependent diabetes mellitus. J Clin Endocrinol Metab 1991; 72: 920-6.
58. Bloch CA, Clemons P, Sperling MA. Puberty decreases insulin sensitivity. J Pediatr 1987; 110: 481-7.
59. Nielsen S, Borner H, Kabel M. Anorexia nervosa/bulimia in diabetes mellitus: a review and presentation of five cases. Acta Psychiatr Scand 1987:75; 464-73.
60. Jones JM, Lawson ML, Daneman D, Olmsted MP, Rodin G. Eating disorders in adolescent females with and without type 1 diabetes: cross sectional study. BMJ 2000;320:1563-6.

61. Rodin GM, Daneman D. Eating disorders and IDDM. A problematic association. Diabetes Care 1992 Oct;15:1402-12
62. Daneman D, Olmsted M, Rydall A, Maharaj S, Rodin G Eating disorders in young women with type 1 diabetes. Prevalence, problems and prevention. Horm Res 1998;50 Suppl 1:79-86.
63. Bryden KS, Neil A, Mayou RA, Peveler RC, Fairburn CG, Dunger DB. Eating habits, body weight, and insulin misuse. A longitudinal study of teenagers and young adults with type 1 diabetes. Diabetes Care 1999 Dec;22:1956-60.
64. Hoffman RP Eating disorders in adolescents with type 1 diabetes. A closer look at a complicated condition. Postgrad Med 2001 Apr;109:67-9, 73-4.
65. Strauch H, Wirth I, Geserick G. Fatal accidents due to train surfing in `Berlin.Forensic Sci Int 1998;94:119-27.
66. Marshall C, Boyd KT, Moran CG. Injuries related to car crime: the joy-riding epidemic Injury 1996;27:79-80.
67. Hauenstein E, Martin R, Snyder A and Clarke W. (1989) Stress in parents of children with diabetes mellitus. *Diabetes Care*, 12:18-23.
68. Schafer L, McCaul K, Glasgow R. (1986) Supportive and non-supportive family behaviors: relationships to adherence and metabolic control in persons with type 1 diabetes. *Diabetes Care*, 9: 179-185.
69. Jacobsen A, Hauser S, Wertlieb D, Wolsdorf J, Orleans J, Vieyra M. (1986) Pychological adjustment of children with recently diagnosed diabetes mellitus. *Diabetes Care*, 9: 323-329.
70. Northam E.A., Anderson P.J., Werther G.A., Warne G.L., Adler R.G., Andrewes D. (1998). Neuropsychological complications of IDDM in children with 2 years after disease onset. *Diabetes Care*, 21: 379-84.
71. Northam E.A., Anderson P.J., Werther G.A., Warne G.L., Andrewes D. (1999). Predictors of change in the neuropsychological profiles of children with type 1 diabetes 2 years after disease onset. *Diabetes Care*, 22: 1438-44.47.
72. Northam EA, Anderson P, Jacobs R, Hughes M, Warne GL, Werther GA. Diabetes Care (2001) In press
73. Becker DJ 1991. Management of insulin-dependent diabetes mellitus in children and adolescents. *Current opinion in Pediatrics*, 3: 710-723.
74. Hanson CL, Henggeler SW, Harris MA, Mitchell KA, Carle DL, Burghen GA. (1988) Associations between family members' perceptions of the health care system and the health of youths with insulin-dependent diabetes mellitus. J Pediatr Psychol;13:543-54.

75. The Diabetes Control and Complications Trial Research Group: The effect of intensive treatment of diabetes on the development and progression of long-term complications in insulin-dependent diabetes mellitus. *New Engl J Med* 329:977-986, 1993.
76. Wake M, Hesketh K, Cameron FJ. The functional health status of children with diabetes. *Diab Med* 2000; 17(10): 700-707.
77. The DCCT Research Group. Reliability and validity of a diabetes quality-of-life measure for the diabetes control and complications trial (DCCT). Diabetes Care 1988 Oct;11(9):725-32.
78. Parkerson,GR, Connis,RT, Broadhead, WE, Patrick,DL, Taylor,TR, Tse,CKJ: Disease-specific versus generic measurement of health-related quality of life in insulin-dependent diabetic patients. *Med Care* 31:629-639, 1993.
79. Ingersoll GM, Marrero DG A modified quality-of-life measure for youths: psychometric properties. Diabetes Educ 1991 Mar-Apr;17(2):114-8.
80. No authors Influence of intensive diabetes treatment on quality-of-life outcomes in the diabetes control and complications trial. Diabetes Care 1996 Mar;19(3):195-203
81. Olsson C, Toumborurou J, Bowes G, Walsh B. Therapeutic peer support. In: *Diabetes and the adolescent.* GA Werther and JM Court (eds), pp217-230. Melbourne, 1998 Miranova.Publishers
82. Court JM. Camping for youth with diabetes. In: *Diabetes and the adolescent.* GA Werther and JM Court (eds), pp271-280. Melbourne, 1998 Miranova Publishers
83. "*Keep your life online- teenagers and young adults living positively with diabetes*". Educational video. ERC Media, Educational Resource Centre, Royal Children's Hospital, Melbourne.
84. Warner DP, McKinney PA, Law GR, Bodansky HJ. Mortality and diabetes from a population based register in Yorkshire. 1978-93.Arch Dis Child 1998; 78:435-8.
85. Court JM. Issues of transition to adult care. J Paediatr Child Health 1993;29 Suppl 1:S53-5

Chapter 16
THE DCCT AND ITS IMPLICATIONS FOR MANAGEMENT OF DIABETES IN CHILDREN AND ADOLESCENTS

Neil H. White, M.D., CDE
Washington University School of Medicine in St. Louis, St. Louis, Missouri

INTRODUCTION AND RATIONALE

Diabetes mellitus is defined as a group of closely related disorders manifest by hyperglycemia as a result of impaired insulin secretion and/or impaired insulin action associated with long-term complications. These complications include the microvascular and neuropathic complications of diabetic retinopathy, nephropathy and neuropathy as well as a marked increase in the risk of macrovascular disease resulting in coronary artery disease and myocardial infarction, cerebrovascular disease and stroke, and peripheral vascular disease and limb amputation. Indeed, diabetes mellitus is a leading cause of new-onset blindness, renal failure and non-traumatic amputations in adults. A relationship between hyperglycemia and diabetes complications has long been suspected, but until near the end of the 20th century specific evidence of direct benefit of improving glycemic control on the development and progression of diabetes complications was lacking. Methods to safely establish and maintain the level of glycemic control necessary to impact on diabetes complications, and techniques for reliable, unequivocal and nonbiased measurement of glycemic control and of diabetes complications became available in the late 1970's and were further refined during the early 1980's. Implementation of these methods during the early 1980's enabled the development and performance of clinical trials to determine whether intervention to lower blood glucose would actually reduce the development and/or slow the progression of diabetes complications. However, because of the long time course for the development of diabetes complications, definitive results of these studies only became available in the early to mid-1990's.

During the decade of the 1990's, results of the Diabetes Control and Complications Trial (DCCT),[1-6] the Stockholm Diabetes Intervention Trial (SDIT)[7] and the United Kingdom Prospective Diabetes Study (UKPDS)[8] were reported and clearly demonstrated that intervention to reduce blood glucose delayed the development and/or slowed the progression of retinopathy, nephropathy and neuropathy in subjects with diabetes and appeared to reduce the risk factors for development of macrovascular disease. The DCCT and the SDIT were performed in subjects with type 1 diabetes and the UKPDS in subjects with type 2 diabetes. The purpose of this chapter is to summarize and discuss the results and implications of the DCCT, especially as they relate to adolescents and children.

Why should the implications of the DCCT be considered separately for children and adolescents than for the adults? Firstly, management strategies and results of therapy could be different in children and teenagers than in young adults. Young children are dependent upon their parents and caretakers to implement daily diabetes management tasks. Meal and activity schedules in children and especially in teenagers may vary widely from day to day. Establishing and maintaining optimal glycemic control in teenagers can be especially problematic as a result of both the physiologic and psychosocial and family factors occurring during this time of life. Secondly, there has been some suggestion that puberty could play an important role in the development of diabetes complications[9-11]. Although this concept is not universally accepted, these reports could indicate that glycemic control during the years before puberty is a less important contributor to the occurrence of diabetes complications later in life than is glycemic control during the years after the onset of puberty. Even if puberty is not a necessary component in the development of diabetes complications, it could serve as a modifying factor in the risk:benefit ratio of glycemic control[29].

Although the major results of the DCCT were reported in 1993[1] and the results of the adolescent cohort in 1994,[2] the entire DCCT cohort continues to be followed as part of a non-randomized observational study known as the Epidemiology of Diabetes Interventions and Complications (EDIC, see below)[12]. EDIC is attempting to address the durability of the benefits demonstrated during the DCCT and whether the interventions implemented during the DCCT had significant impact on more advanced and life-threatening diabetes-related complications, such as renal insufficiency and end-stage renal disease (ESRD) or coronary artery disease and its risk factors. The results of EDIC as reported to date[13,14] will also be discussed in this chapter.

DCCT STUDY DESIGN

The Diabetes Control and Complications Trial (DCCT) was a randomized, controlled, multicenter clinical trial designed to address the hypothesis that the use of intensive diabetes therapy to reduce the blood glucose to as close to the normal range as was safely possible would result in a statistically significant and clinically meaningful reduction in the development and progression of diabetes complications. Retinopathy was chosen as the primary outcome for two reasons. Firstly, well-established and relatively noninvasive and reproducible techniques for determination of retinopathy were available. Secondly, preliminary data about the incidence and rate of progression of diabetic retinopathy were available to enable a reliable determination of the sample size needed for a full-scale clinical trial.

The DCCT was performed as a multicenter collaborative effort between 29 clinical centers (initially 29 centers during Phase II), 7 central laboratory or reading units, a common Coordinating Center and the NIH/NIDDK. (A complete listing of the centers and investigators and staff responsible for performance of the DCCT can be found in the Appendix to reference 1). After submission of competitive applications and selection of the initial study group, the trial was divided into three phases. Phase I consisted of a one-year planning period during which representatives from all of the initial 21 clinical centers and the reading/laboratory units, Coordinating Center and NIH developed a common protocol to address the study's primary hypothesis and secondary hypotheses. Phase II consisted of a 1-2 year feasibility phase during which the study group recruited subjects and implemented the protocol in a relatively small cohort of subjects. The purpose of the feasibility phase was to determine the ability of the study group to: 1) recruit eligible subjects, including adolescents; 2) randomly assign them to one of two different treatment groups designed to establish different levels of glycemic control; 3) assess control and outcomes using standardized common measures that would be sent to central laboratories and reading centers; and 4) maintain subjects in their assigned treatment groups and testing and follow-up frequency for a two-year period. Another important purpose of the feasibility phase was to determine that the two treatment groups did indeed result in a statistically significant and clinically meaningful difference in glycemic control.

To accomplish this, during Phase II, each of the 21 centers was expected to recruit at least 12 eligible subjects of whom at least four were to be "adolescents." Adolescents were considered to be those who were <18 years old at the time of randomization. As noted below, all DCCT subjects had to be at least 13 years old and at least Tanner stage II. It should be noted that during Phase II, adolescents were randomized independently of the remainder of the cohort. This was to assure that the feasibility goals could be independently assessed for adolescents as well as adults. One potential outcome of the feasibility phase could have been an inability to recruit and follow teenage subjects and/or an inability to establish the different levels of glycemic control in teenagers using the treatment modalities selected for use in the DCCT. Had this been the case, the study group could have decided not to include adolescents in the full-scale clinical trial. Indeed, despite the fact that recruitment and management of adolescents was more difficult and more time-consuming than for the adult subjects, adolescent subjects were recruited in the necessary numbers, maintained follow-up and did demonstrate different levels of glycemic control between the two groups during the feasibility phase of the DCCT[15]. Therefore, the study group decided to include adolescents in the phase III full-scale clinical trial, thus enabling the determination of the risks and benefits (summarized herein) of intensive diabetes therapy in this important group of subjects.

After the successful completion of phase II, the phase III full-scale clinical trial commenced in 1985. The full-scale trial included a total of 1441 subjects at 29 clinical centers (including continued follow-up of the 278 enrolled during phase II). 195 of the 1441 DCCT subjects were adolescents (13-17 years of age and at least Tanner stage II puberty) at the time of randomization. It should be noted that although during phase II adolescents had been randomized separately from adults and equally into the intensive treatment group and the conventional treatment group, randomization during phase III was not stratified by age. Nonetheless, among the adolescents in both the primary intervention and the secondary intervention groups (see below), those assigned to the intensive treatment group and the conventional treatment group were similar in all measures at baseline evaluation (see Table 1).

Eligibility and Recruitment

Subjects recruited for participation in the DCCT were selected from those identified as potentially eligible within the clinics or practices of the participating investigators and by word of mouth and advertising in the communities where DCCT centers were based. Recruitment was a multistage process to insure both the selection of appropriate subjects and fully informed consent for this complex and long-duration clinical trial.

The basic eligibility criteria for participation in the DCCT were: 1) age 13-39 years old; 2) type 1 diabetes for at least 5 years, or for at least one year and a Sustacal® stimulated C-peptide<0.2 pmol/ml (<0.5 pmol/ml if duration of diabetes <5 years); 3) willingness to be randomized to either the intensive or the conventional treatment group (see below); 4) absence of significant other medical illnesses; and 5) absence of advanced diabetes complications (proliferative diabetic retinopathy or clinically-significant macular edema, albuminuria >200 mg/day, clinically manifest neuropathy, hypertension, or clinically significant heart disease). A complete listing of excluding and allowable medical conditions and medications can be found in the protocol[16].

Subjects were recruited for participation in a primary prevention arm and a secondary intervention arm of the trial. Those representing the primary prevention cohort had diabetes for 1-5 years, no retinopathy, and urinary albumin <40 mg/day (<28 μg/min). Those in the secondary intervention cohort had to have early background retinopathy (at least microaneurysms, but no evidence of proliferative retinopathy or clinically-significant macular edema). They could have diabetes for 1-15 years and up to 200 mg/day (139 μg/min) of albuminuria. By design, and based on sample size considerations, there were approximately equal numbers of subjects recruited into each cohort. Subjects were randomized to the intensive therapy group (IT) or the conventional therapy group (CT) within each cohort. The demographic and baseline characteristics for the entire study population were similar between the IT and the CT groups within each cohort (primary prevention and secondary intervention) and can be found in the published literature[1]. The demographic and baseline characteristics for the adolescent cohort (N=195; <18 years old at randomization) are shown in Table 1 below.

Treatment groups

After recruitment, obtaining of a multistaged informed consent and eligibility screening, subjects were randomized to either the intensive treatment group (IT) or the conventional treatment group (CT). In the CT group, subjects were expected to manage their diabetes by methods considered standard of care for the time (1983-1989). This included either one or two injections of insulin per day, at least daily monitoring of either blood or urine glucose, maintenance of a meal plan appropriate for people with type 1 diabetes, and quarterly visits with the health care team. The goal was the absence of symptomatic hyperglycemia, symptomatic hypoglycemia, ketosis or ketoacidosis, and a hemoglobin A1c (HbA1c) that was not markedly elevated (>13.1%).

Those assigned to the IT group were provided a regimen that was meant to achieve a blood glucose and HbA1c as close to the normal (non-diabetic) range as was safely possible, that is, as close to normal without significant hypoglycemia. The specific glycemic targets in the IT group were 70-120 mg/dl (3.8-6.9 mM) before meals, <180 mg/dl (<10 mM) after meals, >65 mg/dl (>3.6 mM) at 2 AM, an HbA1c <6.05% (mean + 2 standard deviations for the nondiabetic population) and absence of severe hypoglycemia. In order to accomplish this, subjects administered insulin by multiple (≥3) daily injections or by continuous subcutaneous insulin infusion (CSII or the insulin pump). The regimen of choice in the IT group included premeal bolus doses of short acting insulin plus basal insulin delivery. In addition, treatment in the IT group included self-blood glucose monitoring (SBGM) at least four times each day and at least once a week at 2 AM; ongoing daily insulin dose adjustments based on blood glucose determinations, anticipated dietary intake and anticipated activity; and at least monthly visits to the health care team. In both the IT and the CT group, the primary measure of glycemic control during the DCCT was a hemoglobin A1c (HbA1c) measured quarterly by HPLC in a central laboratory. Seven-point per day blood glucose profiles at home were also recorded for one day prior to each quarterly visit. In the IT group, HbA1c was determined monthly. These additional values were used only to assist the subject and the health care team in diabetes management and were not used in data analysis. Episodes of severe hypoglycemia were recorded at each visit and it is felt that ascertainment of severe hypoglycemia episodes during the DCCT was nearly complete.

Outcomes

The primary outcome of the DCCT was retinopathy as assessed by 7-field stereoscopic fundus photographs taken locally by certified photographers and graded centrally using the Early Treatment Diabetic Retinopathy Study (ETDRS) criteria by graders who were unaware of the treatment group assignment. A 3-step change in retinopathy or progression from no retinopathy to any retinopathy or from mild background retinopathy to clinical-significant macular edema, proliferative retinopathy or the need for laser photocoagulation were considered clinically important progression of retinopathy. Diabetic nephropathy was assessed using serum creatinine and the albumin excretion rate (in mg/24 hours) extrapolated from a standardized 4-hour urine collection. Microalbuminuria was defined at ≥40 mg/24 hours and albuminuria as ≥300 mg/24 hours. Neuropathy was assessed by a standardized examination, nerve conduction studies and an autonomic nerve study. Clinical neuropathy was defined as an abnormal neurologic examination consistent with peripheral sensorimotor neuropathy

Table 1
Baseline Characteristics of Subjects in the DCCT Adolescent Cohort

Characteristics	Primary IT (N=55)	Prevention CT (N=70)	Secondary IT (N=37)	Intervention CT (N=33)
Age (yr)	15±1	15±1	15±1	15±1
Females (%)	44	53	51	61
Caucasian (%)	98	97	95	85
Diabetes Duration (mo):				
Total	38±20	37±20	89±43	97±42
Postpubertal	32±12	31±13	49±18	48±18
Insulin dose (Units/kg/day)	0.89±0.24	0.92±0.30	1.03±0.30	1.06±0.32
Severe hypoglycemia in preceding year (% of subjects)				
Requiring assistance	0.0	4.3	2.7	0.0
Loss of consciousness	3.6	15.7*	8.1	3.0
Stimulated C-peptide (pmol/ml)	0.11±0.11	0.12±0.13	0.05±0.07	0.03±0.03
HbA1c (%)	9.3±1.9	9.2±1.8	9.8±1.8	10.1±1.8
Systolic BP (mm Hg)	109±8	110±12	111±13	109±10
Diastolic BP (mm Hg)	69±7	69±10	71±11	71±9
BMI (kg/m^2): Male	22±2	21±2	21±2	20±3
Female	22±3	22±3	24±2	22±3*
Cholesterol (mg/dl)	159±28	159±31	176±33	174±33
Triglycerides (mg/dl)	91±74	71±29	100±59	92±34
HDL-cholesterol (mg/dl)	46±10	49±11	43±9	49±13
LDL-cholesterol (mg/dl)	94±22	96±28	114±34	106±29
Smoker (%)	5	3	3	0
No retinopathy (%)	100	100	0	0
Microaneuryms (%)	0	0	84*	61
Mild NPDR (%)	0	0	14	27
Moderate NPDR (%)	0	0	3	12
Urine albumin excretion (mg/24 hrs)	15±15	15±9	26±32	29±40
Serum creatinine (mg/dl)	0.72±0.15	0.72±0.15	0.74±0.13*	0.66±0.11
Creatinine clearance (ml/min per 1.73 m^2)	142±42	137±31	141±49	135±28

Mean±SD unless otherwise stated.
* p<0.05 between groups in this strata
BMI, body mass index; NPDR, nonproliferative diabetic retinopathy; HDL, high-density lipoprotein; LDL; low-density lipoprotein. *Table adapted from reference 2.*

along with either abnormal nerve conduction or abnormal autonomic nerve testing. Whenever possible, those assessing the outcomes were masked to the subject's treatment group assignment and level of glycemic control.

RESULTS

The results of the DCCT were masked to the investigators during the trial, which was initially planned to continue until 10 years after randomization of the first subject. However, the external review committees of the DCCT requested termination of the trial one year before the designated study end and the trial was terminated and the overall results were reported in 1993, approximately 9 years after enrollment of the first participant and about 3 years after enrollment of the last participant. Mean follow-up in the DCCT was 6.5 years with a total of more than 9300 patient-years. Ninety-nine percent (99%) of the subjects completed the trial and more than 95% of the scheduled evaluations were completed.[1] Eleven subjects died and 32 were made inactive for purposes of the study. Overall, subjects implemented therapy according to the guidelines of their treatment group assignment 97% of the time[1,3].

There were 195 subjects that comprised the adolescent cohort (<18 years old at the time of randomization)[2]. At the conclusion of the DCCT, these 195 subjects had been followed for a mean of 7.4 years (range 4-9) and a total of 1448 patient-years. The adolescent cohort represented 13.5% of the subjects and 15.6% of the total follow-up during the DCCT. Two adolescent subjects died and two were assigned to inactive status during the DCCT. None voluntarily withdrew from the study and more than 95% of the scheduled visits were completed for the adolescent cohort. Among the adolescent cohort, more than 95% of the study time was spent within the assigned treatment group. Hence, despite initial concerns of some during phase II that adolescents would be hard to recruit, would not adhere to the protocol and would drop out of the study, this proved not to be the case and the adolescent cohort represented a substantial component of the overall DCCT experience and results. The experience within the adolescent group was adequate to allow performance of an independent statistical analysis in this group.

Glycemic control

The target for glycemic control in the IT group was to achieve an HbA1c within the normal range for non-diabetic subjects, that is, below 6.05% (mean + 2 standard deviations of the control population) without severe hypoglycemia. Although this goal could be achieved at some point during the study by nearly half the subjects, few subjects were able to maintain the HbA1c <6.05% throughout the DCCT. The group mean HbA1c for the IT group fell to its lowest point six months after randomization and was maintained about 1.90% below that of the CT group throughout the entire study period (7.12±0.03% in IT vs. 9.02±0.05% in CT; p<0.001). A comparable difference was found in the mean blood glucose obtained quarterly using a 7-point capillary blood glucose profiles (231±55 mg/dL [12.8±3.1 mM] in CT vs. 155±30 mg/dL [8.6±1.7 mM] in IT; p<0.001)[1].

Although mean HbA1c and blood glucose was higher in the adolescents than in the adults, similar differences in glycemic control were found between groups in the adolescent subjects in the DCCT[2]. In the adolescent cohort, HbA1c fell in the IT group during the first 3-6 months and was then maintained about 1.70% lower than in the CT group for the remainder of the study (8.06±0.13% in IT vs. 9.79±0.12% in CT; p<0.001). The mean of the 7-point blood glucose profiles were also slightly higher in both groups of the adolescent cohort than in the adults (177±31 mg/dL [9.8±1.7 mM] in IT vs. 260±52 mg/dL [14.4±2.9 mM] in CT; p<0.001). Thus, although overall adolescent subjects had higher HbA1c and mean blood glucose than adults, treatment group differences were achieved and maintained in this cohort as well as in the adult cohort(see Table 2)[2]. Assuming similar effects of improving glycemic control in adolescents on the development or delay of diabetes complications, the DCCT results should also be able to demonstrate these benefits among teenage subjects.

Hypoglycemia

It had been anticipated that hypoglycemia would be an important risk associated with attempts to lower glucose to near the euglycemic range during the DCCT. Prior and subsequent studies have demonstrated the risks of severe hypoglycemia associated with intensive diabetes therapy especially in those with defective glucose counterregulation,[17-19] hypoglycemia unawareness[20-21] and hypoglycemia-associated autonomic failure (HAAF)[22,23]. The DCCT utilized a standardized definition of severe hypoglycemia and implemented attempts to accomplish complete ascertainment of all episodes of severe hypoglycemia during the DCCT[1,24,25]. Indeed, in the DCCT, severe hypoglycemia was the most significant adverse event associated with IT[1,24,25]. Overall, severe hypoglycemia occurred 3.3 times more frequently in the IT group (62 episodes/100 patient-years) than in the CT group (19 episodes/100 patient-years) and hypoglycemia associated with seizure or coma occurred 3.2 times more frequent in the IT group than the CT group (16 vs. 5 episodes/100 patient-years). Although this higher rate of severe hypoglycemia was not associated with a significant excess of hospitalizations, motor vehicle accidents, or deaths, and was not associated with clinically manifest changes in neuropsychological function,[1,26] other populations, for example children[27] or the elderly, could be at greater risk from hypoglycemia[28,29]. In addition, unlike during the feasibility phase (phase II), during the full-scale trial (Phase III), subjects were excluded if prior to enrollment they had more than two episodes of seizure or coma due to hypoglycemia or more than one episode of severe neurologic impairment secondary to hypoglycemia but without warning symptoms. Thus, subjects recruited for the DCCT were selected to minimize the risk of severe hypoglycemia.

As in the overall study cohort, in the adolescent cohort severe hypoglycemia occurred 2.93 times more frequently in the IT group (85.7 episodes/100 patient-years) than in the CT group (27.8 episodes/100 patient-years; $p<0.001$) and hypoglycemia associated with seizure or coma occurred 2.96 times more frequent in the IT group than the CT group (26.7 vs. 9.7 episodes/100 patient-years; $p<0.001$)[2]. Thus, although the rates of severe hypoglycemia and of severe hypoglycemia associated with seizure or coma were higher in the adolescents than in the adults for both groups, the relative risk of having hypoglycemia in the IT group compared to the CT group was similar for the adolescents as for the adults (see Table 2).

Retinopathy

By study design, the primary outcome of the DCCT was the development or progression of diabetic retinopathy. In the DCCT, IT resulted in a highly significant 76% reduction in development of retinopathy in the primary prevention cohort and a 47-54% reduction in progression of retinopathy and a 56% reduction in the need laser therapy for proliferative retinopathy or macular edema in the IT group compared to the CT group[1,4]. These reductions in cumulative incidence of retinopathy in the IT group compared to the CT group were consistent among all subgroups of subjects in both the primary prevention and the secondary intervention cohorts.

For the adolescent subjects alone, these findings were similar[2]. There was a 53% (Figure 1) and a 70% (Figure 2) reduction in 3-step or more progression of retinopathy in the IT vs. the CT groups for the adolescent primary prevention and the adolescent secondary intervention cohorts, respectively. These between group results were statistically significant and there was no significant difference between the adolescent and the adult cohorts in the level of risk reduction (see Table 2).

Nephropathy

Overall, IT reduced microalbuminuria by 34% (p=0.04) in the primary prevention cohort and by 43% (p=0.001) in the secondary intervention cohort. Albuminuria was reduced by 56% (p<0.01) in the secondary intervention cohort[1]. In the primary prevention cohort (urinary albumin <40 mg/day at baseline), there were too few cases of albuminuria to allow for statistical analysis. Nephropathy results were similar for the adolescent cohort[2]. Although not statistically significant because there were too few events, in the adolescent primary prevention cohort, there were 5.8 episodes of microalbuminuria per 100 patient-years in the IT group compared to 7.1 episodes per 100 patient-years in the CT group (10% reduction, 95% CI:70% to 52%; p=0.745). In the adolescent secondary intervention group, IT significantly reduced the risk of microalbuminuria by 55% (95% CI: 3-79%; p=0.042). (Figure 3) Too few adolescent subjects in either the primary prevention or the secondary intervention cohorts developed albuminuria (≥300 mg/day) to allow any conclusions to be drawn and none developed impaired renal function. As noted in Table 2, although the risk reduction for microalbuminuria in the adolescent cohort did not achieve statistical significance, the magnitude of the risk reduction in the

Table 2

Comparison of Outcomes of IT Between Adolescents and Adults

	Adolescents	Adult	p*
HbA1c (%; mean ±SE)			
IT group	8.06±0.13	7.12±0.03	<0.001
CT group	9.76±0.12	9.02±0.05	<0.001
Difference between IT & CT	1.70±0.18	1.90±0.06	0.134
Risk reduction (%) (95% CI)†			
Any retinopathy	30 (–9, 55)	27 (9, 41)	0.819
3-step change in retinopathy	61 (30,78)	63 (51, 71)	0.802
Albuminuria ≥40 mg/day	35 (–7, 60)	45 (20, 55)	0.886
All severe hypoglycemia in IT			
Rate (per 100 patient-years)	85.7	56.9	0.004
Relative risk (IT vs. CT)	2.93	3.30	0.753
SH with seizure/coma in IT			
Rate (per 100 patient-years)	26.7	14.4	0.001
Relative risk (IT vs. CT)	2.96	3.10	0.678

* p-value for difference between the adolescent and the adult cohort

† Risk reduction for IT vs. CT

Adapted from data in reference 2.

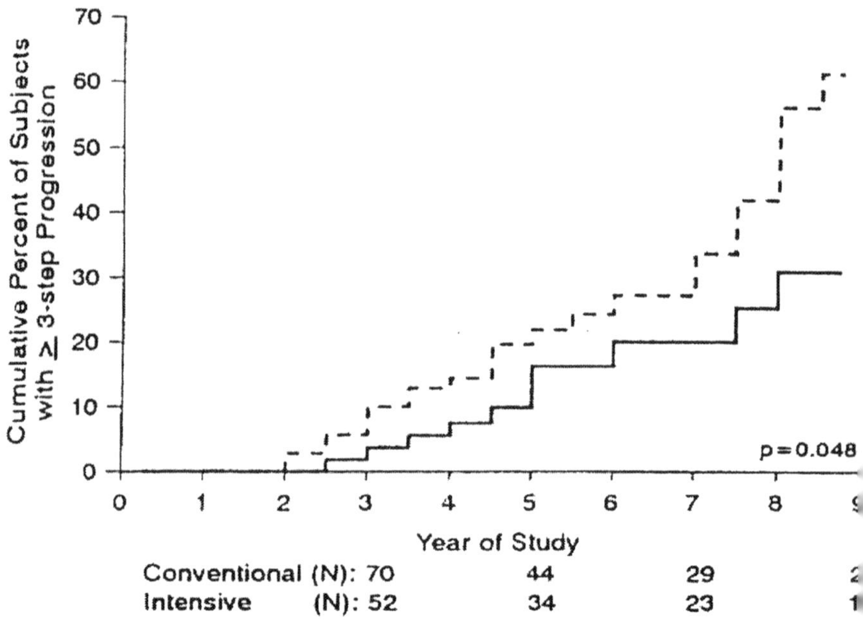

Figure 1: Cumulative incidence plot of a 3-step progression from no retinopathy in the IT group (solid line) and the CT group (dashed line) for the adolescent primary prevention cohort. Numbers at the base of the figure represent the number of subjects at each designated time point. The average adjusted risk reduction associated with intensive therapy is 53% (p=0.048). *Reprinted, with permission, from The Journal of Pediatrics 1994; 125:177-188 (reference 2).*

adolescents was similar (and not statistically different) to that of the adult cohort. Hence, the failure to achieve statistical significance may represent a situation in which there were too few events. Longer follow-up withto accumulate more events (development of microalbuminuria or albuminuria) in the adolescent cohort may be necessary to clarify these results (see EDIC below)[12].

Neuropathy

In the overall cohort, IT reduced the appearance of clinical neuropathy by 60% (95% CI: 38-74%) with significant risk reduction in both the primary prevention cohort (69%; 95% CI: 24-87) and the secondary intervention cohort (57%; 95% CI: 38-74).[1] IT resulted in significant risk reduction for each of the three components defining clinical neuropathy;

neurologic examination (p<0.001), nerve conduction velocity (p<0.001) and autonomic nerve testing (p<0.04).

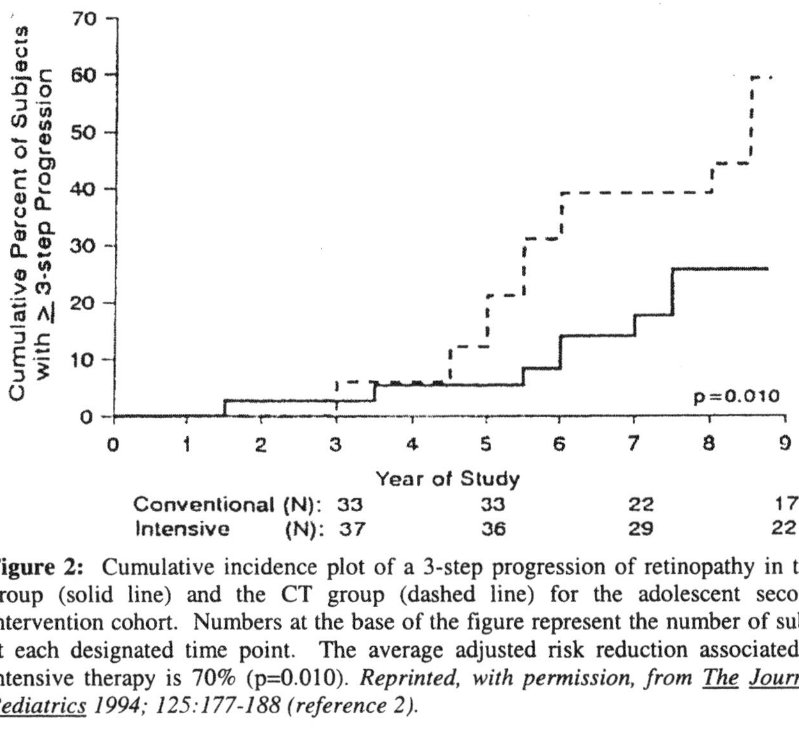

Figure 2: Cumulative incidence plot of a 3-step progression of retinopathy in the IT group (solid line) and the CT group (dashed line) for the adolescent secondary intervention cohort. Numbers at the base of the figure represent the number of subjects at each designated time point. The average adjusted risk reduction associated with intensive therapy is 70% (p=0.010). *Reprinted, with permission, from The Journal of Pediatrics 1994; 125:177-188 (reference 2).*

In the adolescent cohort, seven CT subjects and three IT subjects developed clinical neuropathy[2]. Although this would appear similar to the risk reduction in the overall cohort, there were too few subjects in the adolescent cohort who developed clinical neuropathy for this to be statistically significant. However, nerve conduction velocities, which were similar between IT and CT at baseline, were slower in the CT group than in the IT group at five years for all nerves tested (median motor, p<0.003; median sensory, p=0.04; peroneal, p<0.001; sural, p<0.004)[2].

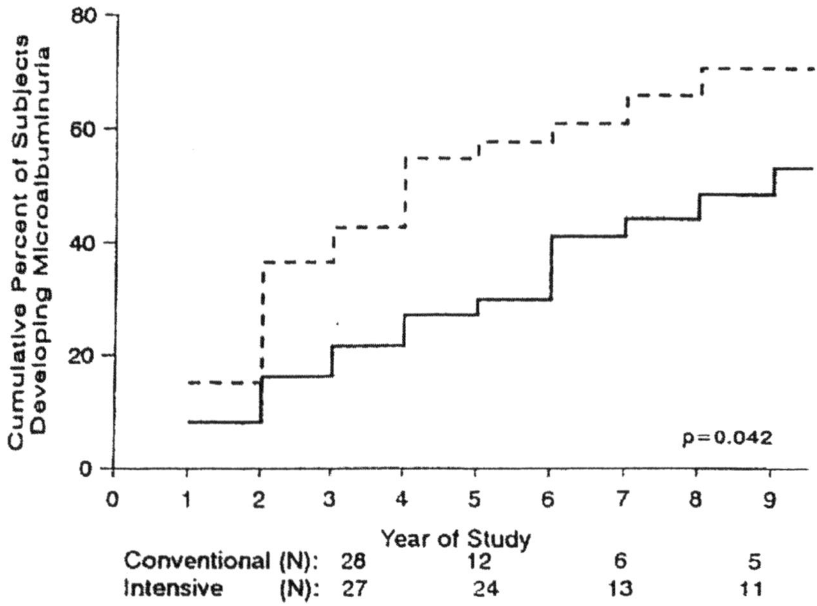

Figure 3: Cumulative incidence plot of microalbuminuria (albumin excretion rate>40 mg/24 hours) in the IT group (solid line) and the CT group (dashed line) for the adolescent secondary intervention cohort. Numbers at the base of the figure represent the number of subjects at each designated time point. The average adjusted risk reduction associated with intensive therapy is 55% ($p=0.042$). *Reprinted, with permission, from The Journal of Pediatrics 1994; 125:177-188 (reference 2).*

Other adverse events

Another anticipated adverse effect of IT was excess weight gain relative to CT. In the entire DCCT cohort, those in the IT group gained a mean of 4.6 kg more than those in the CT group after five years in the DCCT.[1,5] The risk of becoming overweight (defined at >120% above ideal) was 33% higher in the IT than the CT group (12.7 vs. 9.3 cases per 100 patient-years in the IT and the CT groups, respectively). Assessment of weight was a more problematic in the adolescent cohort since many of these subjects were still growing[2]. At the time of their five-year DCCT evaluation, adolescent subjects in the IT group had gained 4.04 kg for males and 3.25 kg for females more than those in the CT group. Treatment group assignment did not influence linear growth. Those in the IT group had a significantly ($p<0.001$ for males; $p<0.019$ for females) greater increase in body mass index (BMI; kg/m^2) and a nearly 2-fold greater risk of becoming overweight (BMI$\geq$27.8 kg/m^2 in boys and BMI$\geq$27.3 kg./m^2 in girls) than those in the CT group.

During the DCCT, the event rate for diabetic ketoacidosis (DKA) in the adolescent cohort was similar between the IT and the CT groups (2.8 vs. 4.7 episodes per 100 patient-years for IT and CT, respectively; $p=0.174$).[2] The rate of DKA in the adolescents was higher than that for the adults (1.8 vs. 1.3 episodes per 100 patient-years for IT vs. CT, respectively). Two adolescent subjects died during the DCCT; one IT subject had a fatal motor vehicle accident unrelated to hypoglycemia and one CT subject committed suicide[2]. In the overall DCCT cohort and in the adolescent cohort, there were no significant differences between groups in the rates of diabetic ketoacidosis, hospitalization, motor vehicle or other accidents, or self-reported quality-of-life[1,2].

Relationship between glycemic control and complications

The primary results and conclusions of the DCCT were based on intention-to-treat analyses comparing the IT to the CT groups. However, in an attempt to address the issue of whether there was a glycemic threshold that could be used to maximize benefits and minimize the risks of IT, a secondary analysis was performed to determine the relation between the development of retinopathy and the glycemic exposure during the DCCT. For this analysis, the risk of complications was determined as the rate of a sustained 3-step or greater progression of retinopathy and glycemic exposure was expressed as the mean of HbA1c values in the subjects obtained at six-month intervals to correspond to the stereo fundus photographs obtained for retinopathy determination.[1] As can be seen in Figure 4, in the IT group there is a continuously increasing rate of retinopathy as mean HbA1c increases. In addition, substantial benefit occurs by lowering HbA1c from high values (such as 10%) down to lower, but not normal, values (such as 9% or 8%). That is, even if the patient cannot get and maintain the HbA1c in the near normal range, any lowering of the HbA1c is likely to result in benefit manifest as reducing or slowing the progression of microvascular complications. Indeed, similar analyses performed for other complications and in both the IT and CT groups and across the combined cohort showed similar results. For every 10% reduction in HbA1c (that is, 10% to 9%; 9% to 8.1%; 8% to 7.2%; 7% to

6.3%) there was a 35-39% reduction in retinopathy risk, a 36-44% reduction in nephropathy, and a 30% reduction in confirmed clinical neuropathy[4]. There was no threshold below which there is no additional benefit of lowering HbA1c[6]. Likewise, there was no threshold above which the benefit of lowering HbA1c was lost. A similar analysis for severe hypoglycemia showed a continuously increasing risk of severe hypoglycemia in the IT group as the mean of monthly HbA1c's declined[1].

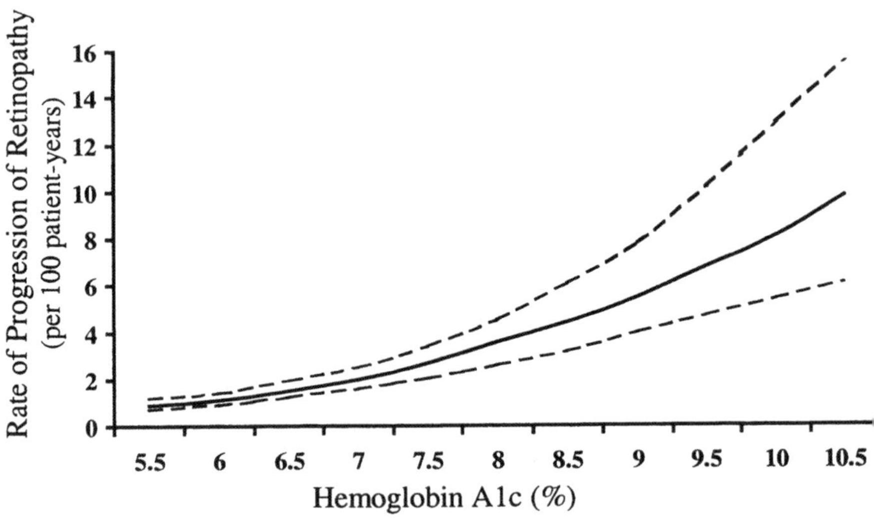

Figure 4: Risk of a sustained progression of retinopathy (3-step or more change from baseline sustained for at least six months; expressed in events per 100 patient-years) in the intensive therapy group plotted versus the mean hemoglobin A1c (HbA1c) obtained every six months during the DCCT. The solid line represents the regression line estimated as a function of the log of the mean HbA1c. The dashed lines represent the 95% confidence interval.
This figure adapted from Figure 5 in reference 1.

EPIDEMIOLOGY OF DIABETES INTERVENTIONS AND CONTROL (EDIC)

The DCCT clearly and unequivocally demonstrated the benefits of IT in reducing diabetes complications based on retinopathy, which had been designated as the primary endpoint. These results for retinopathy were highly statistically significant and clinically meaningful. In the overall DCCT cohort, IT also resulted in statistically significant reduction in the development and progression of albuminuria and in the incidence of diabetic neuropathy. The clinical significance of these latter findings may be likely to also be important, but the event rates for the development of albuminuria and early neuropathy are lower and significant disability resulting from nephropathy and neuropathy usually come later in the course of the disease process. Hence, the clinical meaning of these latter findings is less apparent. In addition, although there was a significant reduction in cardiovascular risk factors (reduced total cholesterol, LDL-cholesterol and triglycerides and increased HDL-cholesterol) with IT,[30] this was a relatively healthy and relatively young cohort; there were too few cardiovascular events (myocardial infarction, stroke) to document reduction in this aspect of diabetes-related morbidity and mortality. Hence, although the results of the DCCT were released to the study group and the public in 1993, and continued maintenance of randomization of subjects to different treatment modalities could not ethically continue, the DCCT Research Group decided that this cohort of subjects should continue to be followed in order to assess the development and progression of more advanced complications over time after conclusion of the DCCT. In addition, it was felt to be important to determine the persistence of the benefits of IT observed during the DCCT. It is for these reasons that the study group developed a follow-up study called the Epidemiology of Diabetes Interventions and Complications (EDIC)[12]. EDIC began in 1994.

Rationale

Although it is reasonable to expect that the reduction of early stages of diabetes complications, as demonstrated during the DCCT, would be expected to slow the development of end-stage complications, such as visual loss and renal failure, too few of these later manifestations of complications occurred during the DCCT to demonstrate this conclusion. In addition, there were too few cardiovascular events in either group during the DCCT to be able to make definitive conclusions about the effect of IT and improved glycemic control on heart disease, stroke and peripheral vascular disease, clearly very important and significant complications of diabetes. Since these later-stage microvascular and macrovascular complications of diabetes usually occur after 15-25 years of diabetes, and the mean duration of diabetes at the end of the DCCT was only about 12 years, it was felt that longer follow-up of this cohort for another 10 years (to a mean duration of 22 years) would likely result in enough events to assess the benefits of prior IT on these later-stage complications.

The objectives of EDIC were:[12]

1) To describe the development and progression of cardiovascular disease in type 1 diabetes.
2) To study the interactions of various risk factors for cardiovascular disease in type 1 diabetes.
3) To examine the long-term effects of prior intervention to lower blood glucose on the development and progression of cardiovascular disease.
4) To follow the development of lipid abnormalities over time and their relationship to diabetes complications.
5) To relate the development of microalbuminuria and other complications and risk factors to clinically significant nephropathy.
6) To study the development of clinically significant neuropathy over time and relate it to prior glycemic control and other risk factors and complications.
7) To examine the progression from background retinopathy to more severe and vision-threatening retinopathy and its relationship to other risk factors and complications.
8) To examine the long-term effects and persistence of the differences in glycemic control achieved during the DCCT on development and progression of diabetes complications.
9) To examine the effect of genetic factors with the development and progression of diabetes complications.
10) To examine health care practices among the former DCCT subjects as it relates to the health care system in which they participate.
11) To examine quality of life in diabetic subjects and the relationship between quality of life and complications.

To date, only data related to objectives 7 & 8 are available and will be summarized herein.

Design of EDIC

EIDC was designed as an epidemiologic observational study to follow the DCCT cohort for another 10 years[12]. Annual evaluations include a standardized history and physical examination along with standardized tests to assess diabetes control, plasma lipids and lipoproteins, diabetes complications, cardiovascular disease and risk factors, current health care and diabetes care practices, and quality of life. EDIC is not an interventional study. At the close of the DCCT and before official start-up of EDIC (1993-1994), all DCCT participants, regardless of study group, were informed of the DCCT study results and encouraged to initiate intensive diabetes therapy. This initiation of intensive therapy was done by DCCT staff during the six months immediately following the release of the DCCT results. Subsequently, all subjects were discharged from the DCCT clinic to return to the care of their primary physician or endocrinologist. They were seen by the DCCT/EDIC staff only for their scheduled evaluation visits, not for their health care or for management of their diabetes. It should be noted, however, that many subjects continue to be seen by the DCCT physicians and/or staff for their routine diabetes care outside of the research study setting.

Of the 1425 surviving members of the DCCT original cohort, 1,375 (96%) agreed to participate in EDIC and 50 were either no longer available or refused further follow-up. The overall EDIC cohort was 33.6±7.0 years old, had diabetes for 12.2±4.8 years, were 48% female and equally represented from the IT group and the CT group of the DCCT[13].

Of the original 195 DCCT adolescents, 191 were surviving at the start of EDIC and 175 (92%) agreed to participate in EDIC[14]. At the start of EDIC in 1994, these subjects had an average age of 23 years (range: 19-28), an average duration of diabetes of about 12-13 years, and an average of 7.4 years (range: 4-9) of follow-up during the DCCT. Slightly more than half (54%) were female and nearly two-thirds (62%) were from the primary prevention arm of the DCCT. Overall, the adolescent EDIC cohort had a longer duration of follow-up within the DCCT/EDIC study and had more primary prevention subjects (that is, no retinopathy and duration <5 years at beginning of DCCT) than the adult cohort.

Glycemic control and diabetes treatment during EDIC

As noted above, after completion of the formal, randomized controlled trial portion of the DCCT, it was recommended, based on the results of the DCCT, that all participants continue or initiate intensive insulin therapy with the goal of reducing mean blood glucose and HbA1c to the DCCT IT group target in order to achieve the demonstrated benefits of intensive therapy. Most chose to undertake IT and were instructed in such and remained under the care of the DCCT staff for the next six months. Subsequently, their care and follow-up was transferred back to their primary physician or endocrinologist. Annual follow-up for determination of research endpoints, but not for treatment, was performed at the DCCT/EDIC center. At present, data has been carefully analyzed and reported out to the fourth year of EDIC, which would have occurred mostly in 1998[13,14].

EDIC 4-year overall study data

Evaluations for retinopathy were available at EDIC year 4 from 1208 of the originally enrolled 1375 EDIC subjects[13]. Renal evaluations were available during EDIC year 3 or 4 on 1302 subjects[13]. Among the subjects evaluated as part of EDIC at these time point, approximately the same number had been in the original DCCT IT group and the DCCT CT group and the age, gender, duration of diabetes and duration of follow-up during the DCCT were similar between those previously assigned to the IT group and those previously assigned to the CT group. Of course, at the baseline EDIC evaluation (which was essentially the closeout DCCT evaluation), those who had been in the IT group had less retinopathy and microalbuminuria than those who had been in the CT group, as reflected in the primary results of the DCCT.

Those previously assigned to the IT group experienced a decline in their adherence to the complex and time-consuming IT regimen and an increase in their HbA1c once the support of the DCCT staff was no longer available. Those previously assigned to the CT group during the DCCT experienced a fall in their HbA1c as they implemented IT for the first time. However, the HbA1c did not fall to the level accomplished by the IT group during the DCCT since after the first six months, DCCT research staff support was no longer available. As a result, subsequent to the first year of EDIC (the first year post-DCCT), treatment regimens and glycemic control were similar between those previously assigned to IT and those previously assigned to CT. The median HbA1c at EDIC year 1 was 7.7% in the former IT group and 8.1% in the former CT group. Mean HbA1c at EDIC year 4 and the overall glycemic exposure during the four years of EDIC was similar between the two groups (median 4-year average 7.9% in the former IT and 8.2% in the former CT groups, respectively).

Despite the similar glycemic exposure of the two groups during the first four years of EDIC, progression of retinopathy was reduced in the former IT group subjects compared to the former CT group subjects. This was true even after adjustment for the differences observed at the end of the DCCT. There was a 75% (95% CI: 67-81%; $p<0.001$) adjusted odds reduction for a 3-step progression in retinopathy from DCCT closeout despite the similar HbA1c's during EDIC. Likewise, there was a 69% (95% CI: 48-82%; $p<0.001$) adjusted odds reduction for progression to proliferative or severe nonproliferative retinopathy, a 58% (95% CI: 31-74%; $p<0.001$) adjusted odds reduction for development of clinically-significant macular edema, and a 52% (95% CI: 19-71%; $p<0.007$) adjusted odds reduction for the need for photocoagulation therapy. Thus, the benefits of IT to reduce the development and progression of retinopathy persisted for at least four years after differences in treatment and glycemic control no longer existed.

Similarly, after adjusting for albuminuria at DCCT closeout, there was a 53% (95% CI: 26-70%; $p<0.002$) adjusted odds reduction in new-onset microalbuminuria, an 86% (95% CI: 60-95%; $p<0.001$) adjusted odds reduction for new-onset albuminuria, and an 80% (95% CI: 27-95%; $p<0.006$) adjusted odds reduction for progression of microalbuminuria to albuminuria during the first three to four years of EDIC.

Overall, these data obtained at EDIC year 3 and 4 indicate that the beneficial effects on risk reduction for retinopathy and nephropathy resulting from lowering the mean HbA1c for an average of 6.5 years during the DCCT persists and carries over for at least the next four years despite increasing hyperglycemia in the former IT group and equalization of glycemic control between the groups. Subsequent evaluations that are not yet available will be necessary to determine whether these beneficial effects persist for longer periods of time.

EDIC 4-year adolescent study data

These results are echoed in the adolescent cohort of DCCT/EDIC[14]. The adolescent cohort evaluated at year 4 of the EDIC study consisted of 170 former DCCT subjects, 81 from the IT group and 89 from the CT group. The characteristics of these 170 subjects at the EDIC baseline examination mirrored those of the 193 subjects (2 adolescents died during the DCCT) at DCCT closeout. Characteristics of the EDIC adolescent cohort at the time of their 4-year evaluation are shown in Table 3.

As was the case for the entire DCCT/EDIC cohort, after the end of the DCCT, therapy available to the two groups was equalized and the glycemic exposure (as reflected by HbA1c) during the first four years of EDIC was similar between the former IT group and the former CT group (see Figure 5).

Table 3
Characteristics of EDIC Adolescent Cohort at EDIC Year 4 by Original DCCT Group Assignment

	Intensive N = 81	**Conventional N= 89**
Age (yr) at EDIC year 4†	27.2±2.4	26.3±2.2
Primary Prevention Cohort (%)	57	67
Diabetes duration (yr) at EDIC year 4†	17.4±4.2	16.3±4.3
Duration (yr) since entry in DCCT†	12.0±1.9	11.3±1.9
Female (%)	48	60
Insulin regimen at EDIC year 4		
1 or 2 injections per day (%)	10	31
MDII* (%)	69	52
CSII* (%)	22	17
Total daily insulin dose (U/kg/day)†	0.82±0.28	0.80±0.22
SMBG* ≥4/day (%) at EDIC year 4	24	29
HbA1c (%) at EDIC year 4†	8.4±1.7	8.5±1.6
SH* during EDIC (events/100 pt-yrs)		
All SH events	51.0	57.0
Events with seizure or coma	16.6	26.8

† Values represent mean±SD unless otherwise indicated.
* MDII, multiple daily insulin injections; CSII, continuous subcutaneous insulin infusion (insulin pump therapy); SMBG, self-monitoring blood glucose; SH, severe hypoglycemia
Table adapted from data in reference 14.

During the first four years of EDIC, there were similar rates of severe hypoglycemia in the former IT and CT groups. In the IT group, 24.7% of the subjects experienced severe hypoglycemia at an event rate of 51.0 episodes per 100 patient-years. In the CT group, 24.2% of the subjects experienced severe hypoglycemia at an event rate of 57.0 episodes per 100 patient-years. There was no significant difference between these event rates (relative risk for severe hypoglycemia in IT was 0.90; p=0.749). Results were similar when including only episodes associated with seizure or coma. There were 16.6 events of seizure or coma per 100 patient-years in the IT group and 26.8 in the CT group (relative risk of IT 0.62; p=0.358). As in the DCCT, the adult cohort had lower rates of severe hypoglycemia during EDIC, but there was no difference between the event rates in the former IT and CT groups.

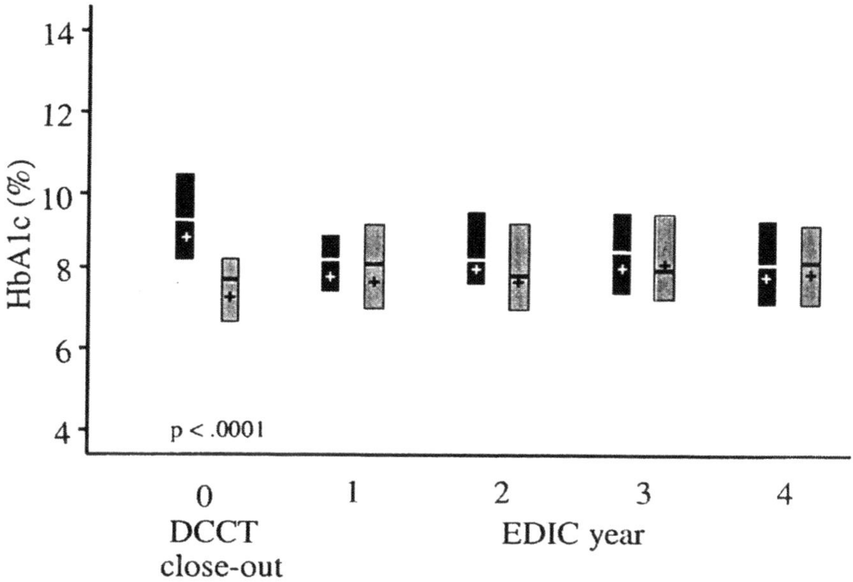

Figure 5: Distribution of hemoglobin A1c (HbA1c) Values in the Conventional Therapy Group (dark bars) and the Intensive Therapy Group (light bars) at the closeout of the DCCT and each year of EDIC. Boxes represent the second and third quartiles (25-75 percentiles). The center line represents the median and the plus sign represents the mean. HbA1c was significantly different between the groups only at the closeout of the DCCT which is equivalent to baseline for EDIC. Subsequently, there was no significant difference between the groups.

As for the entire study cohort, despite the similar levels glycemic control for the two groups during EDIC, progression of retinopathy during the first four years of EDIC was reduced in the former IT group subjects compared to the former CT group subjects. This was true even after adjustment for the differences observed at the end of the DCCT. There was a 74% (95% CI: 49-87%; p<0.001) adjusted odds reduction for a 3-step progression in retinopathy from DCCT closeout despite the similar HbA1c's during EDIC. (see Figure 6)

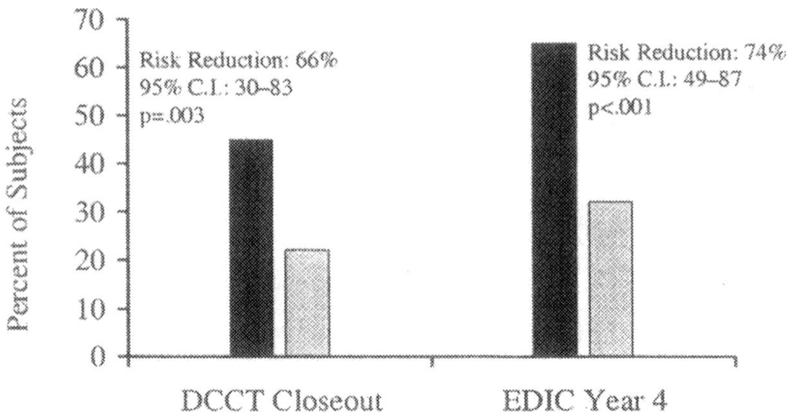

Figure 6: Prevalence of a 3-step or more progression of retinopathy at DCCT closeout and EDIC year 4 in the former DCCT conventional group (dark bars) and the former DCCT intensive group (light bars). Risk reduction by intensive therapy during the DCCT was 66% (95% CI, 30-83; p=0.003). At EDIC year 4, after controlling for retinopathy status at DCCT closeout, the risk reduction for a 3-step progression during EDIC in the former intensive therapy group was 74% (95% CI, 49-87; p<0.001). *This figure is adapted from Figure 1 in reference 14.*

Likewise, there was a 78% (95% CI: 34-92%; p<0.007) adjusted odds reduction for progression to proliferative or severe nonproliferative retinopathy (see Figure 7). These results for progression of retinopathy in the adolescent cohort during the first four years of EDIC were nearly identical to those observed for the study cohort as a whole and for the adult cohort (see Table 5)[14].

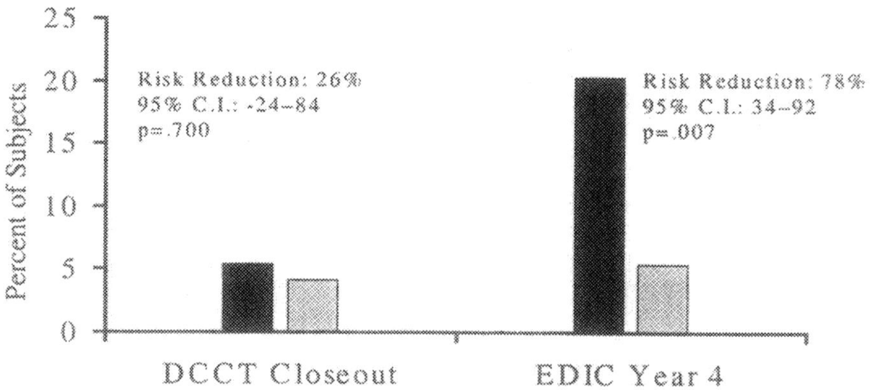

Figure 7: Prevalence of progression to proliferative or severe nonproliferative retinopathy at DCCT closeout and EDIC year 4 in the former DCCT conventional group (dark bars) and the former DCCT intensive group (light bars). Risk reduction by intensive therapy during the DCCT was 26% (95% CI, –24-48; p=0.70). At EDIC year 4, after controlling for retinopathy status at DCCT closeout, the risk reduction in the former intensive therapy group was 78% (95% CI, 34-92; p<0.007). *This figure is adapted from Figure 2 in reference 14.*

Similarly, for those free of microalbuminuria at DCCT closeout (N=128), 13.6% of the former CT group and 8.1% of the former IT group had microalbuminuria (urinary albumin >40 mg/day) at EDIC year 3 or 4[14]. This represented a 48% (95% CI: –69 to 84%; p=0.28) adjusted odds reduction in new-onset microalbuminuria. For those without albuminuria (urinary albumin >300 mg/day) at DCCT closeout (N=156), the prevalence of albuminuria at EDIC year 3 or 4 was 9.9% in the former CT group and only 1.3% in the former IT group. This represents an 85% (95% CI: –28 to 98%; p=0.08) adjusted odds reduction for new-onset albuminuria. (see Table 4) Although there were to few subjects and events for these adjusted odds reductions to be statistically significant for the adolescent cohort alone, they were nearly identical to those observed for the study cohort as a whole and for the adult cohort (see Table 5). No subjects in the adolescent cohor developed renal failure or required dialysis or transplantation during th DCCT or until EDIC year 4.

Table 4
Progression of Microalbuminuria and Albuminuria During EDIC in the Adolescent Cohort

	N	% affected	Adjusted Odds Ratio (%)	95% CI	p-val
AER>40 mg/day (%)*	128				
IT group	62	8.1	48	–69, 84	0.2
CT group	66	13.6			
AER>300 mg/day (%)†	156				
IT group	75	1.3	85	–28, 98	0.0
CT group	81	9.9			

AER, albumin excretion rate; IT, intensive therapy group; CT, conventional therapy grou 95% CI, 95% confidence interval.
* Based on subjects with AER<40 mg/day at DCCT closeout.
† Based on subjects with AER<300 mg/day at DCCT closeout.

Overall, these data obtained at EDIC year 3 and 4 indicate that th beneficial effects on risk reduction for both retinopathy and nephropath resulting from improved glycemic control in adolescents during the DCCT

Table 5
Comparison of Efficacy and Safety of Intensive versus Conventional Therapy in DCCT Adolescents at EDIC Year 4

		Adolescents	Adults	p-value*
HbA1c (%):†	**IT group**	8.4±0.2	8.0±0.1	0.058
	CT group	8.5±0.1	8.3±0.1	0.269
Odds Reduction (%; 95% CI)				
3-step change in retinopathy		72% (33,88)	71% (58,80)	0.929
Albuminuria>208 μg/min		88% (27,98)	92% (76,97)	0.737
Severe Hypoglycemia				
All events (per 100 pt-yrs)		59.3	43.4	0.708
Relative risk (IT vs. CT)		1.00	1.16	
Seizure/coma (per 100 pt-yrs)		18.9	11.2	0.337
Relative risk (IT vs. CT)		0.68	1.21	

† Mean±SEM
* p-value for adolescents vs. adults

persist and carries over for at least the next four years despite increasin hyperglycemia in the former IT group and equalization of glycemic contro between the groups.

IMPLICATIONS OF DCCT AND EDIC IN PEDIATRICS

The results of the DCCT are clear for young adults and adolescents. Improved glycemic control delays the onset and slows the progression of retinopathy, nephropathy and neuropathy. This is true even though teenagers might not be as successful as their adult counterparts. Lowering HbA1c by 10% over an average of 6.5 years reduces complications by 30-50% and any degree of lowering of HbA1c would be expected to yield some benefit in reduction of diabetes-related microvascular and neuropathic complications.

The results of four additional years of observation in the DCCT/EDIC cohort are also clear. The beneficial effects of improved glycemic control for a period of time during adolescence and young adulthood persist even if not sustained indefinitely. The beneficial effects appear to be cumulative over time and do not disappear as soon as blood glucose control worsens again. These results are in agreement with the studies of Engerman and Kern[31] in diabetic dogs. Presumably, subsequent periods of improved control would yield additional benefit. This insight into the benefits of improved glycemic control is particularly applicable to teenagers who may be able to improve their control for short periods of time even though they may not be able to maintain HbA1c values near to the normal range for extended periods. Geffner, in his editorials following the reports of the DCCT[32] and EDIC[33] adolescent results, sums up the benefits of improved glycemic control as "Some is better than none and a little bit goes a long way." That is, any lowering of HbA1c is beneficial; the lower the better. Any duration of improved glycemic control yields some benefit; the longer the duration the greater the benefit.

Of course, using the currently available therapeutic options, hypoglycemia remains an important adverse effect of intensive diabetes therapy and continues to be a limiting factor in the ability to lower the blood sugar in people with type 1 diabetes[19]. Although the results of the DCCT seem to warrant the conclusions that the benefits of intensive therapy outweigh the risks associated with hypoglycemia, the level of risk (and benefit) must be assessed individually for each subject. The risks of hypoglycemia may be greater in some individuals, such as those with defective glucose counterregulation,[17-19] hypoglycemia unawareness,[20,21] or hypoglycemia-associated autonomic failure (HAAF)[22,23]. Indeed, HAAF may be the result of recurrent (sometimes only a few) episodes of treatment-induced hypoglycemia[23] and the associated development of defective glucose counterregulation and hypoglycemia unawareness will increase the likelihood of severe hypoglycemia and in doing so increase the risks associated with hypoglycemia[29]. Hypoglycemia cannot be considered a benign side effect of diabetes therapy,[27-29,34-36] and must be taken seriously with every effort made to avoid severe and recurrent hypoglycemia. Research related to the pathogenesis and prevention of hypoglycemia in insulin-treated subjects must continue with the aim of reducing the risk of hypoglycemia.

Although the goal of good glycemic control is certainly appropriate at any age, extreme caution must be taken in extrapolating the results of the DCCT to the population of young children, toddlers and infants. Successful therapy must take into account factors other than simply the HbA1c and the target for blood glucose often needs to be modified in children[37]. The risks of hypoglycemia are likely to be greater in children, especially those that are younger than 5-6 years old[27]. In addition, young children are often unable to identify and localize symptoms adequately to recognize hypoglycemia and, therefore, have a diminished ability to act independently or verbalize their needs. This places them at an increased level of dependence on their parents and caretakers. Parents are often fearful of hypoglycemia in their young children and may feel more comfortable maintaining mild degrees of hyperglycemia[29]. Families should not be faulted for this attitude and approach. In addition, since lower mean blood glucose and HbA1c could play a less important role in the development of diabetes complications before puberty,[9-11] the benefits of intensive therapy may be weakened in younger children relative to those demonstrated in the DCCT/EDIC study population. Hence, the risk:benefit ratio could be substantially different for young children than for adolescents and young adults.

Management of diabetes should be goal oriented. Individualized and age-specific target blood glucoses ranges are still appropriate[32,37] and quality-of-life, normal growth and development and long-term social, educational and behavioral outcomes must also be considered when setting goals. No one goal or treatment strategy is right for all. However, the results of DCCT/EDIC clearly indicate that in our practice of medicine and the care of our patients with diabetes, and in our academic, research and advocacy endeavors, we must continue to strive for better glycemic control and improved methods and technology to accomplish this goal. We cannot rest our efforts until we can cure or prevent diabetes or at least prevent its complications.

ACKNOWLEDGEMENTS:

Dr. White's efforts toward implementation of the DCCT/EDIC protocol and preparation of this chapter are supported by grants from the U.S.P.H.S. U01 DK 30653 (DCCT/EDIC), M01 RR00036 (GCRC), R01 DK 50860 (Tim Wysocki, PhD—PI) and P60 DK 20579 (DRTC), and by funding from the Juvenile Diabetes Research Foundation.

REFERENCES

1. Diabetes Control and Complications Trial Research Group. The effect of intensive treatment of diabetes on the development and progression of long-term complications in insulin-dependent diabetes mellitus. N Engl J Med 1993: 329:977-986.
2. Diabetes Control and Complications Trial Research Group. Effect of intensive diabetes treatment on the development and progression of long-term complications in adolescents with insulin-dependent diabetes mellitus: Diabetes Control and Complications Trial. J Peds 1994; 125:177-188.
3. Diabetes Control and Complications Trial Research Group. Implementation of treatment protocols in the Diabetes Control and Complications Trial. Diabetes Care 1995; 18:361-376.
4. Diabetes Control and Complications Research Group. The relationship of glycemic exposure (HbA1c) to the risk of development and progression of retinopathy in the Diabetes Control and Complications Trial. Diabetes 1995; 44:968-983.
5. Diabetes Control and Complications Trial Research Group. Adverse events and their association with treatment regimens in the Diabetes Control and Complications Trial. Diabetes Care 1995; 18:1415-1427.
6. Diabetes Control and Complications Trial Research Group. The absence of a glycemic threshold for the development of long-term complications: The perspective of the Diabetes Control and Complications Trial. Diabetes 1996; 45:1289-1296.
7. Reichard P, Nilsson B-Y, Rosenqvist U. The effect of long-term intensified insulin treatment on the development of microvascular complications of diabetes mellitus. N Engl J Med 1993: 329:304-309.
8. UK Prospective Diabetes Study (UKPDS) Group. Intensive blood-glucose control with sulphonylureas or insulin compared with conventional treatment and risk of complications in patients with type 2 diabetes (UKPDS 33). Lancet 1998; 352:837-853.

9. Dahlquist G, Rudberg S. The prevalence of microalbuminuria in diabetic children and adolescents and its relation to puberty. Acta Paediatr Scand 1987; 76:795-800.
10. Kostraba JN, Dorman JS, Orchard TJ, Becker DJ, Ohki Y, Ellis D, Doft BH, Lobes LA, LaPorte RE, Drash AL. Contribution of diabetes duration before puberty to development of microvascular complications of IDDM. Diabetes Care 1989; 12:686-693.
11. Rogers DG, White NH, Shalwitz RA, Palmberg P, Smith ME, Santiago JV. The effect of puberty on the development of early diabetic microvascular disease in insulin-dependent diabetes. Diabetes Res Clin Pract 1987; 3:39-44.
12. Epidemiology of Diabetes Interventions and Complications (EDIC) Research Group. Epidemiology of Diabetes Interventions and Complications (EDIC): Design, implementation, and preliminary results of a long-term follow-up of the Diabetes Control and Complications Trial cohort. Diabetes Care 1999; 22:99-111.
13. Diabetes Control and Complications Trial/Epidemiology of Diabetes Interventions and Complications Research Group. Retinopathy and nephropathy in patients with type 1 diabetes four years after a trial of intensive therapy. N Engl J Med 2000; 342:381-389.
14. Diabetes Control and Complications Trial/Epidemiology of Diabetes Interventions and Complications Research Group. Beneficial effects of intensive therapy of diabetes during adolescence: Outcomes after the conclusion of the Diabetes Control and Complications Trial (DCCT). J Peds 2001; 139:804-812.
15. Diabetes Control and Complications Trial Research Group. Diabetes Control and Complications Trial (DCCT): Results of feasibility study. Diabetes Care 1987; 10:1-19.
16. Diabetes Control and Complications Trial Research Group. DCCT protocol. Springfield, VA: Department of Commerce, National Technical Information Service, 1988. (Publication no. 88-116462-AS).
17. White NH, Skor DA, Cryer PE, Bier DM, Levandoski L, Santiago JV. Identification of type 1 diabetic patients at increased risk for hypoglycemia during intensive therapy. N Engl J Med 1983; 308:485-491.
18. Bolli GB, DeFeo P, DeCosmo S, Perriello G, Ventura MM, Benedetti MM, Santeisanio F, Gerich JE, Brunetti P. A reliable and reproducible test for abnormal glucose counterregulation in type I diabetes mellitus. Diabetes 1983; 32:134-141.

19. Santiago JV, White NH, Skor DA, Levandoski LA, Bier DM, Cryer PE. Defective glucose counterregulation limits intensive therapy of diabetes mellitus. Am J Physiol 1984; 247:E215-E220.
20. Hoeldtke RD, Boden G, Shuman CR, Owen OE. Reduced epinephrine secretion and hypoglycemia unawareness in diabetic autonomic neuropathy. Ann Int Med 1982; 96:459-462.
21. Hoeldtke RD, Boden G. Epinephrine secretion, hypoglycemia unawareness, and diabetic autonomic neuropathy. Ann Int Med 1994; 120:512-517.
22. Cryer PE. Iatrogenic hypoglycemia as a cause of hypoglycemia-associated autonomic failure in IDDM. Diabetes 1992; 41:255-260.
23. Dagogo-Jack S, Craft S, Cryer P. Hypoglycemia-associated autonomic failure in insulin-dependent diabetes mellitus: recent antecedent hypoglycemia reduces autonomic response to, symptoms of, and defense against subsequent hypoglycemia. J Clin Invest 1993: 91:819-828.
24. DCCT Research Group. Epidemiology of severe hypoglycemia in the Diabetes Control and Complications Trial. Am J Med 1991; 90:450-459.
25. Diabetes Control and Complications Trial Research Group. Hypoglycemia in the Diabetes Control and Complications Trial. Diabetes 1997; 46:271-286.
26. Diabetes Control and Complications Trial Research Group. Effects of intensive diabetes therapy on neuropsychological function in adults in the Diabetes Control and Complications Trial. Ann Int Med 1996; 124:379-388.
27. Ryan CM, Atchison J, Puczynski S, Puczynski M, Arslanian S, Becker D. Mild hypoglycemia associated with deterioration of mental efficiency in children with insulin-dependent diabetes mellitus. J Peds 1990; 117:32-38.
28. Cox DJ, Gonder-Frederick L, Clarke W. Driving decrements in type I diabetes during moderate hypoglycemia. Diabetes 1988; 40:680-685.
29. White NH: Hypoglycemia in Diabetic Patients. In Current Review of Diabetes, Simeon I. Taylor (editor), Current Medicine, Inc., Philadelphia, 1999. Pages 35-47.
30. Diabetes Control and Complications Trial (DCCT) Research Group. Effect of intensive diabetes management on macrovascular events and risk factors in the Diabetes Control and Complications Trial. Am J Card 1995; 75:894-903.

31. Engerman RL, Kern TS. Progression of incipient diabetic retinopathy during good glycemic control. Diabetes 1987; 36:808-812.
32. Geffner ME. Reviewing the Diabetes Control and Complications Trial: One member of the "control panel" speaks. J Peds 1994; 125:229-229.
33. Geffner ME. From the control tower: Some is better than none and a little bit goes a long way. J Peds 2001; 139:766-768.
34. Hershey T, Craft S, Bhargava N, White NH. Memory and insulin dependent diabetes mellitus (IDDM): Effects of childhood onset and severe hypoglycemia. Journal of the International Neuropsychological Society 1997; 3:509-520.
35. Hershey T, Bhargava N, Sadler M, White NH, Craft S. Conventional versus intensive insulin therapy in children with type 1 diabetes mellitus: Effects on memory and motor speed. Diabetes Care 1999; 22:1318-1324.
36. Hershey T, Lillie R, Sadler M, White NH. Relationship between severe hypoglycemia (SH) and spatial delayed response (SDR) performance in children with type 1 diabetes. Diabetes 2001; 50 (Suppl. 2):A399.
37. White NH: Management of the young child with diabetes mellitus: How do we measure success? Mayo Clinic Proceedings 1999; 74:309-311.

Chapter 17
HYPOGLYCEMIA

Timothy W. Jones, Elizabeth A. Davis
Princess Margaret Hospital and Western Australian Institute of Child Health Research. Perth, Australia

Insulin induced hypoglycemia has been long recognised as a critical problem in the management of Type 1 diabetes. However, the post DCCT era of tight metabolic control has seen hypoglycemia become established as a key factor limiting the achievement of euglycaemia[1-3]. This is especially the case in children and adolescents since at this age hypoglycemia is not only more frequent[4,5] but potentially has more far reaching implications[6,7].

Hypoglycemia interferes with day to day life by inducing distressing symptoms as well as through its acute affects on the brain and cognition. For the younger child, behavioural and mood changes may be prominent. In addition, in this young age group there is potential for long term impact of severe hypoglycemia on the developing brain. Of more immediate effect, the fear of hypoglycemia in patients and parents is very common and may of itself result in poor diabetes control. The dilemma between, on the one hand, good glycemic control and on the other, episodes of hypoglycemia, adds to the considerable psychosocial burden of diabetes. The aetiology, impact and management of hypoglycemia in pediatric diabetes have been recently reviewed[8-10].

Improved understanding of the pathophysiological mechanisms leading to hypoglycemia in Type 1 diabetes, offers the potential for avoiding this complication of insulin therapy. Furthermore, the introduction of new glucose monitoring technologies, analog insulins and more expert insulin therapy modalities and approaches have contributed to the future likelihood of improving glycaemic control without the expected increased risk of severe hypoglycemia.

DEFINITIONS

In non-diabetic individuals blood glucose levels are closely regulated within a narrow range and hypoglycemia is rare. In individuals with Type 1 diabetes, insulin induced hypoglycemia is common and is characterised according to severity. With the exception of asymptomatic hypoglycemia, this classification is based on clinical findings rather than biochemical glucose values. Commonly accepted categories are:

a) Asymptomatic or biochemical hypoglycemia, in which blood glucose is below a defined but arbitrary concentration.
b) Mild symptomatic hypoglycemia.
c) Severe hypoglycemia in which the patient requires help from another individual.

This latter category includes those events that cause a coma or seizure. Because in very young children the need for external assistance may apply to all forms of hypoglycemia, many published reports, for consistency, limit the use of severe hypoglycemia in children to those episodes resulting in a loss of consciousness (coma or convulsion).

To a certain extent these categories are arbitrary and represent a continuum of severity. They are useful however for descriptive and comparative purposes provided the definitions are carefully documented.

PREVALENCE OF HYPOGLYCEMIA

Symptomatic

The profusion of publications over the last thirty years that have described the epidemiology of hypoglycemia in patients with Type 1 diabetes reflects the high impact of this complication on the management of the disease. Notably, there is considerable variability in the reported frequency of significant hypoglycemia between studies[9-17]. These differences are likely to reflect differences in clinic populations studied, therapeutic approaches, definitions of episode severity and other methodological factors. More recent reports have employed a prospective study design: an approach stimulated by the DCCT experience and likely to remove some of the inaccuracies of retrospective cross-sectional studies[18-25].

Overall, studies in children and adolescents have shown alarmingly high rates of severe hypoglycemia increasing with improved glycaemic control[21,25]. Indeed, young patients appear at particular risk of hypoglycemia. This finding was highlighted in the DCCT study in which the adolescent subgroup had significantly more severe hypoglycemia than the adult subgroup irrespective of whether they were in the intensive or conventional treatment group[4].

Table 1 summarizes recent reports. In a large prospective population based survey of children or adolescents, Davis and colleagues in the mid-nineties reported the rate of coma/seizure to be 4.8 episodes per 100 patient years[24]. In a subsequent review, following intensification of therapy in the same clinic, the event rate for severe hypoglycemia had increased to 15.6 per 100 patient years[25]. Also of interest in this study, were the findings of reduced rates in the first year from diagnosis, increased rates in children less than six years of age and significantly increased rates in children with lower HbA1c values (threefold increase with HbA1c in lower quartile compared to mean frequency).

Table 1: Incidence of severe (coma/convulsion) hypoglycemia in children and adolescents

Study	Incidence (events/100 pt yrs)	Mean HbA1C (%)	Methodology
DCCT (1993) Intensive Conventional	 26.9 9.7	 8.3 9.3	 prospective
Davis et al (1997)	4.8	9.1	Prospective/population based
Davis et al (1999)	15.6	8.6	Prospective/population based
Hvidore (1997)	22.0	8.6	Cross sectional / international
Nordfedlt (1999)	17.0		Prospective
Rewers et al (2002)	19.0		prospective

In another large prospective survey published recently, Rewers and colleagues reported a rate of coma/convulsion at 19 per 100 patient years in a group of children and adolescents with Type 1 diabetes[21]. Tight glycaemic control and increasing diabetes duration were found to be significant risk factors for hypoglycemia. The international cross sectional Hvidore study found the overall incidence of coma/convulsion to be at 22 per 100 patient years in a large sample of children and adolescents with diabetes[26]. In this study, young age was also found to be a particular risk factor.

Recently new therapeutic strategies including continuous subcutaneous insulin infusion, short and long acting insulins, behavioural educational approaches and continuous glucose monitoring have been introduced more widely[27-31]. It has been suggested these may associated with reduced rates of severe hypoglycemia, however, given the variation in reported frequency of hypoglycemia, the impact of such new therapeutic strategies needs to be carefully evaluated. Clearly, the systematic monitoring of hypoglycemia frequency is particularly important in the current era, as changes occur in the management that are aimed at achieving tighter glycaemic control.

Asymptomatic hypoglycemia

Asymptomatic hypoglycemia is important especially when it develops nocturnally. It may lead to counterregulatory hormone failure and contribute to the cycle of hypoglycemia unawareness and further hypoglycemia[31-35]. In addition there are concerns that it may be a cause of CNS damage in the young if prolonged or profound[36].

The incidence of asymptomatic hypoglycemia has been reported as 14-35% in various reports in adults[37-40] and it is likely to be higher in children[41,42]. Many studies have been limited by being performed in hospital rather than in the home setting and by reliance on reflectance meter analysis of blood glucose. Recent reports have described very high rates of hypoglycemia at night in children on conventional insulin therapy[43-45]. Up to 50% of young children may experience asymptomatic hypoglycemia overnight that at times may be prolonged. Several studies suggest it may be difficult to predict the likelihood of hypoglycemia based on prebed readings. Newly available techniques of continuous glucose monitoring have also documented the high prevalence of nocturnal hypoglycemia in diabetic children[46].

CAUSES OF HYPOGLYCEMIA

Hypoglycemia develops when the consumption of glucose exceeds its supply, whether that supply is from endogenous (glucogenolysis and gluconeogenesis) or exogenous (carbohydrate consumption) sources. In the Type I diabetic, the ultimate cause of hypoglycemia is excessive insulin action as a result of imperfect insulin replacement. However it is important to recognise that the predisposition to hypoglycemia in the patient with Type I diabetes is also a result of defects in the counter-regulatory mechanisms that normally protect against reductions in circulating glucose. These counter-regulatory deficiencies are described below.

Observational studies have described a number of clinical factors and comorbid diseases that are associated with the occurrence of hypoglycemia.

Certain patients are at increased risk, including the young, those with tight metabolic control, those who have recently experienced a severe episode and those with hypoglycemia unawareness. Other clinical situations may lead to hypoglycemia such as mistakes in insulin administration, following exercise, inadequate carbohydrate intake or missed meals and alcohol consumption. In a significant proportion of cases, no predisposing factors are identified in patients who experience severe hypoglycemia.

The non-physiologic nature of insulin replacement therapy is of central importance when considering the risk of hypoglycemia in insulin treated diabetic patients. All regimens result, on the one hand, in periods of insufficient insulin compared to requirements with resultant hyperglycaemia. On the other hand periods of excess insulin relative to physiological demands are inevitable with a consequent hypoglycaemic tendency. This is particularly likely at night when insulin requirements are minimal. Until recently twice daily insulin was the standard therapy in children. Newer insulins and insulin pump therapy, although imperfect, offer potential to significantly improve the accuracy of insulin replacement.

GLUCOSE COUNTER-REGULATION

Multiple mechanisms exist to protect the individual from a fall in circulating blood glucose[47-50]. In the non-diabetic, these may be summarised as follows:

1. A reduction in endogenous insulin production. This results in an increase in glucose output from the liver.
2. The generation of counterregulatory hormones (glucagon, adrenaline). These increase circulating glucose by promoting increased glucose release by the liver and reduced glucose uptake in the muscle.
3. The generation of symptoms that may result in hunger and carbohydrate ingestion.

Additional mechanisms are also activated during profound hypoglycemia.

It remains to be definitively established how glucose is sensed and how the counterregulatory response is coordinated and effected. Evidence suggests that neurons in the central nervous system, in particular the ventro-medial hypothalamus play a critical role[51].

Patients with Type I diabetes are characterised not only by insulin deficiency, but also by an impairment of the hierarchy of responses to counteract insulin induced hypoglycemia. Glucagon responses to hypoglycemia are lost in the course of diabetes[52] and there is preliminary evidence that in adolescents, this may occur in the first twelve months from diagnosis[53]. Interestingly, the pancreatic α cell is still present in the pancreatic islet and is responsive to alternative stimuli. For example, infusion of Arginine results in the release of glucagon into the circulation. The precise mechanism by which these cells lose their responsiveness to hypoglycemia is not known.

As a result of the loss of the glucagon hormonal response to hypoglycemia, the patient with Type 1 diabetes has increased dependency on the sympatho-adrenal responses to hypoglycemia. Unfortunately, these responses may also become attenuated and this places the diabetic patient at even greater risk of hypoglycemia. The degree to which children and adolescents lose their adrenergic responsiveness, is not clear.

Glycemic thresholds initiating counter-regulation may be altered. Strict glycemic control and antecedent hypoglycemia has been repeatedly observed to alter the threshold at which counter-regulation is initiated, resulting in a lower plasma glucose value, at which the hormonal response is observed[3]. Conversely, it has been observed in adolescents with poorly controlled diabetes, that counter regulation may be initiated at higher glucose values than normally expected[54]. The cellular adaptations by which chronic hyperglycaemia alters these thresholds are unclear.

Other factors that may influence the counter-regulatory response include gender[55] and sleep[60]. Despite initial concerns to the contrary, there is no evidence that insulin species (ie human vs pork) modifies the counter-regulatory response[56].

Table 2: Top 6 hypoglycemic symptoms in a survey of 456 children and parents

PARENTS	CHILDREN
Pale	Shaky
Irritable	Weak
Hungry	Dizzy
Weak	Feeling tired
Sweaty	Hungry
Aggressive	Sweating

SYMPTOMS OF HYPOGLYCEMIA

The symptoms of hypoglycemia are usually classified into those generated by activation of the autonomic nervous system ("neurogenic") and those resulting from cerebral glucose deficit ("neuroglycopaenic")[50]. Neurogenic symptoms may be adrenergic (catecholamine mediated symptoms) or cholinergic (eg sweating). In children, a third clinical constellation of symptoms may be added that may be classified as behavioural however these may result from the combined effects of neuroglycopaenia and adrenergic activation[57]. Results of a survey of parents in our clinic are shown in Table 2. The symptom profile does not differ substantially from a comprehensive report from reported by McCrimmon[58].

Typically, the neurogenic symptoms occur at a slightly higher glucose level than the neuroglycopaenic symptoms. In children symptoms develop at a higher glucose value than in adults (approximately 0.5 mmol/L above adult values)[54]. Hypoglycemic symptomatology may be further altered in patients with Type I diabetes. For example, persistent hyperglycaemia may result in hypoglycemic symptoms occurring at a higher glucose level than normal[59]. Conversely, frequent hypoglycemia may result in hypoglycemic symptoms occurring at a lower glucose level[3].

HYPOGLYCEMIA UNAWARENESS

Hypoglycemia unawareness has been extensively studied in adult patients. In hypoglycemia unawareness, patients may not experience the perception of their usual hypoglycemic symptoms. In adults, this may be associated with a reduced autonomic response to hypoglycemia. This specific counterregulatory hormone deficit and hypoglycemia unawareness has been described as hypoglycemia associated autonomic failure, a functional disorder not linked to diabetic autonomic neuropathy[50].

An episode of hypoglycemia may reduce the symptomatic and autonomic response to subsequent hypoglycemia[33]. Based on this observation, it is considered likely that hypoglycemia *per se* may underly the development of hypoglycemia unawareness[35]. The physiological and biochemical mechanisms underlying this are not clear. Hypoglycemia unawareness places patients at a particular risk of severe hypoglycaemic episodes. Studies in adults have shown that hypoglycemia unawareness may be reversible within weeks with meticulous avoidance of hypoglycemia[59].

Nocturnal Hypoglycemia

Most severe episodes of hypoglycemia occur at night and in studies in which plasma glucose has been measured at night in patients with diabetes, asymptomatic hypoglycemia is common and its duration often prolonged for more than four hours[44-46]. This propensity to nocturnal hypoglycemia results from several factors including a mismatch between the action of insulin administered overnight and the increased hepatic sensitivity to insulin that occurs during the night. In addition to these factors, sleep per se impairs counterregulatory hormone responses to hypoglycemia in both nondiabetic and diabetic individuals[61]. This sleep induced blunting of responses may contribute to the propensity to nocturnal hypoglycemia in insulin treated patients.

Nocturnal hypoglycemia has serious implications including neurological as well as psychosocial morbidity. The common occurrence of asymptomatic hypoglycemia may contribute to further deficits in counterregulatory responses as well as hypoglycemia unawareness. Resultant severe episodes may be important reasons for the failure of patients to follow and their physicians to prescribe insulin therapy aimed at optimising glycemic control.

Acute Hypoglycemia And Cognitive Function

Because the brain is dependent on glucose as its primary metabolic fuel, the most important acute adverse effect of hypoglycemia is neurological dysfunction. Many studies have documented impairments of cognitive function as plasmic glucose is lowered[62-65]. A number of these studies have relied on the hypoglycemic glucose clamp technique, and although his does not mimic accurately the development of hypoglycemia in a patient with diabetes, it does allow controlled studies to be performed with a reproducible hypoglycemic stimulus. A variety of tests have been employed to evaluate various aspects of cognitive function. In brief, these studies have implied that with mild hypoglycemia, those functions that are more complex may be preferentially impaired[66]. Recently, attention has focussed on memory function, as the hippocampus appears to be particularly susceptible to hypoglycemic dysfunction[66,67].

The impact of hypoglycemia on cognitive function is particularly important for children and adolescents. Hypoglycemia may be one of a number of factors responsible for the impaired academic performance that is frequently observed in diabetic children[6,7,75,76]. Studies in children have shown cognitive function may be impaired with arterialised glucose plasma values between 3 and 3.5 mmol/L[63,68]. Whether the thresholds for cognitive dysfunction are different in children compared to adults is, as yet, not established but there is preliminary evidence to suggest greater susceptibility in the young[68]. An observation in keeping with the higher glucose level that generates the counterregulatory response in children. The high variability in the effect of hypoglycemia on the brain between individuals complicates the interpretation of studies[69]. There remains controversy as to whether prior hypoglycemia can alter thresholds for cognitive impairment. On the one hand, studies have shown a resistance neuroglycopaenia in patients with tight glycemic control[70-72]. Other studies have shown no effect of prior hypoglycemia[73,74]. These differences may be explained by different experimental techniques, as well as patient sub-groups.

LONG-TERM SEQUELAE OF HYPOGLYCEMIA

The DCCT identified young age as an independent risk factor for hypoglycemia[4]. In addition, as described above, several paediatric studies have noted that younger children (<6 yrs) are at an even greater risk of severe hypoglycemic events[24,26]. This is of concern since there is evidence to suggest that the developing brain is more sensitive to long term damage from hypoglycemic insult. It is well recognised that severe and prolonged hypoglycemia may induce neuronal injury but studies in patients with T1DM have not found convincing evidence of neurological sequelae of the hypoglycemic events that are the inevitable complication of insulin therapy.

A number of studies have documented cognitive impairment and academic difficulties in children and adolescents with type 1 diabetes[6,7,75-77]. In particular children with long-term diabetes, especially those diagnosed before 6 years, appear to be at greatest risk of impairment[78]. Global intellectual deficits have been described as well as specific neurocognitive difficulties in for example such functions as memory, visuospatial skills and attention[78-80]. A recent prospective study found evidence for neuropsychological complications within two years of diabetes onset in a cohort of children with the greatest effect seen in those of younger onset[75,76]. These effects may be the result of factors specific to diabetes such as metabolic disturbance, hyperglycemia and hypoglycemia as well as the less specific long term psychosocial effects of a chronic disease. The relative importance of these different influences on cognition in the child with diabetes, however, remain unclear.

There is little direct evidence linking hypoglycemia to the neuropsychological defects described in children with diabetes. One study has identified specific defects associated with a positive history of severe hypoglycemic events[78]. A separate study found no association with severe episodes and suggested that asymptomatic hypoglycemia may be more important[81]. Recent reports have also failed to support an impact of hypoglycemia on cognition[82]. The latter although observing cognitive impairment provided data to suggest this to be more likely associated with chronic hyperglycaemia than a history of hypoglycemia. Difficulties in obtaining an accurate history of hypoglycemia, measuring cognitive function prospectively in the young, controlling for the other factors that may affect cognition and small sample sizes, have been difficult to overcome.

The effect of repeated episodes of severe hypoglycemia in adults with type 1 diabetes is also unclear and controversial. Although the DCCT failed to find an adverse effect of recurrent severe hypoglycemia over the course of the study other reports have been less reassuring. For example Deary found verbal IQ deficits in patients with diabetes compared to nondiabetic controls, a difference that was abolished when a history of severe hypoglycemia was controlled for[83-85].

PRE-SCHOOLERS

Young children can present some particular issues in diabetes management for both the parents and the diabetes teams. The incidence of severe hypoglycemia in this age group has been reported to be higher than other age groups. Hypoglycemia can be troublesome in young children for a number of reasons. Young children are less likely to recognise the symptoms of hypoglycemia, and even if they do recognise them, will not reliably seek help. For the parent or carer the signs of hypoglycemia can be difficult to detect, and change in the behaviour or pallor are two of the most frequently used signs, to assist in recognition of hypoglycemia. Because young children are less likely to present for help, and detection of hypoglycemia is difficult, recognition of hypoglycemia in these young children is frequently delayed and can result in a more severe episode. Other contributors to the frequency of hypoglycemia in this age group are difficulties with erratic eating behaviours, the lack of routine and sporadic bursts of activity. The availability of analog insulin has helped decrease incidence of hypoglycemia in this age group. The rapid acting analog insulins offer the advantage of being able to be given once the child has completed the meal, so the dose can be tailored to the intake. Other approaches which are useful in decreasing nocturnal hypoglycemia, is the splitting of the night time insulin, that is giving analog insulin at dinner and long acting insulin as the young child goes to bed. This approach reduces the overlap of short and intermediate acting insulins and may reduce nocturnal hypoglycemia[86].

RECURRENT HYPOGLYCEMIA

Every diabetes clinic has a handful of children who present with recurrent episodes of hypoglycemia. These patients tend to be adolescents and this pattern is more frequent in girls than in boys. It can be difficult to determine the cause of these episodes of recurrent hypoglycemia. For the physician it is important to exclude comorbid conditions such as Addison's disease and coeliac disease. Other causes which need to be considered are excess periods of exercise without insulin adjustment, incorrect administration of insulin dosage, alcohol use, eating disorders, and also the syndrome of self-administration of insulin. The involvement of the team psychologist or social worker at recognition of recurrent episodes can be beneficial, as it has been our experience that this latter presentation is frequently a marker of family stress or social dysfunction in the adolescent. One of the side-effects of recurrent hypoglycemia is the loss of hypoglycemia awareness and it is important to explore the signs and symptoms in these patients with recurrent hypoglycemia.

ADOLESCENTS

It is accepted that good strict control is more difficult to achieve in adolescents and likewise hypoglycemia becomes important in diabetes management in this age group. Fear of hypoglycemia has been shown to adversely affect glycemic control, as a number of adolescents choose higher glycemia despite their knowledge of the risk of complications. Certain situations are associated with a particular increased fear of hypoglycemia such as school, jobs and social situations with peers. Conversely, there are a number of adolescent lifestyle behaviours which increase the risk of hypoglycemia. These include dietary manipulation and alcohol (which suppresses hepatic gluconeogenesis) and can result in delayed hypoglycemia. Prolonged episodes of activity (see exercise) is also a recognised cause of hypoglycemia.

Driving with diabetes is a critical issue for adolescents. Driving can be impaired by moderate hypoglycemia[87]. Requirements between countries and states vary but most require medical assessment as part of the driver's licence application, and some require regular medical review to maintain a valid license. For the physician these decisions are helped by assessing the frequency of hypoglycemia and, importantly, the hypoglycemia awareness of the patient. All patients should be reminded to test blood glucose before driving and to carry food at all times in the car for hypoglycemia treatment.

EXERCISE

Exercise has been a focus of much recent research activity in diabetes. It is generally recognised that regular activity for anyone is healthy and is encouraged in the diabetic individual . With planning and regular blood glucose testing patients should be able to participate in sport and exercise. Fear of hypoglycemia tempts many parents to remove their children from strenuous activities. Hypoglycemia is relatively unusual during the time of exercise and occurs much more frequently a period of time after the exercise, this delayed hypoglycemia often presents as a nocturnal event. This is thought to be related to glycogen depletion secondary to excess activity. The patient at greatest risk is the one who has exercised above and beyond their usual activity level. Management approaches include identifying the exercise patterns of individual and determining what their blood glucose levels usually do with exercise and in the time period following activity. Approaches can be individualised but include insulin adjustments such as decreasing nocturnal night time insulin following extra activity, (or the night time basal rate on the pump therapy) this combined with increasing carbohydrate intake with the night time meal may prevent post exercise hypoglycemia. Insulin pump therapy can be considered in patients who continue to have hypoglycemia with sport, or whose activity levels vary greatly from day to day. Sports which have potential to be dangerous such as surfing, motorbike racing and water sports require rigorous blood glucose monitoring, carrying glucose tablets or equivalent at all times and regular assessments, to ensure hypoglycemia awareness is intact.

Continuous Subcutaneous Insulin Infusion Therapy

Hypoglycemia results from a mismatch between insulin and food. The use of the insulin pump potentially allows the insulin pattern to more closely mimic physiological requirements. The basal rates can be set to accommodate a wide range of requirements from, for example, those patients with minimal nocturnal insulin requirements through to the insulin resistant adolescent. The bolus function enables the calculated dose for the carbohydrate of the meal or snack to be accurately determined and given at the correct time. Theoretically this closer match to normal physiology should reduce hypoglycemia rates impressively. In our clinic, in which hypoglycemia is monitored prospectively, we have observed rates of severe events falling to a third of rates of patients treated with injection therapy. This experience is not unusual and has been reported from other centres[88].

The pump has the facility to deliver different insulin rates on different days and this can be advantageous in children who have varying exercise patterns or who have a major disparity between numbers of hypoglycemia events on weekends vs. school days.

REFERENCES

1 The Diabetes Control and Complication Trial Research Group. The effect of intensive treatment of diabetes on the development and progression of long term complications in insulin-dependent diabetes mellitus. N Engl J Med. 329:977-986,1993.

2 The Diabetes Control and Complication Trial Research Group. Hypoglycemia in the Diabetes Control and Complication Trial. Diabetes 46:271-286, 1997.

3 Amiel SA: Risks of strict glycaemic control. *In Hypoglycemia in Clinical Diabetes.* 1st ed. Frier BM, Fisher BM, Eds. Chichester. U.K. Wiley, P. 147-166, 1999..

4 The DCCT Research Group: Effect of intensive diabetes treatment on the development and progression of long term complications in adolescents with insulin dependent diabetes mellitus: Diabetes Control and Complications Trial. J Pediatr;125:177-88,1994

5 Rosenbloom AL. Schatz DA. Krischer JP. Skyler JS. Becker DJ. Laporte RE. Libman I. Pietropaolo M. Dosch HM. Finberg L. Muir A. Tamborlane WV. Grey M. Silverstein JH. Malone JI. Therapeutic controversy; prevention and treatment of diabetes in children (Review) (286 refs). Journal of Clinical Endocrinology & Metabolism 85(2):494-522, 2000.

6 Ryan C, Vega A, Drash A: Cognitive deficits in adolescents who developed diabetes early in life. Pediatrics 75:921-927,1985

7 Rovet J, Ehrlich RM, Hoppe M: Intellectual deficits associated with early onset of insulin dependent diabetes mellitus in children. Diabetes Care 10:510-15, 1987.

8 Becker D, Ryan C. Hypoglycemia: a complication of diabetes therapy in children. TEM 11:198-202, 2000

9 Ryan C, Becker D. Hypoglycemia in children with Type 1 diabetes mellitus.Risk factors, cognitive function and management. Endocrinology and Metabolism Clinics NA, 883-900, 1999

10 *In Hypoglycemia in Clinical Diabetes.* 1st ed. Frier BM, Fisher BM, Eds. Chichester. U.K. Wiley, 1999..

11 Goldstein D. et al: A Prospective Study of Symptomatic Hypoglycemia in Young Diabetic Patients. Diabetes Care:4:601-605, 1981.

12 Daneman D.,Perlman K.,Ehrlich R.: Severe hypoglycemia in children with insulin dependent diabetes-mellitus:Frequency and predisposing factors. Peds:115:681-685, 1989.

13 Bhatia V., Wolfsdorf J.: Severe Hypoglycemia in Youth With Insulin-Dependent Diabetes Mellitus: Frequency and Causative Factors. Pediatrics:88,1187-1192, 1991.

14 Goldgewicht C, Slama G, Papoz L, Tchobroutsky G: Hypoglycemic reactions in 172 type 1 (insulin dependent) diabetic patients. Diabetologia 24:95-99, 1983.

15 MacLeod KM, Hepburn DA, Frier BM: Frequency and morbidity of severe hypoglycemia in insulin treated diabetic patients. Diabetic Med 10:238-245, 1993.
16 Pramming S, Thorstieinsson B, Bendston I, Binder C: Symptomatic hypoglycemia in 411 type 1 diabetic patients. Diabetic Med 8:217-222,1990.
17 Bognetti F, Brunelli A, Meschi F, Viscardi M, Bonfanti R, Chiumello G Frequency and correlates of severe hypoglycemia in children and adolescents with diabetes mellitus. Eur J Paediatr 156(8):589-91, 1997
18 Barkai L, Vamosi I, Lukacs K. Prospective assessment of severe hypoglycemia in diabetic children and adolescents with impaired and normal awareness. Diabetologia 41(8):898-903, 1998.
19 The DCCT Research Group: Epidemiology of Severe Hypoglycemia in the Diabetes Control and Complications Trial. The American Journal of Medicine: 90,450-459,1991.
20 Nordfelt S, Ludvigsson J Adverse events in intensively treated children and adolescents with type 1 diabetes. Acta Paediatrica 88(11): 1184-93, 1999.
21 Rewers A, Chase HP, Mackenzie T et al. Predictors of acute complications in children with Type 1 diabetes. JAMA 287:2511-2518, 2002
22 Chase HP, Lockspeiser T, Peery B. The impact of the Diabetes Control and Complications Trial and Humalog insulin on Glycohemoglobin levels and severe hypoglycemia in Type 1 Diabetes. Diabetes Care 24:430-434, 2001
23 Allen C, LeCaire T, Palta M. Risk factors for frequent and severe hypoglycemia in Type 1 diabetes. Diabetes Care 24:1878-1881, 2001
24 Davis E.A., Keating B, Byrne GC, Russell M, Jones TW, Hypoglycemia: Incidence and Clinical predictors in a large population based sample of children and adolescents with IDDM. Diabetes Care 20:22-25,1997.
25 Davis E.A., Keating B, Byrne GC, Russell M, Jones TW , The impact of improved glycaemic control on rates of hypoglycemia in patients with IDDM. Archives of Disease in childhood 78:111-115m, 1998.
26 Mortensen HB, Hohngaard P, for the Hvidore Study Group on Childhood diabetes: Persistent differences among centers over 3 years in glycaemic control and hypoglycemia in a study of 3805 children and adolescents with Type 1 diabetes from the Hvidore study group. Diabetes Care 24:1340-1347, 2001

27 Heller SR. Amiel SA. Mansell P: Effect of the fast-acting insulin analog lispro on the risk of nocturnal hypoglycemia during intensified insulin therapy: U.K. Lispro Study Group Diabetes Care 22:1607-1611, 1999.

28 Ratmer RE. Hirsch IB. Neifing JL. Garg SK. Mecca TE. Wilson CA: Less hypoglycemia with insulin glargine in intensive insulin therapy for type 1 diabetes: U.S. Study Group of Insulin Glargine in Type 1 Diabetes. Diabetes Care 23:639-643, 2000.

29 Schiel R. Ulbrick S. Muller UA: Quality of diabetes care, diabetes knowledge and risk of severe hypoglycemia one and four years after participation in a 5-day structured treatment and teaching program for intensified insulin therapy. Diabetes Metab. Rev 24:509-514, 1998.

30 Kaufman FR, Gibson LC, Halvorson M et al. A pilot study of the continuous glucose monitoring system: clinical decisions and glycemic control after its use in pediatric type 1 diabetic subjects. Diabetes Care 24 (12): 2030-4, 2001

31 Miniatis AK, Kligensmith GJ, Slover RH et al. Continuous subcutaneous insulin infusion therapy for children and adolescents: an option for routine care. Pediatrics 107, 351-6, 2001

32 Vaneman T, Mitrakou A, Mokeu M, Cryer P, Gerich J. Hypoglycemia unawareness by asymptomatic nocturnal hypoglycemia. Diabetes 42: 1233-37, 1993.

33 Heller SR, Cryer PE: Reduced neuroendocrine and symptomatic responses to subsequent hypoglycemia after 1 episode of hypoglycemia in nondiabetic humans. Diabetes 40:223-226, 1991.

34 Lingenfelser T. Renn W. Sommerwerck U. Jung MF. Buettner UW. Zaiser-Kaschel H. Kaschel R. Eggstein M. Jakober B: Compromised hormonal counterregulation, symptom awareness, and neurophysiological function after recent short-term episodes of insulin-induced hypoglycemia in IDDM patients. Diabetes 42:610-618, 1993.

35 Cryer PE Iatrogenic hypoglycemia as a cause of hypoglycemia-associated autonomic failure in IDDM: A vicious cycle. Diabetes 41:255-260, 1992.

36. Golden MP, Ingersoll GM, Brack CJ, Russel BA, Wright JC, Huberty TJ: Longitudinal relationship of asymptomatic hypoglycemia to cognitive function in IDDM. Diabetes Care 12:89-93, 1989.

37 Gale E, Tattersall R: Unrecognized nocturnal hypoglycemia in insulin treated diabetics. Lancet, I:1049-52, 1979.

38 Dornan T, Peckar C, Mayon-White V, Knight A, Moore R, Hockaday T, Bron A, Turner R: Unsuspected hypoglycemia, hemoglobinA1, and diabetic control. Quart J Med, 197:31-38, 1981.

39 Pramming S, Thorteinsson B, Bendtson I, Ronn B, Binder C: Nocturnal hypoglycemia in patients receiving conventional treatment with insulin. Br Med J, 291:376-79, 1985.

40 Bendtson I, Kverneland A, Pramming S, Binder C: Incidence of nocturnal hypoglycemia in insulin-dependent diabetic patients on intensive therapy. Acta Med Scan, 223:543-48, 1988.

41 Whincup G, Milner RD. Prediction and management of nocturnal hypoglycemia in diabetes. Arch Dis Childhood 62:333-337, 1987.

42 Shalwitz RA, Farkas-Hirsch R, White NH, Santiago JV. Prevalence and consequences of nocturnal hypoglycemia in conventionally treated children with diabetes mellitus. J Pediatr 116:685-89, 1990.

43 Matyka KA, Crowne EC, Havel PJ, Macdonald IA, Matthews D Dunger DB. Counterregulation during spontaneous nocturnal hypoglycemia in prepubertal children with type 1 diabetes. Diabetes Care 22:1144-50, 1999.

44 Matyka KA, Crawford C, Wiggs L, Dunger D, Stores G, Alterations in sleep physiology in young children with insulin dependent diabetes mellitus: relationship to nocturnal hypoglycemia. Journal of Pediatrics 137:233-8, 2000

45 Porter P., Keating B., Byrne G.C., Jones T.W., Incidence and Predictive Criteria of Nocturnal Hypoglycemia in young Children with Insulin Dependent Diabetes Mellitus. J. Paediatrics 130:366-72, 1997.

46 Boland E , Monsod T, Delucia M. Limitations of conventional methods of self monitoring of blood glucose: lessons learned from 3 days of continuous glucose sensing in pediatric patients with type 1 diabetes. Diabetes Care 24(11), 1858-62, 2001

47 Cryer PE, Fisher JN, Shamoon H. Hypoglycemia. Diabetes Care:17,734-755, 1994.

48 Cryer PE, Binder C, Bolli GB, Cherrington AD, Gale EAM, Gerich JE, Sherwin RS. Hypoglycemia in IDDM. Diabetes 1989; 38:1193-1199.

49 Hypoglycemia *in Clinical Diabetes:* 1st ed. Frier BM, Fisher BM, eds. Chichester, UK Wiley, 1999.

50 Cryer PE. *Hypoglycemia: Pathophysiology, Diagnosis and Treatment,* Oxford University Press, 1999

51 Borg WP, Sherwin RS. During MJ. Borg MA. Shulman GI: Local ventro-medial hypothalamus glucopenia triggers counterregulatory hormone release. Diabetes, 44:180-184, 1995.

52 Gerich J, Langlois M, Noacco C, Karam J, Forsham P. Lack of glucagon response to hypoglycemia in diabetes: evidence for an intrinsic pancreatic alpha-cell defect, Science. 182:171-173, 1973.

53 Caplin N, Jones TW, Davis EA. Loss of glucagon responses to hypoglycemia is earlier than expected in adolescents with Type 1 diabetes (abstract). JPEM, vol 13, suppl3, p1186, 2000

54 Jones, T.W., Boulware, S.D., Kramer, D.K., Caprio, S., Sherwin, R.S. and Tamborlane, W.V. Independent effects of youth and poor diabetes control on responses to hypoglycemia in children. Diabetes, 40:358-63, 1991.

55 Davis SN, Fowler S, Costa F. Hypoglycemic counterregulatory responses differ between men and women with Type 1 diabetes. Diabetes 49:65-72, 2000

56 Colagiuri S, Miller JJ, Peetocz P. Double-blind crossover comparison of human and porcine insulins in patients reporting lack of hypoglycemia awareness. Lancet 339:1432-5, 1992.

57 McAulay V, Deary I, Frier BM. Symptoms of hypoglycemia in people with diabetes. Diabetic Medicine 18(9): 690-705, 2001

58 McCrimmon RJ, Gold AE, Deary I et al. Symptoms of hypoglycemia in children with IDDM. Diabetes Care 18:858-861, 1995.

59 Boyle PJ. Schwartz NS, Shah SD, Clutter WE, Cryer PE: Plasma glucose concentrations at the onset of hypoglycemic symptoms in patients with poorly controlled diabetes and in nondiabetics. N.Engl J Med 318.1487-92. 1988

60 Cranston I, Lomas J, Maran A, Macdonald I, Amiel SA. Restoration of hypoglycemia aweareness in patients with long duration insulin dependent diabetes. Lancet344(8918):283-7, 1994

61 Jones,T.W., Porter P, Sherwin RS, Davis EA, O'Leary P, Stick S, Fraser F, Byrne G, Tamborlane WV Decreased epinephrine responses to hypoglycemia during sleep. N Eng J Med 338:1657-62, 1998.

62 Blackman JD, Towle VL, Sturis J, Lewis GF, Spire JP, Polonsky KS. Hypoglycemic thresholds for cognitive dysfunction in IDDM. Diabetes 41:392-399, 1992.

63 Ryan C, Atchison J, Puczynski S, Puczynski M, Arslanian S, Becker D: Mild hypoglycemia associated with deterioration of mental efficiency in children with insulin dependent diabetes mellitus. J Pediatrics 117:32-38, 1990.

64 Gschwend S, Ryan C, Atchinson J, Arslanian S, Becker D. Effects of acute hyperglycemia on mental efficiency and counterregulatory hormones in adolescents with insulin dependent diabetes mellitus. J Pediatrics 126:178-84, 1995.

65 McAulay V, Feguson S, Deary I, Frier B. Acute hypoglycemia in humans causes attentional dysfunction while nonverbal intelligence is preserved Diabetes Care 24:1745-1750,2001

66 Deary IJ. Symptoms of hypoglycemia and effects on mental performance and emotions. In Hypoglycemia in Clinical Diabetes. Frier BM, Fisher BM Eds. Chichester, John Wiley and Sons, 1999, p29-54.

67 McNay E, Fries TM, Gold PE. Decreases in rat extracellular hippocampal glucose concentration associated with cognitive demand during a spatial task. PMAS 97:2881-2885,2000

68 Jones T.W., Borg, W.P., Boulware, S., McCarthy G., Sherwin, R.S., Tamborlane W.V. Enhanced adrenomedullary response and increased susceptibility to neuroglycopenia: mechanisms underlying the adverse effects of sugar ingestion in healthy children. J. Pediatr 126:171-7, 1995.

69 Amiel SA. Cognitive function testing in studies of acute hypoglycemia rights and wrongs? Diabetologia 41:713-719, 1998.

70 Jones T.W., Borg W.P., Borg M, Silver D, Boulware S.D., McCarthy.G, Tamborlane WV., Sherwin RS. Resistance to Neuroglycopenia: An Adaptive Response During Intensive Insulin Treatment of Diabetes. J Clin Endocrinol Metab 82:1713-1718, 1997.

71 Boyle PJ, Nagy RJ, O'Connor AM, Kempers SF, Yeo RA, Qualls C. Adaptation in brain glucose uptake following recurrent hypoglycemia. Proc Natl Acad Sci USA. 91:9352-9356, 1994.

72 Fruehwald-Schultes B, Born J, et al. Adaptation of cognitive function to hypoglycemia in healthy men. Diabetes Care 23:1059-1066, 2000.

73 Widom B, Simonson D. Glycemic control and neuropsychologic function during hypoglycemia in patients with insulin dependent diabetes mellitus. Ann Intern Med 112:904-912, 1990.

74 Amiel SA, Pottinger RC, Archibald HR et al. Effect of antecedent glucose control on cerebral function during hypoglycemia. Diabetes Care 14:109-118, 1991.

75 Northam E, Anderson P. Werther GA. Warne GL. Adler RG. Andrews D. Neuropsychological Complications of IDDM in children 2 years after disease onset. Diabetes Care 21 (3, 379-384, 1998.

76 Northam E, Anderson P, Jacobs P, Hughes M, Warne G, Werther GA. Neuropsychological profiles of children with diabetes 6 years after disease onset. Diabetes Care 24: 1541-1546, 2001

77 Scoenle EJ, Schoenle D, Molinari L, Largo RH. Impaired intellectual development in children with type 1 diabetes: association with HbA1c, age at diagnosis and sex. Diabetologia 45:108-114, 2002

78 Rovet JF, Ehrlich RM. Hoppe M: Specific intellectual deficits in children with early onset diabetes mellitus. Child Dev 59:226-34, 1988.

79 Rovet J. Neuropsychological sequelae of paediatric diabetes. In *Paediatric Neuropsychologicy Research, Theory and practice.* Yeates K, Ris M. Taylor H, eds, New York, Guildford press, 1999, p336-365.

80 Rovet J, Alvarez M. Attentional functioning in children and adolescents with IDDM. Diabetes Care 20(5) 803-810, 1997.

81 Golden MP, Ingersoll GM, Brack CJ et al. Longitudinal relationship of asymptomatic hypoglycemia to cognitive function. Diabetes care 12:89-93, 1989

82 Ferguson SC, Blane A, Perros P et al. Cognitive ability and brain structure in Type 1 diabetes: relation to microangiopathy and preceding severe hypoglycemia. Diabetes 52:149-156, 2003

83 Deary I, Crawford JR, Hepburn DA et al. Severe hypoglycemia and intelligence in adult patients with insulin treated diabetes. Diabetes 42:341-44, 1993

84 Wredling R. Levander S. Adamson U. Lins PE: Permanent neuropsychological impairment after recurrent episodes of severe hypoglycemia in man. Diabetologia 33: 152-157, 1990.

85 Langan SJ. Deary IJ. Hepburn DA. Frier BM: Cumulative cognitive impairment following recurrent severe hypoglycemia in adult patients with insulin-treated diabetes mellitus. Diabetologia 34:337-344, 1991.

86 Amin R, Ross K, Acerini CL.et al Hypoglycemia prevalence in prepubertal children with Type 1 diabetes on standard insulin

regimen: use of continuous glucose monitoring system. Diabetes Care, 26:662-7, 2003

87 Cox D, Clarke W, Gonder-Frederick L,Kovatchev B. Driving mishaps and hypoglycemia; risk and prevention. Int journal of Clinical Practice (suppl) (123):38-42,2001.

88 Ahern J, Boland E, Doane R et al . Insulin pump therapy in pediatrics: a therapeutic alternative to safely lower HbA1c levels across all age groups. Pediatric Diabetes 3:10-15, 2002

Chapter 18
DIABETIC NEPHROPATHY

Denis Daneman MB BCh FRCPC and Etienne Sochett MB ChB FRCPC
Division of Endocrinology, Department of Pediatrics, The Hospital for Sick Children and University of Toronto, Toronto, Ontario, Canada

INTRODUCTION

Type 1 diabetes poses serious health risks, particularly as a result of its chronic or long-term complications, specifically diabetes-related micro- and macrovascular disease. Most of the excess mortality associated with type 1 diabetes resides within the group of patients that develops overt diabetic nephropathy[1].Overt nephropathy is almost unknown before puberty and exceptionally rare even in teens with long-standing diabetes[2-4].Nevertheless, the key changes that lead to overt diabetic nephropathy appear to be initiated very early in the course of the diabetes, perhaps even at disease onset. The earliest stages of nephropathy may be detectable histologically within 2-5 years after diagnosis[2-6]. Health care professionals involved in the care of children and teens with type 1 diabetes must be aware of these early changes both to provide education on the risk factors for nephropathy, as well as to carry out appropriate surveillance and intervention.

In type 1 diabetes, the cumulative risk of diabetic nephropathy after 40 years duration of disease is between 30-40%, and is greatest in those whose diabetes develops in early childhood[7-9]. There are some recent reports that the cumulative incidence may be declining with improvements in diabetes care, specifically control of hyperglycemia and hypertension[10]. Nonetheless, even with these improvements in care, end-stage renal disease (ESRD) resulting from diabetic nephropathy remains the most common reason for new patients entering renal dialysis and transplantation programs in developed countries[11].

This chapter will address the following issues relevant to early diabetic nephropathy:

(i) stages of diabetic nephropathy highlighting clinical and pathological correlates;
(ii) pathogenetic mechanisms;

(iii) risk factors for the development or progression of diabetic nephropathy;

(iv) natural history of early nephropathy in children and teens, and the importance of the pubertal years in this process; and

(v) screening and intervention strategies.

STAGES OF NEPHROPATHY: MORPHOLOGIC/CLINICAL CORRELATES:

Diabetic nephropathy results from structural changes in all renal compartments, including the glomeruli, tubules, interstitium and extraglomerular blood vessels. The clinical course is determined by the severity of these changes. The pathological findings follow a similar pathway in all those developing nephropathy. It is of note, however, that not all individuals with type 1 diabetes are destined to develop progressive diabetic nephropathy. This suggests that there are both individual susceptibility factors (e.g. specific genes) as well as modifiable risk factors (e.g. metabolic control) that either put some at risk or protect others from developing overt nephropathy.

Five stages of diabetic nephropathy can be identified:

i. Stage 1: At the time of diagnosis of diabetes, kidney size and the glomerular filtration rate (GFR) are often elevated. Generally, these abnormalities are reversible with the institution of effective insulin therapy and blood glucose control. However, in some individuals, both nephromegaly and the raised GFR may persist.

ii. Stage 2 develops in virtually all individuals with type 1 diabetes in the first 2-5 years after diagnosis. Although no functional impairment other than a raised GFR may be found, characteristic pathologic changes are evident. These include mesangial matrix expansion and thickening of the glomerular basement membrane[14-16]. The mesangial changes appear to correlate more closely with later functional deterioration than do the changes in glomerular basement membrane thickening[15,16]. Progression of nephropathy beyond this second stage occurs in some 30-40% of individuals with type 1 diabetes. This progression and can be prevented or slowed by establishment and maintenance of excellent glycemic control[17].

iii. Stage 3 is heralded by the appearance of **microalbuminuria**, defined by an albumin excretion rate (AER) in at least two of three timed urine specimens (either 24-hour or overnight) greater than 15-20 μg/min and less than 200 μg/min. Usually microalbuminuria develops in the latter part of the first decade of diabetes, although a small number of individuals develop it earlier[18,19]. In adults with type 1 diabetes those with microalbuminuria in the second decade of their diabetes are highly likely (75-100%) to progress to overt nephropathy or ESRD over the subsequent 10-15 years[18, 20-25]. Studies in adults show that this stage is highly amenable to intervention with both intensive diabetes management and angiotensin converting enzyme inhibition or angiotensin II receptor blockade[17, 26-30]. There is some uncertainty whether microalbuminuria found in adolescents with type 1 diabetes of less than 10 years' duration has the same predictive value[4, 31,32]. The AER in nondiabetic children and teens does not exceed 6.9-7.2 μg/min (95th percent confidence limits of AERs in nondiabetic children)[33,34].

In general, the pathological findings demonstrate advancement in the glomerular lesions. However, there is considerable variation: some studies show significant differences in glomerular pathology between normo- and microalbuminuric individuals[35,36].

iv. Stage 4 is marked by the presence of (dipstick positive) **overt proteinuria**. This equates to an AER over 200 μg/min or 300 mg/24 hr. This stage is characterized by decreasing GFR and a high prevalence of systemic hypertension. There is frequently evidence of other microvascular complications, particularly retinopathy, as well as macrovascular complications, namely cardiovascular, cerebrovascular and peripheral vascular disease. The relative mortality is forty-fold higher in those patients with type 1 diabetes who develop overt proteinuria compared to those that do not[37,38]. This progression from overt proteinuria to ESRD can be slowed with antihypertensive agents, particularly ACE inhibitors[39-41].

v. Stage 5 occurs with the progression to **ESRD** that usually develops 5-10 years after the onset of overt proteinuria. Treatment interventions include dialysis and transplantation; however, these are associated with poorer outcomes in patients with diabetes than in their nondiabetic peers. The major reason for the poorer prognosis is the high frequency of associated macrovascular disease[42].

PATHOGENESIS OF DIABETIC NEPHROPATHY:

The characteristic lesions of diabetic nephropathy are found independent of the type of diabetes suggesting that it is the diabetic milieu itself that accounts for these lesions rather than an intrinsic mechanism associated with the etiology of the diabetes. Furthermore, correction of the hyperglycemia significantly decreases the likelihood of onset or progression of nephropathy, providing further evidence for a pivotal role for chronic hyperglycemia in the pathogenesis of diabetic nephropathy[17].

Any comprehensive hypothesis for the development of diabetic nephropathy must of necessity explain both the functional and structural changes that characterize the condition, specifically the changes in glomerular filtration, mesangial cell hypertrophy and matrix accumulation, glomerular basement membrane thickening, glomerular hypertrophy and nephromegaly[43]. Although a unifying hypothesis remains elusive, data derived from both in vitro and in vivo studies have implicated a number of interrelated factors in the pathogenesis of diabetic nephropathy. These include hemodynamic alterations; chronic hyperglycemia, increased protein glycation with accumulation of advanced glycation end-products (AGE's), derangement in the polyol pathway, protein kinase C activation and increased growth factors and/or cytokines.

i. **Hemodynamic alterations**: Hyperfiltration is a consistent finding in both experimental and human diabetes at the time of onset of diabetes[44]. Many of the derangements brought about by the diabetic milieu are also mediators of hyperfiltration. These include metabolites and hormones such as glucose, ketone bodies, insulin deficiency, growth hormone excess, glucagon excess, high protein diets, and a host of mediators such as activation of the sodium-lithium countertransporter, elevated nitrous oxide, prostaglandins and atrial natriuretic peptide[45-59]. Correction of the hyperglycemia will ameliorate the hyperfiltration in some but not all individuals. There may be specific genetic factors that predispose certain individuals to persistent hyperfiltration and possibly earlier progression of diabetic nephropathy. There is some evidence that the concomitant glomerular hypertension may be more responsible for the progression of nephropathy than the hyperfiltration per se. This is seen in nondiabetic animal models of glomerular hyperfiltration/hypertension where ACE inhibition reduces systemic BP, glomerular capillary pressure and the rate of progression of glomerulosclerosis, without altering the GFR [60].

ii. **Chronic hyperglycemia** is associated with alterations in endothelial and mesangial cell structure, synthetic capacity and function. In the endothelial cells, hyperglycemia reduces life-span, and leads to changes in cell shape, basement membrane thickness and vasoconstriction[61-65]. The mesangial cells synthesize increased amounts of extracellular matrix and become unresponsive to modulation by vasoconstrictors, e.g. angiotensin ll[66,67].

iii. **Advanced Glycation End Products** (AGEs) form in the presence of sustained hyperglycemia. AGEs result in extensive cross-linking of proteins and have a long biological half-life[68]. Receptors for AGEs are present on endothelial and mesangial cells, the initial targets of diabetic nephropathy. Activation of these receptors causes alterations in endothelial and mesangial cell function consistent with the findings in diabetic nephropathy[69,70]. Further evidence for the support of the role of AGE's comes from trials with the drug, aminoglutethimide, which inhibits AGE formation. These studies have shown that the development of the classical lesions of diabetic nephropathy in animals with diabetes can be inhibited with this agent[71].

iv. **Polyol pathway derangements**: An excess of intracellular glucose in the kidney and other organs results in increased sorbitol production, a reaction mediated by the enzyme aldose reductase. The accumulation of sorbitol is associated with reduced intracellular *myo*-inositol concentrations which, in turn, triggers changes in the structure and function of the endothelial and mesangial cells[72]. Several trials with aldose reductase inhibitors, both in animals and humans with diabetes, however, have failed to have a significant impact on diabetic nephropathy[73].

v. **Protein Kinase C (PKC) activation**, specifically of the β–isoform, has been proposed as another possible factor associated with the pathogenesis of diabetic nephropathy[74]. Hyperglycemia both in vitro and in vivo increases PKC activity in vascular smooth muscle cells, again leading to characteristic changes of diabetic nephropathy. Use of a PKC inhibitor in diabetic animals has shown promising results [75].

vi. **Growth factors and cytokines**: A variety of cell types present in the kidney, including mesangial, endothelial and epithelial cells, produce a host of growth factors and cytokines which interfere with cellular functions and may be involved in the pathogenesis of the characteristic lesions of diabetic nephropathy. These include: growth hormone and IGF-l, transforming growth factor-β (TGF-β), tumor necrosis factor-α (TNF-α), platelet-derived growth factor (PDGF), and a host of other cytokines, the local and systemic renin-angiotensin system (RAS), and arachidonic acid products, such as prostaglandins and thromboxanes[76-81].

DIABETIC NEPHROPATHY: RISK FACTORS AND MODULATORS

Certain factors have been identified that influence the onset and /or progression of diabetic nephropathy. Some, such as disease duration, are not modifiable and will not be discussed in this section. Others, such as metabolic control, systemic hypertension, hyperlipidemia, and smoking, may be amenable to highly effective intervention strategies. Still others, such as dietary protein intake, are of uncertain importance in the earliest stages of nephropathy development.

i. **Metabolic control**:

Epidemiologic studies as well as randomized control trials, have demonstrated unequivocally the close relationship between the degree of metabolic control achieved throughout the life of an individual with type 1 diabetes and their risk for the development and progression of microvascular complications (nephropathy, retinopathy and neuropathy)[17, 82-85]. Most of the intervention trials have been conducted in adults, although the Diabetes Control and Complications Trial (DCCT) did include an adolescent cohort [86]. The DCCT compared complication onset or progression in two groups of subjects: one treated conventionally (mean HbA1c in adult cohort 8.9%, adolescent cohort 9.8%), the other with intensive diabetes management using multiple daily insulin injections or continuous subcutaneous insulin infusion pumps (mean HbA1c in adults 7.2%, adolescents 8.1%)[87]. The almost 2% difference in HbA1c levels between the two treatment groups was associated with an almost 50% lower risk of the development or progression of microalbuminuria and macroalbuminuria over the mean 6.5 year duration of the trial. Of note, this same difference in complication risk between the conventional and intensive treatment groups was present in the adolescents despite the fact that mean HbA1c levels were about 1% higher than in the adult cohort[86].

There have been no prospective intervention studies evaluating the impact of glycemic control on development of nephropathy in prepubertal children. However, there are at least 5 studies of the natural history of microalbuminuria in teens with type 1 diabetes that show that the level of metabolic control is the most consistent predictor of progression or regression of microalbuminuria[4,9,31,32,88]. Furthermore, epidemiologic data suggest that children who develop diabetes at the youngest ages may be at the highest risk[9]. These studies argue strongly for institution of good metabolic control for even the youngest children with type 1 diabetes. Clearly, attempts to achieve excellent control in the youngest children need to be balanced against the risk of severe hypoglycemia and its potential impact on the developing brain.

Furthermore, recent data suggest that there may be a degree of hyperglycemia "memory." That is to say that, although improved metabolic control does decrease relative risk of complication development or progression if it is instituted prior to overt proteinuria, it appears that the preceding period of poor metabolic control continues to contribute significantly to ongoing risk. This has been well demonstrated in the follow-on phase of the DCCT, called the Epidemiology of Diabetes Interventions and Complications (EDIC), in which both the initially conventionally and intensively treated cohorts have achieved similar mean HbA1c levels (8.1%) over the 6 years following completion of the trial[89]. Despite this, new cases of microalbuminuria and macroalbuminuria have accrued at a significantly slower rate in those treated intensively during the active phase of the DCCT. After 6 years of EDIC, new microalbuminuria and clinical proteinuria were diagnosed in 4.2% and 0.6% respectively of the intensive group compared to 12.7% and 5.4% respectively of the conventional group. Thus, intensive management during the active phase of the DCCT continued to confer a reduced odds of 69% for microalbuminuria and 87% for clinical albuminuria over the subsequent 6 years.

The level of HbA1c that must be maintained in order to prevent or slow the progression of nephropathy has not been determined. Results of the DCCT showed a linear relationship between metabolic control and relative risk of complications, including nephropathy[87]. In this study there was decreasing risk with lower HbA1c levels even into the nondiabetic range. Our observations in adolescents with type 1 diabetes with and without microalbuminuria support this finding[31]. Krolewski and colleagues, however, reported a threshold effect with nephropathy risk rising sharply above an HbA1c level of about 8.1%[90]. The occasional occurrence of complications in teens and adults in excellent metabolic control suggests that other factors also play an important role in the pathophysiology of diabetic nephropathy.

ii. **Hypertension**:

An association between systemic hypertension and progression of both microalbuminuria and overt diabetic nephropathy has been well demonstrated[91,92]. Nevertheless, it is uncommon to find blood pressure measurements exceeding the 97th percentile for age and gender in either preadolescents or adolescents with type 1 diabetes[2,93]. Clinic BP readings are statistically higher in microalbuminuric adolescents with type 1 diabetes than those who are normoalbuminuric, although these levels are still mostly within the normal range[92].

Twenty four-hour ambulatory blood pressure monitoring (ABPM) has been extremely informative in documenting early changes in BP in adolescents with diabetes[94]. Prior to the onset of microalbuminuria, some adolescents show loss of the nocturnal decrease in BP ('nondippers'), as well as an increased systolic and diastolic pressure burden (defined by the frequency of BP readings >97th percentile for age and gender). These changes may precede and, in fact, contribute to development of both micro- and macrovascular disease. In adults with type 1 diabetes, 'nondipping' status in those with microalbuminuria or overt proteinuria is highly correlated with cardiovascular morbidity and mortality. The significance of nondipping in normoalbuminuric individuals remains to be established.

ABPM is proving very useful in assessing the significance of clinic BP measurements above the 97th centile for age and gender, by separating real from "white coat" hypertension. Many clinicians use ABPM in deciding whether to recommend ACE-inhibitor therapy to an adolescent with mild microalbuminuria.

iii. **Genetics**:

There is strong epidemiologic evidence that diabetes-related complications in general, and diabetic nephropathy in particular, occur on a background of genetic susceptibility[95,96]. First, there is a tendency for diabetic nephropathy to cluster in families[95]. For example, in multiplex families, the presence of nephropathy in one sibling with diabetes signals a higher likelihood of nephropathy in their diabetic sibling(s). Second, several studies have shown that patients with diabetic nephropathy are more likely to have a history of essential hypertension in one or both parents [96].

Candidate genes include those involved in the renin-angiotensin-aldosterone system, such as the angiotensin converting enzyme or angiotensin II receptor genes[97-100] .The linkage between polymorphisms in these and a host of other genes and the risk for nephropathy has been extensively studied with conflicting results.

iv. **Smoking**:

Adults with diabetes appear as likely as their nondiabetic peers to start smoking. The frequency of smoking in adolescents with type 1 diabetes has been reported between 7 and 48%[101-103]. There is now good evidence that smoking is a strong risk factor for the onset and progression of both diabetic nephropathy and retinopathy. Furthermore, smoking is also an independent predictor for augmented progression of renal disease in severe essential hypertension[104]. Studies of the relationship between smoking and diabetes-related complications have all involved adults; however, it is in the teen years that smoking begins and prevention programs are likely to be more effective when targeted at this population.

In the EURODIAB IDDM Complications Study of 3250 men and women aged 15-60 years of age, current smokers were more likely to be in poor metabolic control and have evidence of nephropathy and retinopathy than were either previous or non-smokers[105]. In those with short duration diabetes, both cigarette smoking and family history of hypertension were risk factors for the early development of nephropathy. Gay and co-workers compared 241 adults with type 1 diabetes to 5876 controls: morbidity was ten times more frequent in smokers with diabetes than nonsmoking controls and two to three times more frequent than nonsmokers with diabetes[106]. The smoking versus diabetes interaction was more than multiplicative for all morbidity measures.

Smoking may contribute to the development of nephropathy through one of several mechanisms: sympathetic activation, increased endothelin production, impaired endothelial-dependent vasodilatation.[107] Cessation of smoking does slow progression to more advanced nephropathy.

v. **Dietary protein**:

Whether dietary protein intake can be implicated in the pathogenesis of diabetic nephropathy remains unresolved. In diabetic rats, protein restriction has been shown to reduce glomerular capillary pressure and flow, albuminuria and structural glomerular lesions when compared to their high protein-fed littermates. In a meta-analysis of studies in adults with diabetes, Pedrini and colleagues concluded that dietary protein restriction slows progression of nephropathy in individuals with either type 1 or type 2 diabetes[108]. In a cross-sectional study of normo- and microalbuminuric children and adolescents with diabetes, we found no correlation between dietary protein intake and either kidney size or albumin excretion rates, but a positive correlation to GFR[109]. These findings prior to the onset of nephropathy do not provide support for the restriction of dietary protein intake in children and teens with type 1 diabetes. However, longitudinal studies of the relationship between protein intake and the onset and progression of nephropathy are needed to provide a definitive answer.

vi. **Hyperlipidemia**:

While there is a close relationship between disturbances in lipid metabolism and the macrovascular complications of diabetes, the relationship between lipid abnormalities and the onset and/or progression of diabetes-related microvascular disease is much less clear[110,111]. In the Berlin Retinopathy Study there was a correlation between the presence of retinopathy and raised triglyceride and lowered HDL-cholesterol concentrations[110]. In experimental diabetes, a relationship has also been demonstrated between lipid abnormalities and diabetic nephropathy, and a similar relationship to the progression of nephropathy has been noted in humans[111].

Further support for a role of lipid abnormalities in the onset or progression of diabetic nephropathy can be found in the studies of the effect of HMG-CoA reductase inhibitors both in vitro and in vivo[112-116]. One such agent, pravastatin suppresses induction of TGFβ1 in cultured mesangial cells exposed to hyperglycemia, while rats given atorvastatin following subtotal nephrectomy show a decrease in both TGFβ1 gene expression and proteinuria[115]. However, it has been suggested that these effects may operate through pathways independent of their lipid-lowering effect, given that lovastatin suppresses TGFβ1 expression and delays the onset of nephropathy in streptozotocin-induced diabetic rats independent of changes in lipid levels[114]. There have been no reports linking lipid abnormalities to the onset of microalbuminuria in humans with diabetes.

PUBERTY AS A RISK FACTOR FOR DIABETIC NEPHROPATHY:

Early manifestations of both diabetic nephropathy and retinopathy are exceedingly uncommon in prepubertal children with type 1 diabetes[3,4,111]. Even though a few studies report rare instances of very mild elevations in AER or early background retinopathy in prepubertal children, the long-term consequences of these findings remain to be determined. In none of the studies in which microalbuminuria was detected in such children were either other renal disorders excluded nor long-term observations made on the natural history of these findings.

In contrast to the rarity of complications in the prepubertal age group, the prevalence of both nephropathy and retinopathy accelerate during puberty, independent of the duration of the diabetes[3, 4,111,117]. This has led some investigators to take the view that the prepubertal years do not contribute substantially to the accretion of complication risk[118]. For example, Kostraba et al reported that individuals developing type 1 diabetes after the onset of puberty had higher prevalence rates for microalbuminuria and retinopathy than those with diabetes onset before puberty, when the duration of the diabetes was similar[118]. These differences disappeared when only the postpubertal duration of diabetes was considered. Their findings, however, appears to be at odds with more recent data from a number of sources. It is our contention that the prepubertal years do contribute to complication risk, although not to the same degree as do the pubertal years[117]. In one study, a relationship was found between pubertal duration and both AER and kidney size (both early markers of nephropathy) in a large cohort of children and teens with type 1 diabetes. However, even in the prepubertal group nephromegaly was noted in 14% of the subjects. With respect to retinopathy, Murphy and colleagues reported that the relative risk of the pubertal years was 4.8-fold greater than the prepubertal years[119].

The mediators of the effects of puberty have not been fully determined although changes in the growth hormone-IGF-1 axis, TGFβ and other hormonal factors such as androgens have been implicated[120].

EPIDEMIOLOGY OF EARLY DIABETIC NEPRHOPATHY IN CHILDREN AND TEENS:

i. Prevalence of Microalbuminuria in Children and Teens with Type 1 diabetes:

Numerous studies of the prevalence of microalbuminuria in adolescents with type 1 diabetes have been undertaken[2,3,5-7,9,12]. More recent studies have found microalbuminuria in 8-13% of adolescents after a mean duration of 5-8 years of diabetes using an AER >15-20 μg/min as the cut-off[2,5-7,9]. Those investigators who have used lower cut-off levels (e.g. the 95th percentile or nondiabetic children) have found the prevalence to be 11-38%[3]. Most of the studies show that there is a very small, but not zero, likelihood of finding microalbuminuria in the prepubertal age group[3].

ii. Microalbuminuria Does Not Predict Nephropathy as accurately in teens as in adults:

A number of investigators have found that the presence of microalbuminuria in adults with type 1 diabetes (usually in the second decade of their disease) is highly predictive (75-100%) of progression to overt nephropathy in the following 5-10 years[18-24]. More recent data suggest that, with ongoing improvements in diabetes management, this may be lowered to about 60%[121]. These data imply that microalbuminuria in adolescents ought to be regarded in the same light as in the adult population. This, however, does not appear to be the case.

The natural history of microalbuminuria detected in adolescents and followed for periods of 3-10 years has been reported in five studies[4,9,31,32,88]. In all, 1273 subjects with and without microalbuminuria have been reported with 145 (11%, range of 7-27% depending on the study) having microalbuminuria. At follow-up 3-10 years later, 77 or 53% showed regression of the microalbuminuria, while 65 or 47% were persistent or progressive. Factors that predicted persistence or progression of microalbuminuria included HbA1c in all studies, but also the initial level of

AER (higher levels were more likely to be associated with persistence), age (older age, greater likelihood of persistence), and age of diagnosis (younger age predicted persistence). In none of these studies was blood pressure a significant contributor to microalbuminuria status at follow-up. Given these data, there is a clear difference between adults and adolescents with type 1 diabetes in terms of the natural history of microalbuminuria. Furthermore, the data suggest strongly that excellent metabolic control is the most important predictor of outcome. It is difficult at this time to make general recommendations about the use of ACE inhibitors or angiotensin ll receptor blockers in adolescents with microalbuminuria, given the high rate of apparent remission of microalbuminuria and the paucity of intervention studies in this age group.

iii. Prognosis in Diabetic Nephropathy

In patients with type 1 diabetes diagnosed in the period between 1930 and 1950, those who developed proteinuria had a forty-fold increased relative mortality compared to the group that remained free of proteinuria[10]. The cumulative mortality 10 years after the development of overt proteinuria ranges between 50-77%. At least two groups have shown a significant decrease in the development of overt proteinuria as well as a significant decrease in relative mortality from diabetic nephropathy in the middle of the previous century[10, 122]. This is having a profound effect on the number of new patients with type 1 diabetes entering dialysis and transplantation programs as well as the numbers dying of this complication. The same is not however true for those with type 2 diabetes.

End-stage renal disease accounts for about two-thirds of the deaths in patients with type 1 diabetes who develop diabetic nephropathy[11].The final cause of death is most frequently due to the associated macrovascular disease with cardiovascular disease almost forty times as common in proteinuric type 1 diabetes than in the general population.

SCREENING AND INTERVENTION:

i. Screening tests in children and teens

Surveillance for complications, specifically nephropathy and retinopathy, in children and teens with type 1 diabetes remains a controversial topic. Some groups advise screening for both complications starting early in the course of the disorder, while others recommend starting at a later age and after longer duration. The Guidelines for Diabetes Management in Canada (1998) recommends that screening begins at age 15 years and after 5 years of diabetes duration[123].

In order for a screening or surveillance program to be effective a number of essential criteria must be met: first, that there is a sensitive and specific test to detect the disorder before it becomes irreversible or causes serious morbidity; second, that the test should be cost-effective; and, finally, that effective intervention strategies are in place to prevent or slow progression of these conditions. Surveillance for nephropathy and hypertension meet most, if not all of these criteria. It is the timing of starting surveillance, the types of tests to be used, and the appropriate types of intervention that remain controversial.

We propose that surveillance start at the time of onset of diabetes with the regular performance of HbA1c measurement. Since metabolic control is the best identified mediator of complication risk, it is important to use HbA1c measurement as a test of the effectiveness of diabetes management and a surrogate marker for long-term complication risk. Taken together with other aspects of monitoring, this assists health care professionals in helping these children and teens and their families make appropriate adjustments in the treatment program in order to achieve and maintain the best possible control in each individual with type 1 diabetes. The knowledge of HbA1c levels and their relationship to long-term complications of diabetes should help motivate youngsters and their families to focus on excellent metabolic control.

The data regarding the natural history of diabetic nephropathy in children and teens with type 1 diabetes make the decision regarding when to start urinary albumin measurements much more controversial and difficult[4, 9, 31, 32, 88]. We continue to support the view that screening for nephropathy should begin at the onset of puberty and after 3-5 years' duration of diabetes. Earlier screening may be advisable if there has been poor metabolic control, the presence of hypertension or a strong family history of essential hypertension or diabetic nephropathy.

Screening for nephropathy fulfills all the criteria of a screening program listed above except for the decision regarding the most effective intervention strategies. Almost 50% of teens with microalbuminuria will show regression of AERs into the normal or near normal range over a 3-10 year observation period[4,9,31,32,88]. This makes the routine use of ACE inhibitors in teens with raised AERs debatable.

Also controversial is the most appropriate test(s) to be used in nephropathy surveillance. In adults with diabetes, the recommended screening method is measurement of a random albumin:creatinine ratio in a random daytime urine sample[123]. If values >2.8 for females or >2.0 for males are detected, the test should be repeated and confirmed in 2 of 3 tests performed over a 3 month period. If uncertainty still exists, the microalbuminuria should be confirmed by measurement of AERs in timed (24-hour or overnight) urine collections.

Whether the albumin:creatinine ratio provides the same sensitivity and specificity in children and teens with type 1 diabetes is uncertain. We continue to recommend measurement of AER in timed overnight urine collections. Again, the high day-to-day variability in AER (up to 40% in some studies) makes confirmation of microalbuminuria on multiple specimens over a 3-6 month period essential[124].

The definition of microalbuminuria varies in different studies. Cut-offs for microalbuminuria have been variously set at 15, 20 or 30 μg/min. These are somewhat arbitrary, given the fact that the upper limit of AER in nondiabetic children and teens has been reported in two studies as 6.9 and 7.2 μg/min respectively[125, 126]. Furthermore, in our study of the natural history of microalbuminuria we found that AER was a continuous rather than a dichotomous variable in predicting both the level of the AER or the presence of microalbuminuria at follow-up 6 years later[31].

In patients in whom a normal initial screening test is found, annual follow-up screening is sufficient given the pace of changes in diabetic nephropathy. This presumption is supported by the slow rate of accretion of new cases of microalbuminuria in both the adult and adolescent cohorts in the DCCT[17]. In those positive for microalbuminuria on the initial screen, at least 2 more tests are required over the following 3 months to confirm the presence of persistent microalbuminuria. If persistent microalbuminuria is diagnosed, based on high AERs in two of these three collections, appropriate intervention should be instituted. If the microalbuminuria is intermittent (only one of three tests with an elevated AER) more frequent screening is justified based on the risk for accelerated progression of nephropathy in this group[125].

In addition to HbA1c and AER measurement, all children and teens with type 1 diabetes should be screened for hyperlipidemia and attempts made to correct abnormalities when detected[110,111]. Unlike type 2 diabetes, type 1 diabetes is not a dyslipidemic disorder per se. However, poor metabolic control and familial factors contribute to the possibility of hyperlipidemia. We advise lipid screening about 6 months after diagnosis. In those in whom lipids are normal, a follow-up screening in early to mid-adolescence may be all that is required. In those with hyperlipidemia, more frequent screening and appropriate interventions are indicated. As stated before, such interventions may ameliorate to a degree the risk of nephropathy.

ii. Intervention:

Some reports provide evidence of a striking decline in the prevalence of overt diabetic nephropathy over the past 30-50 years[10, 122]. Two factors appear to have played a major role in lowering the prevalence of diabetic nephropathy: first, recognition of the role of systemic hypertension in the development and progression of nephropathy and its increasingly effective management; and, second, slow but steady improvements in our ability to achieve and maintain near normoglycemia[17, 87, 91, 92]. The fact that these observations predate the development of more intensive diabetes management programs as well as the introduction of ACE inhibitors and angiotensin ll receptor blockers makes it highly likely that further decreases in diabetic nephropathy prevalence will become evident in the next 10-20 years.

Intervention strategies can be divided into those that prevent the onset of the complication, termed primary prevention, and those that ameliorate its course (secondary intervention). The DCCT demonstrated that intensive diabetes management is effective in both primary prevention and secondary intervention in both adults and adolescents[17, 86, 87]. Antihypertensive agents in general and ACE inhibitors in particular have been demonstrated to be highly effective in secondary intervention, decreasing progression of both microalbuminuria to macroalbuminuria and the latter to ESRD[19, 25-30]. These agents have not been studied in the primary prevention of diabetic nephropathy. Other, less well studied approaches including dietary protein restriction, PKC inhibition, aldose reducatse inhibition, prevention of AGE formation, lipid lowering agents (specifically HMG-CoA reducatse inhibitors) also hold promise in preventing nephropathy onset of progression[71, 73, 75,115].

a. Glycemic Control:

The DCCT demonstrated the effectiveness of intensive diabetes management on both primary prevention and secondary intervention in individuals with type 1 diabetes[17, 86, 87]. The UK Prospective Diabetes Study (UKPDS) demonstrated similar outcomes in adults with type 2 diabete[127]. Given the linear relationship between control and complications in both studies as well as the potential for hyperglycemia "memory," it is essential that the best possible glycemic control should be instituted as early as possible in the course of type 1 diabetes[87, 89,127]. These measures, detailed in the chapter "Insulin therapy and comprehensive, outpatient diabetes management", include more intensive insulin administration regimens, more frequent blood glucose monitoring, careful nutritional approaches and appropriate adjustments for nonbasal conditions such as during exercise and intercurrent illnesses.

The detection of microalbuminuria in teens with type 1 diabetes should trigger a more concerted effort to establish excellent metabolic control[86]. Further interventions should only considered if microalbuminuria is not reduced by improving metabolic control or if improvements in metabolic control prove difficult to achieve and maintain or if hypertension is documented.

b. ACE inhibition:

Numerous studies attest to the effectiveness of ACE inhibition and angiotensin II receptor blockade in preventing or slowing the progression of both microalbuminuria and macroproteinuria in adults with types 1 and 2 diabetes[19, 25-30,128-131]. In addition, in adults, correction of hypertension has been well shown to slow the rate of decline in renal function[128-131]. The Microalbuminuria Captopril Study Group reported, in 235 microalbuminuric adults with type 1 diabetes, that only 7% progressed to overt nephropathy in the captopril group, compared to 21% of placebo-treated subjects[19]. Lewis and colleagues studied the effects of captopril on normo- and hypertensive subjects with overt diabetic nephropathy: time–to-doubling of serum creatinine concentration was significantly reduced in the group treated with captopril whose initial serum creatinine concentrations were above 133 mumol/L[128].

Kasiske et al performed a meta-analysis demonstrating that ACE inhibition was superior to other antihypertensive agents in reducing urinary albumin excretion in both normotensive and hypertensive patients with types 1 and 2 diabetes[132]. This superiority was greatest in the normotensives and decreased progressively with greater degrees of BP reduction. There have been only a few studies of ACE inhibitor use in microalbuminuric adolescents with type 1 diabetes. In a placebo-controlled, double blind, randomized control trial in microalbuminuric adolescents with type 1 diabetes, our group demonstrated a significant reduction in AER (~50%) with captopril treatment versus no change with placebo over a 12 week treatment period[133]. In a similar population, Rudberg and Dahlquist were able to demonstrate that ACE inhibition could protect the kidney from progression of renal pathological changes[134].

While there are no obvious contraindications to ACE inhibitor use in microalbuminuric adolescents, most clinicians have been reluctant to use these agents at detection of only mildly elevated AERs because of the very high spontaneous remission in microalbuminuria over 3-10 year observation periods[4, 9, 31, 32, 88]. Many clinicians elect to wait for evidence of rising AER and/or evidence of hypertension before starting these agents.

c. Blood Pressure Control

Hypertension, both systolic and diastolic, markedly accelerates the progression of diabetic nephropathy. Studies demonstrate that aggressive antihypertensive therapy can markedly slow this progression, whether from microalbuminuria to overt proteinuria or from overt proteinuria to ESRD. Such therapy can decrease both the progression to dialysis and transplantation and mortality 16 years after the onset of overt proteinuria.

The primary goal of antihypertensive therapy is to achieve both systolic and diastolic readings within the normal range, e.g. less than 130/85 in the nonpregnant individual over 18 years of age. This level of BP control is based on consensus statements from the American and Canadian Diabetes Associations as well as other organizations[1, 123]. The exact levels to be targeted in adolescents have not been determined, but should be below the 95th percentile for age, sex and body size.

In adolescents with type 1 diabetes and hypertension, lifestyle modifications (weight loss, decreased salt and protein intake, lower alcohol consumption and increased exercise) are unlikely to have as great an effect as in those with type 2 diabetes. The first line of therapy should be addition of an ACE inhibitor (or angiotensin II receptor blocker). If this is unsuccessful in reducing BP to normal over a 4-6 week period, additional antihypertensive therapy should be added. In general, these medications are added in stepwise fashion, providing maximum dose of each medication before adding the next one.

d. Other

A. Dietary Protein Restriction

Animal studies have shown a salutary effect of dietary protein restriction on hyperfiltration and intraglomerular pressure, retarding progression of nephropathy. Studies in humans have been less definitive, although a meta-analysis by Pedrini and colleagues concluded that there is a beneficial effect of protein restriction[108]. There have been no studies in adolescents with type 1 diabetes. In fact, we were unable to show a relationship between dietary protein intake in children and teens with type 1 diabetes and markers of glomerular hypertrophy/hyperfiltration[109].

B. PKC and HMG-Co reductase inhibitors

Both in vitro and in vivo studies in animals have shown beneficial effects of both PKC and HMG-CoA reductase inhibitors on the development and/or progression of diabetic nephropathy[75, 115]. Both may be through suppression of TGF-β and extracellular matrix proteins such as fibronectin and type IV collagen. These agents warrant careful study in those with diabetic nephropathy at different stages.

DIALYSIS AND TRANSPLANTATION

In developed countries diabetic nephropathy accounts for about one-third of all cases of ESRD[11]. The management of the patient with ESRD is difficult given the associated damage to many other organs, including cardiovascular, cerebrovascular and peripheral vascular disease. Renal replacement therapy in those with diabetes-related ESRD can be accomplished with one of three options: hemodialysis, continuous ambulatory peritoneal dialysis, or renal transplantation with or without pancreas (or islet) transplantation. Renal transplantation together with pancreas transplantation offers the best chance for rehabilitation.

SUMMARY AND CONCLUSIONS

Diabetic nephropathy remains the most important factor determining the long-term outlook for people with type 1 diabetes. Recent research has shed light on a number of potential pathophysiologic mechanisms, as well as on the natural history of this complication. However, by far the most important advances have been in the unequivocal demonstration of the role of glycemic control and aggressive hypertension management in delaying the onset or slowing the progression of the early stages of diabetic nephropathy. Prevention of diabetic nephropathy starts with the institution and maintenance of excellent metabolic control from disease onset, and the screening for microalbuminuria and hypertension at the appropriate time. It is to be expected that the prevalence of ESRD due to type 1 diabetes will decrease in the future as a result of aggressive surveillance and interventional strategies.

REFERENCES

1. American Diabetes Association. Clinical Practice Recommendations 2001: Diabetic Nephropathy. Diabetes Care 24 (Supplement 1):S69-72, 2001.
2. Cook J, Daneman D. Microalbuminuria in adolescents with insulin-dependent diabetes mellitus. Am J Dis Child 144:234-237, 1990.
3. Donaghue KC, Fung AT, Hung S, et al. The effect of prepubertal diabetes duration on diabetic microvascular complications in early and late adolescence. Diabetes Care 20:77-80, 1997.
4. Rudberg S, Dahlquist G. Determinants of progression of microalbuminuria in adolescents with IDDM. Diabetes Care 19:369-371, 1996.

5. Dahlquist G, Rudberg S. The prevalence of microalbuminuria in diabetic children and adolescents and its relationship to puberty. Acta Paediatr Scand 79:795-800, 1987.
6. Mathiesen ER, Saubrey N, Hommel E, et al. Prevalence of microalbuminuria in children with type 1 (insulin-dependent) diabetes mellitus. Diabetologia 29:640-643, 1986.
7. Andersen AR, Christiansen JS, Andersen JK, et al. Diabetic nephropathy in type 1 diabetes: an epidemiological study. Diabetologia 25:496-501, 1983.
8. Lapuz MHS. Diabetic nephropathy. Med Clin North Am 81:679-688, 1997.
9. Schultz CJ, Konopelska-Bahu T, Dalton RN, Carroll TA, Stratton I, Gale EA, Neil A, Dunger DB. Microalbuminuria prevalence varies with age, sex, and puberty in children with type 1 diabetes followed from diagnosis in a longitudinal study. Oxford Regional Prospective Study Group. Diabetes Care 22:495-502, 1999.
10. Krolewski AS, Warram JH, Christlieb AR, et al. The changing natural history of nephropathy in type 1 diabetes. Am J Med 78:785-794, 1985.
11. Incidence and causes of treated ESRD [abstract]. *In* Annual Report, Bethesda, MD, United States renal Data System, 1995, pp 25-37.
12. Mathiesen ER, Ronn B, Storm B, et al. The natural history of microalbuminuria in insulin-dependent diabetes mellitus: A 10 year prospective study. Diabet Med 12:482-487, 1995.
13. Mogensen CE. How to protect the kidney in diabetic patients: With special reference to IDDM. Diabetes 46 (Suppl 2):104-111, 1997.
14. Osterby R: Glomerular structural changes in type 1 (insulin-dependent) diabetes mellitus: Causes, consequences, and prevention. Diabetologia 35:803-812, 1992.
15. Steffes MW, Bilous RW, Sutherland DER, et al: Cell and matrix components of the glomerular mesangium in type 1 diabetes. Diabetes 41:679-684, 1992.
16. Mauer SM, Steffes MW, Ellis EN, et al: Structural-functional relationships in diabetic nephropathy. J Clin Invest 74:1143-1155, 1984.
17. DCCT Research Group. The effect of intensive therapy on the development and progression of diabetic nephropathy in the Diabetes Control and Complications Trial. Kidney Int 47:1703-1720, 1995.
18. Mogensen CE, Chistensen CK. Predicting diabetic nephropathy in insulin-dependent patients. New Engl J Med 311:89-93, 1984.

19. The Microalbuminuria Captopril Study group. Captopril reduces risk of nephropathyIDDM patients with microalbuminuria.Diabetologia 39:587-593, 1996.
20. Parving H-H, Oxenboll B, Svendsen PA, et al: Early detection of patients at risk of developing diabetic nephropathy. Acta Endocrinol 100:550-555, 1982.
21. Viberti GC, Hill RD, Jarrett RJ, et al: Microalbuminuria as a predictor of clinical nephropathy in insulin-dependent diabetes mellitus. Lanceti:1430-1432, 1982.
22. Mathiesen ER, Oxenboll B, Johansen K, et al: Incipient nephropathy in type 1 (insulin-dependent) diabetes. Diabetologia 26:406-410, 1984.
23. Mogensen CE: Microalbuminuria predicts clinical proteinuria and early mortality in maturity onset diabetes. N Engl J Med 310:356-360, 1984.
24. Nelson RG, Knowler WC, Pettitt DJ, et al: Assessing risk of overt nephropathy in diabetic patients from albumin excretion in untimed urine specimens. Arch Intern Med 151:1761-1765, 1991.
25. Ravid M, Savin H, Jutrin I, et al: Long-term stabilizing effect of angiotensin-converting enzyme inhibition on plasma creatinine and on proteinuria in normotensive type II diabetic patients. Ann Intern Med 118:577-581, 1993.
26. Marre M, Leblanc H, Suarez L, et al: Converting enzyme inhibition and kidney function in normotensive diabetic patients with persistent microalbuminuria. BMJ 294:1448-1452, 1987.
27. Marre M, Chatellier G, Leblanc H, et al: Prevention of diabetic nephropathy with enalapril normotensive diabetics with microalbuminuria. BMJ 297:1092-5, 1988.
28. Laffel LMB, McGill JB, Gans JD: The beneficial effect of angiotensin-converting enzyme inhibition with captopril on diabetic nephropathy in normotensive IDDM patients with microalbuminuria. Am J Med 99:497-504, 1995.
29. Viberti GC, Mogensen CE, Groop L, et al: Effect of captopril on progression to clinical proteinuria in patients with insulin-dependent diabetes mellitus and microalbuminuria. JAMA 271:275-279, 1994.
30. Mathiesen ER, Hommel E, Giese J, et al: Efficacy of captopril in postponing nephropathy in normotensive diabetic patients with microalbuminuria. BMJ 303:81-87, 1991.
31. Gorman D, Sochett E, Daneman D. The natural history of microalbuminuria in adolescents with type 1 diabetes. J Pediatr 134:333-337, 1999.

32. Shield JP, Hunt LP, Karachliou F, et al. Is microalbuminuria progressive? Arch Dis Child 73:512-514, 1995.
33. Couper JJ, Clarke CF, Byrne GC, Jones TW, Donaghue KC, Nairn J, Boyce D, Russell M, Stephens M, Raymond J, Bates DJ, McCaul K. Progression of borderline increases in albuminuria in adolescents with insulin-dependent diabetes mellitus. Diabet Med.14:766-71, 1997.
34. Lorini R, d'Annunzio G, Vitali L, Scaramuzza A, Bacchella L, Zonta LA. Normal values of overnight albumin excretion rate in a sample of healthy Italian children and adolescents. J Pediatr Endocrinol Metab 11:639-43, 1998.
35. Fioretto P, Steffes MW, Mauer SM: Glomerular structure in nonproteinuric IDDM patients with various levels of albuminuria. Diabetologia 43:1358-1364, 1994.
36. Ellis EN, Warady BA, Wook EG: Renal structural-functional relationship in early diabetes mellitus. Pediatr Nephrol 11:584-591, 1997.
37. Borch-Johnsen K, Andersen PK, Deckert T: The effect of proteinuria on relative mortality type 1(insulin-dependent) diabetes mellitus.Diabetologia 28:590-6, 1985.
38. Borch-Johnsen K: The prognosis of insulin-dependent diabetes mellitus: An epidemiological approach. Dan Med Bull 39:336-349, 1989.
39. Rossing P, Hommel E, Smidt UM, et al: Reduction in albuminuria predicts a beneficial effect on diminishing the progression of human diabetic nephropathy during antihypertensive treatment. Diabetologia 37:511-516, 1994.
40. Parving H-H, Hommel E, Smidt UM: Protection of kidney function and decrease in albuminuria by captopril in insulin dependent diabetics with nephropathy. BMJ 297:1086-1091, 1988.
41. Lewis E, Hunsicker L, Bain R, et al: The effect of angiotensin-converting-enzyme inhibition on diabetic nephropathy. N Engl J Med 329:1456-1462, 1993.
42. Wand SL, Head J, Stevens L, et al. Excess mortality and its relation to hypertension and proteinuria in diabetic patients: The WHO multinational study of vascular disease in diabetes. Diabetes Care 19:305-312, 1996.
43. Steffes MW, Osterby R, Chavers BM, et al: Mesangial expansion as a central mechanism for loss of kidney function diabetic patients.Diabetes 38:1077-81, 1989.

44. Hostetter TH, Troy JL, Brenner BM: Glomerular hemodynamics in experimental diabetes mellitus. Kidney Int 19:410-415, 1981.
45. Christiansen JS, Gammelgaard J, Tronier B, et al: Kidney function and size in diabetics before and during initial insulin treatment. Kidney Int 21:683-688, 1982.
46. Christiansen JS: On the pathogenesis of the increased glomerular filtration rate in short-term insulin-dependent diabetes. Dan Med Bull 31:349-361, 1984.
47. Christiansen JS, Frandsen M, Parving H-H: Effect of intravenous glucose infusion on renal function in normal man and in insulin-dependent diabetics. Diabetologia 21:368-373, 1981.
48. Trevisan R, Nosadini R, Fioretto P, et al: Ketone bodies increase glomerular filtration rate in normal man and in patients with type 1(insulin-dependent) diabetes mellitus. Diabetologia 30:214-221, 1987.
49. Christiansen JS, Frandsen M, Parving H-H: The effect of intravenous insulin infusion on kidney function in insulin-dependent diabetes mellitus. Diabetologia 20:199-204, 1981.
50. Christiansen JS, Gammelgaard J, Orskov H, et al: Kidney function and size in normal subjects before and during growth hormone administration for one week. Eur J Clin Invest 11:487-490, 1981.
51. Christiansen JS, Gammelgaard J, Frandsen M, et al: Kidney function and size in type I diabetic patients before and during growth hormone administration for one week. Diabetologia 22:333-337, 1982.
52. Parving H-H, Christiansen JS, Noer I, et al: The effect of glucagon infusion on kidney function in short-term insulin-dependent juvenile diabetes. Diabetologia 19:350-354, 1980.
53. Kupin WL, Cortes P, Dumler F, et al: Effect on renal function of change from high to moderate protein intake in type I diabetic patients. Diabetes 36:73-79, 1987.
54. Christiansen JS, Rasmussen JF, Parving H-H: Short-term inhibition of prostaglandin synthesis has no effect on the elevated glomerular filtration rate of early insulin-dependent diabetes. Diabetic Med 2:17-20, 1985.
55. Jones SL, Perico N, Benigni A, et al: Glomerular filtration rate, extracellular fluid volume and atrial natriuretic factor in insulin-dependent diabetics. Kidney Int 33:268, 1988.
57. del Castillo E, Fuenzalida R, Uranga J: Increased glomerular filtration rate and glomerulopressin activity in diabetic dogs. Horm Metab Res 2:46-53, 1977.

58. Osterby R, Gundersen HJG: Glomerular size and structure in diabetes mellitus: I. Early abnormalities. Diabetologia 11:225-229, 1975.
59. Lawson ML, Sochett EB, Chait PG, et al: Effect of puberty on markers of glomerular hypertrophy and hypertension in IDDM. Diabetes 45:51-55, 1996.
60. Anderson S, Meyer TW, Rennke HG, et al: Control of glomerular hypertension limits glomerular injury rats with reduced renal mass.J Clin Invest 76:612-9, 1985.
61. Cagliero E, Roth T, Roy S, et al: Characteristics and mechanisms of high-glucose-induced overexpression of basement membrane components in cultured human endothelial cells. Diabetes 40:102-110, 1991.
62. Meraji S, Jayakody L, Senaratne MP, et al: Endothelium-dependent relaxation in aorta from diabetic rats. Diabetes 36:978-981, 1987.
63. Tesfamariam B, Brown ML, Cohen RA: Elevated glucose impairs endothelium-dependent relaxation by activating protein kinase C. J Clin Invest 87:1643-8, 1991.
64. Yamauchi T, Ohnaka K, Takayanagi R, et al: Enhanced secretion of endothelin-1 by elevated glucose levels from cultured bovine aortic endothelial cells. FEBS Lett 267:16-18, 1990.
65. Lorenzi M, Cagliero E, Toledo S: Glucose toxicity for human endothelial cells in culture: Delayed replication, disturbed cell cycle, and accelerated death. Diabetes 34:621-627, 1985.
66. Ayo SH, Radnik RA, Glass WF, et al: Increased extracellular matrix synthesis and mRNA in mesangial cells grown in high-glucose medium. Am J Physiol 260:F185-F191, 1991.
67. Mene P, Pugliese G, Pricci F, et al: High glucose inhibits cytosolic calcium signalling in cultured rat mesangial cells. Kidney Int 43:585-591, 1993.
68. Brownlee M, Cerami A, Vlassara H: Advanced glycosylation end products in tissue and the biochemical basis of diabetic complications. N Engl J Med 318:1315-1321, 1988.
69. Haitglou CS, Tsilibary EC, Brownlee M, et al: Altered cellular interactions between endothelial cells and non-enzymatically glycosylated laminin/type IV collagen. J Biol Chem 267:12404-12407, 1992.
70. Crowley ST, Brownlee M, Edelstein D, et al: Effects of nonenzymatic glycosylation on mesangial matrix on proliferation of mesangial cells. Diabetes 40:540-547, 1991.
71. Soules-Liparota T, Cooper ME, Papazoglou D, et al: Retardation by aminoguanidine of development of albuminuria, mesangial

expansion, and tissue fluorescence in streptozotocin-induced diabetic rat. Diabetes 40:1328-1334, 1991.
72. Greene D: The pathogenesis and prevention of diabetic neuropathy and nephropathy. Metabolism 37:25-29, 1988.
73. Tsai SC, Burnakis TG: Aldose reductase inhibitors: An update. Ann Pharmacol 27:751-754, 1993.
74. Ha H, Kim KH. Pathogenesis of diabetic nephropathy: the role of oxidative stress and protein kinase C. Diab Res Clin Pract 45:147-151, 1999.
75. Koya D, Haneda M, Nakagawa H, Isshiki K, Sato H, Maeda S, Sugimoto T, Yasuda H, Kashiwagi A, Ways DK, King Gl, Kikkawa R. Amelioration of accelerated diabetic mesangial expansion by treatment with a PKC inhibitor in diabetic db/db mice, a rodent model for type 2 diabetes. FASEB J 14:439-447, 2000.
76. Nakamura T, Fukui M, Ebihara I, et al: mRNA expression of growth factors in glomeruli from diabetic rats. Diabetes 42:450-456, 1993.
77. Moran A, Brown DM, Kim Y, et al: Effects of IgF-I and glucose on protein and proteoglycan synthesis by human fetal mesangial cells in culture. Diabetes 40:1346-1354, 1991.
78. Hasegawa G, Nakano K, Sawada M, et al: Possible role of tumor necrosis factor and interleukin-1 in the development of diabetic nephropathy. Kidney Int 40:1007-1012, 1991.
79. Flyvbjerg A, Frystyk J, Osterby R, et al: Kidney IgF-I and renal hypertrophy in GH deficient dwarf rats. Am J Physiol 262:E956-E962, 1992.
80. Gronbaek H, Volmers P, Bjorn SF, et al: Effect of isolated GH and IgF-1 deficiency on long-term renal changes and urinary albumin excretion in streptozotocin diabetic dwarf rats. Am J Physiol 272:E918-E924, 1997.
81. Sharma K, Jin Y, Guo J, et al: Neutralization of TGF-beta by anti-TGF-beta antibody attenuates kidney hypertrophy and the enhanced extracellular matrix gene expression in STZ-induced diabetic mice. Diabetes 45:522-530, 1996.
82. Wang PH, Lau J, Chalmers TC: Meta-analysis of effects of intensive blood-glucose control on late complications of type I diabetes. Lancet 341:1306-1309, 1993.
83. Christensen CK, Christiansen JS, Schmitz A, et al: Effect of continuous subcutaneous insulin infusion on kidney function and size in IDDM patients: A 2 year controlled study. J Diabetes Complications 1:91-95, 1987.

84. Dahl-Jorgensen K, Hanssen KF, Kierulf P, et al: Reduction of urinary albumin excretion after 4 years of continuous subcutaneous insulin infusion in insulin-dependent diabetes mellitus. Acta Endocrinol 117:19-25, 1988.
85. Reichard P, Berglund B, Britz A, et al: Intensified conventional insulin treatment retards the microvascular complications of insulin-dependent diabetes mellitus (IDDM): The Stockholm Diabetes Intervention Study (SDIS) after 5 years. J Intern Med 230:101-108, 1991.
86. DCCT Research Group. Effect of intensive diabetes treatment on the development and progression of long-term complications in adolescents with insulin-dependent diabetes mellitus: Diabetes Control and Complications Trial. J Pediatr 125:177-188, 1994.
87. DCCT Research Group. The effect of intensive treatment of diabetes on the development and progression of long-term complications in insulin-dependent diabetes mellitus. New Engl J Med 329:977-986, 1993.
88. Bojestig M, Arnqvist HJ, Karlberg BE, Ludvigsson J. Glycemic control and prognosis in type I diabetic patients with microalbuminuria. Diabetes Care. 19:313-7, 1996.
89. Steffes MW, Molitch ME, Chavers BM, Cleary PA, Lachin J, The DCCT/EDIC Study group. Sustained reduction in albuminuria six years after the Diabetes Control and Complications Trial. Diabetes 50 (Suppl 2):A63, 2001.
90. Krolewski AS, Laffel LM, Krolewski M, Quinn M, Warram JH. Glycosylated hemoglobin and the risk of microalbuminuria in patients with insulin-dependent diabetes mellitus. New Engl J Med. 332:1251-1255, 1995.
91. Mogensen CE, Hansen KW, Osterby R, et al. Blood pressure elevation versus abnormal albuminuria in the genesis and prediction of renal disease in diabetes. Diabetes Care 15:1192-1220, 1992.
92. Norgaard K, Feldt-Rasmussen B, Borch-Johnsen K, et al. Prevalence of hypertension in type 1 (insulin-dependent) diabetes mellitus. Diabetologia 33:407-410, 1992.
93. Mathieson ER, Saubrey N, Hommel E, et al. Prevalence of microalbuminuria in children with type 1 (insulin-dependent) diabetes mellitus. Diabetologia 29:640-643, 1986.
94. Sochett EB, Poona I, Bale JW, Daneman D. Ambulatory blood pressure monitoring in IDDM adolescents with and without microalbuminuria. J of Diabetes and its Complications, 12:18-23, 1998.

95. Seacoast ER, Goetz FC, Rich S, Barbs J. Familial clustering of diabetic kidney disease. Evidence for genetic susceptibility to diabetic nephropathy. New Engl J Med.320:1161-5, 1985.
96. Quinn M, Angelic MC, Warram JH, Krolewski AS. Familial factors determine the development of diabetic nephropathy in patients with IDDM. Diabetologia. 39:940-5, 1996.
97. Fujisawa T, Ikegami H, Kawaguchi Y, et al: Meta-analysis of association of insertion/deletion polymorphism of angiotensin I-converting enzyme gene with diabetic nephropathy and retinopathy. Diabetologia 41:47-53, 1998.
98. Tarn L, Glued C, Parving H-H: Diabetic nephropathy and the insertion/deletion polymorphism of the angiotensin-converting enzyme gene. Nephrol Dial Transplant 13:1125-1130, 1998.
99. Tarn L, Cabmen F, Rossing P, et al: Angiotensinogen gene polymorphisms in IDDM patients with diabetic nephropathy. Diabetes 45:367-369, 1996.
100. Tarnow L, Cambien F, Rossing P, et al: Angiotensin II type 1 receptor gene polymorphism and diabetic microangiopathy. Nephrol Dial Transplant 11:1019-1023, 1996.
101. Couper JJ, Staples AJ, Cocciolone R, Nairn J, Badcock N, Henning P. Relationship of smoking and albuminuria in children with diabetes. Diabetic Medicine 11:666-669, 1994.
102. Hargrave DR MC, O'Hare MM, Carson DJ. Tobacco smoke exposure in children and adolescents with diabetes mellitus. Diabetic Medicine 16:31-34, 1999.
103. Holl RW, Grabert M, Heinze E, Debatin KM. Objective assessment of smoking habits by urinary cotinine measurement in adolescents and young adults with type 1 diabetes. Reliability of cigarette consumption and relationship to urinary albumin excretion. Diabetes Care 21:787-791, 1998.
104. Regalado M, Yang S, Wesson DE. Cigarette smoking is associated with augmented progression of renal insufficiency in severe essential hypertension. Am J Kidney Dis. 35:687-94, 2000.
105. Chaturvedi N, Stephenson JM, Fuller JH. The relationship between smoking and microvascular complications in the EURODIAB IDDM Complications Study. Diabetes Care. 18:785-792, 1995.
106. Gay EC, Cai Y, Gale SM, Baron A, Cruickshanks KJ, Kostraba JN, Hamman RF.
Smokers with IDDM experience excess morbidity. The Colorado IDDM Registry.
Diabetes Care. 15:947-52, 1992.

107. Ritz E, Ogata H, Orth SR. Smoking: a factor promoting onset and progression of diabetic nephropathy. Diabetes Metab 26 (Suppl 4):54-63, 2000.
108. Pedrini MT, Levey AS, Lau J, Chalmers TC, Wang PH. The effect of dietary protein restriction on the progression of diabetic and nondiabetic renal diseases: a meta-analysis. Ann Intern Med. 124:627-32, 1996.
109. O'Hayon BE, Cummings EA, Daneman D, Ossip MG, Lawson ML, Sochett EB. Does dietary protein intake impact on early nephropathy in children and adolescents with type 1 diabetes? Diabetic Medicine 17:708-12, 2000.
110. Kordonouri O, Danne TH, Hopfenmuller W, et al. Lipid profiles and blood pressure: Are they risk factors for the development of early background retinopathy and incipient nephropathy in children with insulin-dependent diabetes mellitus? Acta Paediatr 85:43-48, 1996.
111. Danne T, Kordonouri O, Hovener G, et al. Diabetic angiopathy in children. Diabet Med 14:1012-1025, 1997.
112. Jandeleit-Dahm K, Cao Z, Cox AJ, Kelly DJ, Gilbert RE, Cooper ME. Role of hyperlipidemia in progressive renal disease: focus on diabetic nephropathy. Kidney Int Suppl. 71:S31-6, 1999.
113. Han DC, Kim JH, Cha MK, Song KI, Hwang SD, Lee HB. Effect of HMG CoA reductase inhibition on TGF-beta 1 mRNA expression in diabetic rat glomeruli. Kidney Int Suppl. 51:S61-5, 1995.
114. Kim SI, Han DC, Lee HB. Lovastatin inhibits transforming growth factor-beta1 expression in diabetic rat glomeruli and cultured rat mesangial cells. J Am Soc Nephrol.11(1):80-7, 2000.
115. Yokota T, Utsunomiya K, Murakawa Y, Kurata H, Tajima N. Mechanism of preventive effect of HMG-CoA reductase inhibitor on diabetic nephropathy. Kidney Int Suppl. 71:S178-81, 1999.
116. Oda H, Keane WF. Recent advances in statins and the kidney. Kidney Int Suppl. 71:S2-5, 1999.
117. Lawson M, Sochett EB, Chait PG, Balfe JW, Daneman D. Effect of puberty on markers of glomerular hypertrophy and hypertension in diabetes. Diabetes 45: 51-55, 1996.
118. Kostraba JN, Dorman JS, Orchard TJ, Becker DJ, Ohki Y, Ellis D, Doft BH, Lobes LA, LaPorte RE, Drash AL. Contribution of diabetes duration before puberty to development of microvascular complications in IDDM subjects. Diabetes Care. 12:686-93, 1989.
119. Murphy RP, Nanda M, Plotnik L, et al. The relationship of puberty to diabetic retinopathy. Arch Ophthalmol 108:215-218, 1990.

120. Cummings EA, Sochett EB, Dekker M, Lawson M, Daneman D. Contribution of growth hormone and IGF-I to early diabetic nephropathy in type 1 diabetes. Diabetes 47:1341-46, 1998.
121. Tabaei BP, Al-Kassab AS, Ilag LL, Zawacki CM, Herman WH. Does microalbuminuria predict diabetic nephropathy? Diabetes Care 24:1560-1566, 2001.
122. Bojestig M, Arnqvist HJ, Hermansson G, Karlberg BE, Ludvigsson J. Declining incidence of nephropathy in insulin-dependent diabetes mellitus. New Engl J Med. 1994 Jan 6;330(1):15-8, 1994.
123. Meltzer S, Leiter L, Daneman D, Gerstein HC, Lau D, Ludwig S, Yale JF, Zinman B, Lillie D. 1998 clinical practice guidelines for the management of diabetes in Canada. Canadian Diabetes Association. CMAJ. 159 Suppl 8:S1-29, 1998.
124. Krolewski AS, Warram JH. Natural history of diabetic nephropathy: How can it be changed? Diabetes Rev 3:446-459, 1995.
125. Couper JJ, Clarke CF, Byrne GC, Jones TW, Donaghue KC, Nairn J, Boyce D, Russell M, Stephens M, Raymond J, Bates DJ, McCaul K. Progression of borderline increases in albuminuria in adolescents with insulin-dependent diabetes mellitus. Diabet Med. 14:766-71, 1997
126. Lorini R, d'Annunzio G, Vitali L, Scaramuzza A, Bacchella L, Zonta LA. Normal values of overnight albumin excretion rate in a sample of healthy Italian children and adolescents. J Pediatr Endocrinol Metab. 11:639-43, 1998.
127. Stratton IM, Adler AI, Neil HA, Matthews DR, Manley SE, Cull CA, Hadden D, Turner RC, Holman RR. Association of glycaemia with macrovascular and microvascular complications of type 2 diabetes (UKPDS 35): prospective observational study. BMJ. 321:405-12, 2000.
128. Lewis EJ, Hunsicker LG, Bain RP, Rohde RD. The effect of angiotensin-converting-enzyme inhibition on diabetic nephropathy. The Collaborative Study Group. New Engl J Med.329:1456-62, 1993.
129. Lewis EJ, Hunsicker LG, Clarke WR, Berl T, Pohl MA, Lewis JB, Ritz E, Atkins RC, Rohde R, Raz I. Renoprotective effect of the angiotensin-receptor antagonist irbesartan in patients with nephropathy due to type 2 diabetes. New Engl J Med.345:851-60, 2001.
130. Brenner BM, Cooper ME, de Zeeuw D, Keane WF, Mitch WE, Parving HH, Remuzzi G, Snapinn SM, Zhang Z, Shahinfar S. Effects of losartan on renal and cardiovascular outcomes in patients

with type 2 diabetes and nephropathy. New Engl J Med. 345:861-9, 2001.

131. Parving HH, Lehnert H, Brochner-Mortensen J, Gomis R, Andersen S, Arner P.
The effect of irbesartan on the development of diabetic nephropathy in patients with type 2 diabetes. New Engl J Med. 345:870-8, 2001.

132. Kasiske BL, Kalil RS, Ma JZ, Liao M, Keane WF. Effect of antihypertensive therapy on the kidney in patients with diabetes: a meta-regression analysis. Ann Intern Med. 118:129-38, 1993.

133. Cook J, Daneman D, Spino M, Sochett E, Perlman K, Balfe JW. Angiotensin converting enzyme inhibitor therapy decreases microalbuminuria in normotensive children with insulin-dependent diabetes mellitus. J. Pediatr. 117: 39-45, 1990

134. Rudberg S, Osterby R, Bangstad HJ, Dahlquist G, Persson B. Effect of angiotensin converting enzyme inhibitor or beta blocker on glomerular structural changes in young microalbuminuric patients with Type I (insulin-dependent) diabetes mellitus. Diabetologia. 42:589-95, 1999.

Chapter 19
DIABETIC RETINOPATHY

Andrew W. Eller, MD
Department of Ophthalmology
Associate Professor of Ophthalmology
The Eye and Ear Institute, University of Pittsburgh School of Medicine, Pittsburgh, PA

This chapter was supported in part by The Eye and Ear Foundation.

INTRODUCTION

The significance of diabetic retinopathy cannot be understated in the pediatric age group. It has been predicted that 72% of patients with type 1 diabetes will eventually develop proliferative diabetic retinopathy.[1] Untreated, this disease has disastrous consequences as it typically leads to blindness. Yet, rarely does diabetic retinopathy require ophthalmic intervention prior to late adolescence. Therefore, it is the role of the pediatric diabetes specialists (not the ophthalmologist) that assumes the greatest importance in the prevention of blindness from diabetic retinopathy in the pediatric population. The Diabetes Control and Complications Trial (DCCT) has shown the value of tight control in reducing the risk of blindness.[2] By implementing intensive glycemic control in their patients, primary diabetes caregivers are on the front line of treating diabetic retinopathy.

Epidemiology

Diabetic retinopathy is the leading cause of new cases of blindness in persons age 20 to 74 years in the United States.[3-8] In patients who have had Type 1 diabetes for 30 or more years (insulin-dependent diabetes for 30 or more years), the prevalence of blindness is 12%. In the United States, blindness due to diabetes is estimated to involve an expense of about $500 million annually due to lost income and public welfare.

In the Wisconsin Epidemiologic Study of Diabetic Retinopathy (WESDR)[9] 10,135 patients with diabetes in an 11-county area were identified, and 1210 patients with Type I diabetes were selected for the survey (all insulin-taking patients diagnosed at age <30 years). As expected, the frequency of visual impairment increased with increasing age, and duration of diabetes. No cases of legal blindness were identified in persons age <25 years. However, the rate of legal blindness increased with age (65 to 74 years) in both males and females reaching peaks of 14% and 20%, respectively. In addition, the WESDR evaluated the rate of progression of retinopathy in this younger-onset group of diabetic patients. The 14-year progression rate was 86%, while progression to proliferative diabetic retinopathy was 37%. The incidence of diabetic macular edema was 26%.[10]

Visual acuity as a predictor of death was studied in the WESDR. After adjusting for age and sex, the younger-onset group of patients with a vision of 20/200 (legal blindness) or poorer in their better eye at baseline had a 6-year survival rate of 57.9%. This was compared with 89.9% in patients whose vision was better than 20/40 in their better eye. The relationship between survival and vision remained after controlling for other factors associated with mortality, such as age, hypertension, higher glycosylated hemoglobin, and cardiovascular disease.

Note that diabetic retinopathy is seldom seen before the age of 13 years, regardless of the duration of diabetes, despite[11] the fact that the prevalence and severity of diabetic retinopathy otherwise increases with age. This may be explained by the effect of puberty on diabetic retinopathy. In the WESDR, postmenarchal subjects were 3.2 times as likely to have diabetic retinopathy as those who were premenarchal.[12] Prior to menarche, the duration of diabetes did not influence the risk of retinopathy, while duration of diabetes did correlate with an increased risk after menarche. A number of possible factors have been implicated in the effect of puberty on diabetic retinopathy. These include increases in insulin-like growth factor I, growth hormone, sex hormones, blood pressure, and worse diabetic control.[13-19]

The Diabetes Control and Complications Trial (DCCT) demonstrated the positive effect of intense blood glucose control. This was a large, randomized controlled clinical trial of 1441 patients with type 1 diabetes. The intensive-therapy group had a reduced incidence and progression of retinopathy, progression to non-proliferative diabetic retinopathy, and proliferative diabetic retinopathy, and incidence of macular edema. In addition, there was a reduced need for panretinal photocoagulation when compared to the group with conventional insulin treatment.[20-21]

Pathophysiology of Diabetic Retinopathy

The retina is comprised of three groups of elements: neural, glial, and vascular. It is thought that in some way, all of these elements are adversely affected in the relatively hyperglycemic environment that is imposed upon them in diabetes mellitus. However, from a clinical point of view, it is the(retina vasculature changes that is) most obviously affected by diabetes.

One of the hallmarks of the retinal vasculature is that of autoregulation, as this is a feature of all blood vessels in the central nervous system. The retinal arteries have smooth muscle, while the arterioles, capillaries, and venules have pericytes which function as modified smooth muscles. In diabetes, presumably due to changes in retinal metabolism there is a demand for increased retinal blood flow. As a result of autoregulation, there is vasodilation, with an increase in blood flow. Although not typically measured, it is thought that increased retinal blood flow may be one of the earliest findings in diabetic retinopathy. Buzney and Weiter have hypothesized that it is damage from chronic vasodilation of the retinal vessels that leads to the formation of the characteristic retinal lesions seen in diabetic retinopathy.[22] Other mechanisms have been postulated to explain retinovascular damage including increased glucose metabolism by the polyol pathway, advanced glycosylation end products that may give rise to basement membrane thickening, and activation of protein kinase C.[23-25]

Diabetic retinopathy can be divided into two phases: non-proliferative, and proliferative. Non-proliferative retinopathy is the development of progressive retinal damage that eventually results in capillary closure, and retinal ischemia. The proliferative phase of retinopathy can be regarded as aberrant repair, or a "healing" response of the retina to ischemic injury. It has been shown that the ischemic retina produces vascular endothelial growth factor (VEGF) which leads to neovascularization of the retina and optic nerve.[26] The neovascular membranes actually proliferate on the surface of the optic nerve and the retina, and grow into the vitreous humor (Figure 1). The vitreous is a gelatinous body that has the appearance and consistency of egg white. When the new blood vessels grow into the vitreous gel, they may rupture and produce a vitreous hemorrhage. As these neovascular membranes mature, they become fibrotic and contract. The vitreous gel serves as a scaffold, and with contraction of the membranes there is tension on the retina, which may result in a traction retinal detachment. Perhaps the most serious complication of proliferative diabetic retinopathy is the formation of a neovascular membrane on the surface of the iris. This is termed rubeosis iridis, and is a result of profound retinal ischemia. When these new vessels occlude the trabecular meshwork (drainage angle of the anterior chamber), the eye pressure becomes elevated, resulting in neovascular glaucoma.

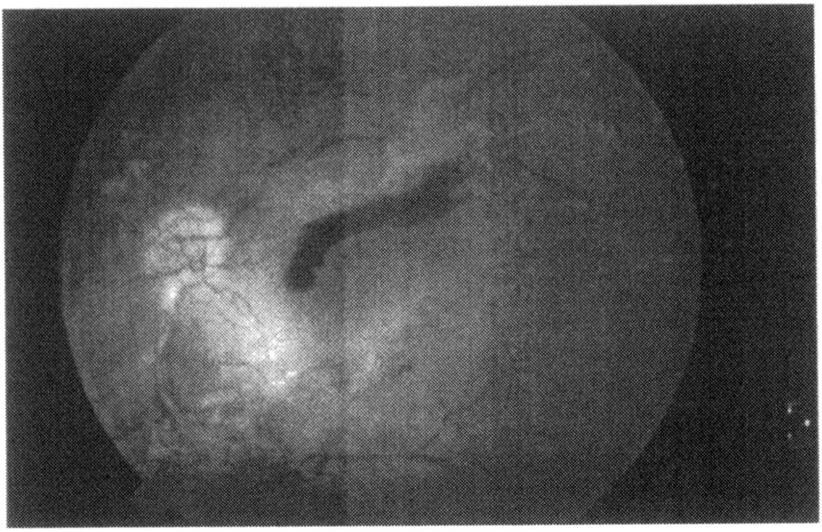

Figure 1: nerve. On the inferior border of the optic nerve, there is a fibroglial membrane that is exerting traction on the retina. A streak of vitreous hemorrhage is seen over the macula. On the right side of the photo, the retina has a dull, featureless appearance, which is indicative of severe retinal Proliferative Diabetic Retinopathy with neovascularization of the optic ischemia.

The macula is the "center" of the retina, and is the region responsible for the most sensitive or best vision. Whenever diabetic changes affect this area of the retina, it is termed diabetic maculopathy. Macular edema occurs as a result of the leakage of serum from microaneurysms, or from broader areas along walls of damaged capillaries.

The retinal pigmented epithelium (RPE) is the outermost layer of the retina. The RPE has a pumping mechanism that attempts to eliminate fluid from the retina. As the fluid is removed from serum, the residual lipoproteinaceous exudates deposit in the retina. When the RPE pump can no longer keep up with the leakage, there is retinal thickening or edema formation in addition to the hard exudates. Damage to the macula is the most common cause of significant vision loss in the diabetic patient. Diabetic maculopathy can coincide with any stage of diabetic retinopathy. Therefore, a patient may have only mild nonproliferative disease, and yet be legally blind from diabetic macular edema. Interestingly, epidemiologic studies have shown that diabetic macular edema is not seen as frequently in type I diabetes mellitus as it is in individuals with type 2 diabetes mellitus.

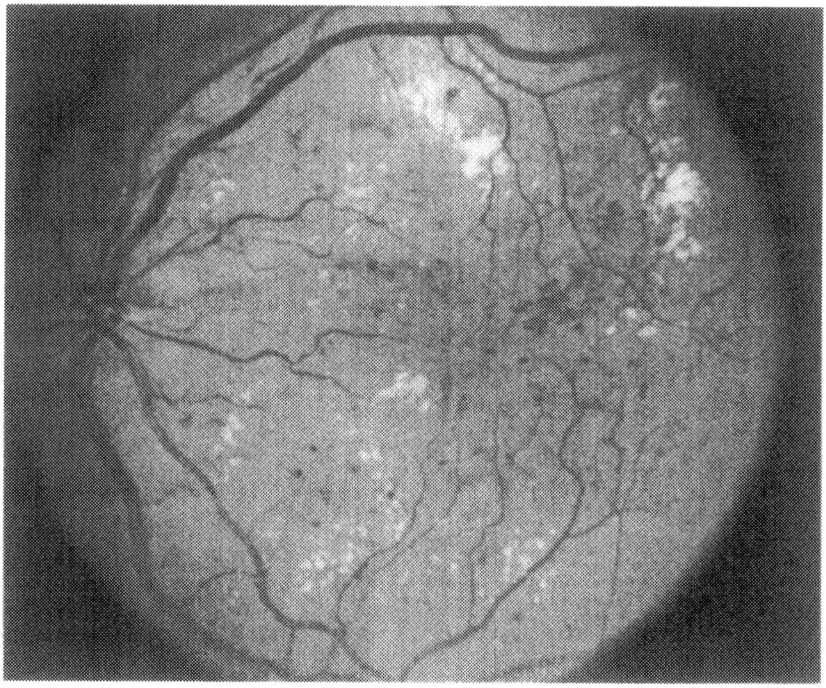

Figure 2: Diabetic Maculopathy with numerous microaneurysms, intraretinal hemorrhages, and clusters of hard exudates. When the center of the macula (fovea) becomes edematous as a result of leakage from the damaged retinal vasculature, this can lead to irreversible loss of central vision.

Classification of Diabetic Retinopathy
Nonproliferative Retinopathy (NPDR)

Mild: This is characterized by the presence of microaneuryms, intraretinal hemorrhages (dot and blot, and flame-shaped), and hard exudates.

Moderate: In addition to the above features, in this stage, nerve fiber layer infarcts (cotton-wool spots) are seen. The later represent focal areas of retinal ischemia.
Severe: As the retina becomes progressively ischemic, the nerve fiber layer infarcts begin to fade, and there are larger areas of retinal non-perfusion due to capillary closure. When this occurs, the larger, surrounding venules become increasing dilated. This is known as "venous beading." Also, some residual capillaries become dilated and serve as collateral vessels to carry blood flow across an area of capillary closure. These collateral vessels are known as intraretinal microvascular abnormalities (IRMA). The Early Treatment Diabetes Retinopathy Study (ETDRS) defined severe NPDR by the 4:2:1 rule: diffuse intraretinal hemorrhages and microaneuryms in 4 quadrants, venous beading in 2 quadrants, and IRMA in 1 quadrant of the retina.[27] Patients in this category had a 15 % chance of progressing to high-risk proliferative diabetic retinopathy in one year.
Very Severe: This was defined as having any two of the above features, and these patients had a 45% chance of progressing to high-risk proliferative diabetic retinopathy in one year.

Proliferative Retinopathy

Non-high Risk: Any retinal neovascularization that does not meet the more advanced criteria of "High Risk" that is discussed below.
High Risk: The Diabetic Retinopathy Study described retinal findings that were termed high risk characteristics of proliferative diabetic retinopathy.[28] These include neovascularization of the optic nerve that is greater than 1/4 to 1/3 of the disc surface area, any neovascularization of the optic nerve with vitreous hemorrhage, and retinal neovascularization that is associated with a vitreous hemorrhage.

Diabetic Maculopathy

Diabetic maculopathy has been classified into three categories.[29] 1) Focal disease results from leakage of microaneuryms in a centrifugal manner leading to a circinate pattern of hard exudates. 2) Diffuse disease occurs when there is more widespread damage to the capillaries. 3) Macular ischemia can follow diffuse disease, as further capillary damage, can result in closure. In some eyes, components of all three types may be identified.

Treatment of Diabetic Retinopathy

The principles of our treatment of diabetic retinopathy are based on the results of two very well designed, multicentered clinical trials. These are the Diabetic Retinopathy Study (DRS), and the Early Treatment Diabetic Retinopathy Study (ETDRS).[30,31]

Proliferative Retinopathy

Since publication of the DRS, panretinal photocoagulation (PRP) has served as the mainstay of treatment for proliferative diabetic retinopathy. **Indications for PRP:** The DRS showed that treatment benefit from PRP was seen in patients with High Risk disease. Later, the ETDRS demonstrated that PRP in severe nonproliferative disease (A-NPDR), and in non-high risk proliferative disease also had a more favorable outcome with PRP. The technique is to place scatter laser burns in the retina, in a polka dot pattern, throughout the entire mid- and far-peripheral retina. In other words, the laser treatment is placed outside the major vascular arcades that delineate the macular region. The inner retina contains a rich supply of capillaries. In diabetic retinopathy, these capillaries become increasingly closed, rendering the inner retina ischemic. The outer retina which contains the photorecptors (rods and cones) is avascular. This area is nourished by diffusion of oxygen from the underlying choroid, which is comprised of fenestrated capillaries. The photoreceptors, which are highly dependent on oxygen, are ablated by the laser treatment. Following PRP, the outer retina, no longer consumes as much oxygen. Therefore, the oxygen continues to diffuse into the ischemic inner retina. In turn, the improved oxygenation of the inner retina, reverses the production of VEGF.

Diabetic Macular Edema

The treatment of diabetic macular edema is based on the results of the ETDRS. The ETDRS introduced the important concept of clinically significant macular edema (CSME). When the macular edema progresses to the "threshold" level of being clinically significant, then laser treatment is indicated.

Laser treatment for macular edema is directed in a focal manner to close the "leaky" microaneurysms. In areas of more diffuse macular edema, a "grid" treatment is placed to stimulate the pumping action of the retinal pigment epithelium.

Vitreous Hemorrhage

To the patient, this is perhaps the most frightening complication of diabetic retinopathy.[32] When there is a spontaneous rupture of disc or retinal neovascularization, there is bleeding within the vitreous cavity. This can be very mild and appear to the patient as reddish smoke, or it may be a substantial hemorrhage with significant loss of vision. If the patient has not had previous PRP, there is reason for concern. In this setting, the proliferative disease can continue to progress resulting in a traction retinal detachment, or neovascular glaucoma. These patients should be followed very carefully. If the blood clears spontaneously, then a PRP should be performed. On the other hand, if the blood does not clear within a period of 2 or 3 months, then surgical evacuation with a vitrectomy is recommended in conjunction with an intraoperative PRP. When the patient has had previous PRP laser treatment, then one can safely wait for clearing of the blood. If the blood fails to clear after 3 months, we consider performing a vitrectomy to remove the blood as well as the vitreous gel from inside the eye. This procedure is commonly performed and is generally quite successful in restoring sight.

Traction Retinal Detachment

As proliferative diabetic retinopathy represents a form of aberrant repair, the production of neovascular membranes is only of the first phase of this "healing or scarring" process. After the neovascular membranes are formed, the glial cell component begins to produce collagen as well as the contractile protein, actin. At the end stage, they appear as white, fibroglial membranes, that may exert significant traction on the retina. As the membranes proliferate on the surface of the retina, they interface with the vitreous gel. The vitreous serves as a scaffold along which the membranes grow. When the membranes eventually contract, depending on their extent and location, the retina may become detached. If the macula is affected, then the vision will be reduced. The only treatment for a traction retinal detachment is vitrectomy in conjunction with dissection or delamination of the membranes from the surface of the retina.

Neovascular glaucoma

Progressive retinal ischemia can result in the growth of a neovascular membrane on the surface of the iris. This is known as rubeosis irides. The trabecular meshwork lines the drainage angle of the anterior chamber. If the neovascular tissue occludes the trabecular meshwork, then the pressure rises in the eye, producing glaucoma. This can be a very serious problem, as not only can it lead to blindness, but the eye can become extremely painful as well. Early treatment with panretinal photocoagulation alone may be sufficient. However, in more advanced cases, a surgical glaucoma procedure may be necessary to ultimately control the eye pressure.

Other Ophthalmic Complications of Diabetes Mellitus

Refractive error

Fluctuations in blood glucose levels can result in changes in refractive error which manifest as blurred vision. It is thought that as the glucose levels rise, the "excess" glucose undergoes reduction by aldose reductase into sorbitol. The sorbitol accumulates within the crystalline lens of the eye, and creates an osmotic gradient drawing water into the lens.[33] As the lens swells, it typically results in a myopic (nearsighted) shift in the refractive error. Less commonly, the refractive shift may be hyperopic (farsighted). When this occurs the vision is always correctable with a new refraction.

From a practical standpoint, it is important to ensure that the blood glucose is in a normal range just prior to prescribing a new pair of glasses. Otherwise, the prescription will be in error when the glucose returns to baseline. It is recommended that the patient check their blood glucose just before having their eyes examined for glasses. If the blood glucose is not stable, then the appointment should be rescheduled.

Cataract

When the crystalline lens of the eye becomes hazy or cloudy, it is termed a cataract. Cataracts are 2 to 4 times more likely to occur in diabetics, than in nondiabetic persons.[34] The risk of developing a cataract increases with duration of diabetes as well as with poor metabolic control. Cataracts secondary to diabetes mellitus are infrequent in the pediatric age-group. Today, cataract surgery is a highly successful procedure, but one must also be aware of the small risk of exacerbation of diabetic retinopathy. Cataract surgery in diabetes must be very carefully planned, and when indicated, pre-operative laser treatment should be performed if there is adequate visualization through the lens to see the retina.

Diabetic papillopathy

An uncommon ocular complication of diabetes mellitus is optic nerve edema, or swelling.[35] This has been called diabetic papillopathy, and is considered to have a good visual prognosis. Interestingly, it can be seen with any stage of retinopathy. It usually presents between the second and fourth decades of life, and tends to occur in poorly controlled diabetes patients. There is bilateral involvement in approximately 50% of cases, although the eyes may not be affected simultaneously. Typically the vision is only reduced to the level of 20/50, but in some cases it may be as poor as 20/200. Recovery to 20/30 or better is seen 2 to 6 weeks after onset.

It is important to distinguish this rather benign condition from papilledema, PDR with neovascularization of the optic disc, and acute ischemic optic neuropathy.

Rapid Initiation of Tight Glycemic Control

When strict glycemic control is rapidly induced, there is evidence of a faster progression of diabetic retinopathy than otherwise anticipated. In the DCCT, it was shown that there was early worsening of retinopathy at the 6- and/or 12-month visit in 13.1% of patients in the intensive treatment group, and in only 7.6% in the conventional treatment group. ($P<.001$)[36] In fact, the higher the Hemoglobin A_{1c}, the more likely it was for worsening to occur with initiation of intensive therapy. On the other hand, there was no evidence of a reduced risk of progression when there was a more gradual reduction of glycemia during the first six months of the study. In the long-term, the two groups were similar, or more favorable for the intensive treatment group.

The long-term benefits of strict glycemic control outweigh any potential worsening of diabetic retinopathy. It is important that patients be screened for any progression of retinopathy at 3 month intervals during the first year after intensive therapy has been induced, because, sight-saving laser therapy can be performed at the appropriate time, if threshold criteria for treatment are identified.

Recommendations for Screening for Diabetic Retinopathy

Screening is an essential tool in the management of diabetic retinopathy. A patient may have a significant degree of diabetic macular edema, or proliferative retinopathy and still have normal vision. If we were to rely on ocular symptoms, such as "floaters", or loss of vision to indicate the presence of diabetic retinopathy, then there would already be a delay in diagnosis. At this point, application of laser treatment is less likely to be effective.

In reviewing the data from two clinical trials, it has been shown that the treatment for diabetic retinopathy may be 90% effective in preventing severe vision loss utilizing present strategies.[37] This underscores the importance of routine screening for diabetic retinopathy so that intervention with laser treatment can be performed in a timely manner. The American Academy of Ophthalmology has published its recommendations for screening eye examinations of diabetic retinopathy.[38] (Table 1)

Table 1

Recommended Eye Examination Schedule
for Patients with Diabetes

Age of Onset of Diabetes Mellitus	Recommended Time of First Exam	Recommended Follow-up
0 - 29	5 years after onset	Yearly
30 and older	At time of diagnosis	Yearly
Prior to pregnancy	Prior to conception or early in the first trimester	No retinopathy to non-severe NPDR: every 3-12 months. Other stages of diabetic retinopathy; every 1-3 months

Exquisite diabetic control is important as it can delay or prevent the onset of clinically evident diabetic retinopathy. The pathophysiologic changes in the retina probably begin soon after the inception of diabetes. Yet, rarely does the diabetic damage accrue to the level of clinical relevance until the patient reaches their late teens or early twenties, and has had diabetes mellitus for at least 10 years. Therefore, it is of utmost importance for the pediatric care providers to help their patients achieve optimal control from the time of diagnosis in order to help prevent blindness from the complications of diabetic retinopathy.

REFERENCES

1. Javitt JC, Canner JK, Sommer: Cost-effectiveness of current approaches to the control of retinopathy in type I diabetics. Ophthalmology. 1989; 96:255-64.
2. Diabetes control and complications Trial Research Group: The effect of intensive diabetes treatment on the progression of diabetic retinopathy in insulin-dependent diabetes mellitus. Arch Ophthalmol. 1995;113:36-51.
3. Vision Problems in the U.S: A Statistical Analysis. New York: National Society to Prevent Blindness; 1980.
4. Kahn HA, Moorhead HB: Statistics on Blindness in the Model Reporting Area, 1969-70. National Eye Institute, National Institutes of Health Publ. No. 73-427. Washington, DC: US Govt Printing Office: 1973.
5. US Department of Health, Education and Welfare (USDHEW): Model Reporting Area-Proceedings of the 2nd Annual Conference of the Model Reporting Area for Blindness Statistics. Public Health Service Publ. No. 1135. Washington, DC: US Govt Printing Office; 1963.
6. Kahn HA, Hiller R: Blindness caused by diabetic retinopathy. Am J Ophthalmology. 1974;78:58-67.
7. Brechner RJ, Crowie CC, Howie LJ, et al: Ophthalmic examination among adults with diagnosed diabetes mellitus. J Am Med Assoc. 1993;270:1714-1718.
8. Hiller R, Krueger DE: Validity of a survey question as a measure of visual impairment. Am J Public Health. 1983;73:93-96.
9. Klein R, Klein BEK, Moss SE: Visual impairment in diabetes. Ophthalmology. 1984;91:1-9.
10. Klein R. Klein BEK, Moss SE, Cruickshanks KJ: The Wisconsin Epidemiologic Study of Diabetic Retinopathy, XVII: the 14-year incidence and progression of diabetic retinopathy and associated risk factors in type 1 diabetes. Ophthalmology. 1998;105:1801-1815.
11. Klein R. Klein BEK, Moss SE, et al: The Wisconsin Epidemiologic Study of Diabetic Retinopathy, II: prevalence and risk of diabetic retinopathy when age at diagnosis is less than 30 years. Arch Ophthalmology. 1984;102:520-526.
12. Klein BEK, Moss SE, Klein R: Is menarche associated with diabetic retinopathy? Diabetes Care. 1990;13:1034-1038.

13. Dills DG, Moss SE, Klein R, et al: Is insulin-like growth factor I associated with diabetic retinopathy? Diabetes. 1990;39:191-195.
14. Pieters GF, Smals AG, Kloppenborg PW: Defective suppression of growth hormone after oral glucose loading in adolescence. J Clin Endocrinol Metab. 1980;51:265-270.
15. Klein R, Klein BEK, Moss SE, DeMets DL: Blood pressure and hypertension in diabetes. Am J Epidemiol. 1985;122:75-89.
16. Blethen SL, Sargeant DT, Whitlow MG, Santiago JV: Effect of pubertal stage and recent blood glucose control on plasma somatomedin C in children with insulin-dependent diabetes mellitus. Diabetes. 1981;30:868-872.
17. Allen C, Zaccaro DJ, Palta M, et al: Glycemic control in early IDDM. The Wisconsin Diabetes Registry. Diabetes Care. 1992;15:980-987.
18. Sizonenko PC: Endocrinology in preadolescents and adolescents, I: hormonal changes during normal puberty. Am J Dis Child. 1978;132:704-712.
19. Haffner SM, Klein R, Dunn JF, et al: Increased testosterone in type I diabetic subjects with severe retinopathy. Ophthalmology. 1990;97:1270-1274.
20. DCCT Research Group; Diabetes Control and Complications Trial (DCCT): results of feasibility study. Diabetes Care. 1987;10:1-19.
21. Diabetes Control and Complications Trial Research Group The effect of intensive treatment of diabetes on the development and progression of long-term complications in insulin-dependent diabetes mellitus. N Engl J Med. 1993;329:977-986.
22. Buzney SM. Weiter JJ: Pathogenesis of diabetic retinal angiopathy: proposed mechanisms and current research. International Ophthalmology Clinics. 1984;24(4):1-12.
23. Greene DA, Lattimer SA, Sima AA: Sorbitol, phosphoinositides, and sodium-potassium-ATPase in the pathogenesis of diabetic complications. N Engl J Med. 1987;316:599-606.
24. Brownlee M: Glycation and diabetic complications. (Lilly Lecture 1993) Diabetes. 1994;43:836-841.
25. Koya D, King GL: Protein kinase C activation and the development of diabetic complications. Diabetes. 1998;47:859-866.
26. Aiello LP, Avery RL, Arrigg Pg, et al: Vascular endothelial growth factor in ocular fluid of patients with diabetic retinopathy and other retinal disorders. N Engl J Med. 1994;331:1480-1487.

27. Early Treatment diabetic Retinopathy Study Research Group. Early photocoagulation for diabetic retinopathy. ETDRS Report 9. Ophthalmology. 1991;98:766-785.

28. Diabetic Retinopathy Study Research Group. Four risk factors for severe visual loss in diabetic retinopathy: DRS Report 3. Arch Ophthalmol. 1979;97:654-655.

29. Blach RK. Whitelocke RA. Hamilton AM: The diabetic maculopathies. Developments in Ophthalmology. 1981;2:243-7.

30. Diabetic Retinopathy Study Research Group. Photocoagulation treatment of proliferative diabetic retinopathy: clinical application of diabetic retinopathy study (DRS) findings. DRS Report 8. Ophthalmology. 198;88;583-600.

31. Early Treatment Diabetic Retinopathy Study Research Group. Photocoagulation for diabetic macular edema. Arch Ophthalmol. 1985;103:1796-1806.

32. Eller AW: Diagnosis and management of vitreous hemorrhage. Focal Points. San Francisco: American Academy of Ophthalmology; 2000;28(10):1-14.

33. Benson WE, Brown GC, Tasman W: Diabetes and Its Ocular Complications. Philadelphia: WB Saunders Co; 1988:27-34.

34. Klein BE, Klein R, Moss SE: Prevalence of cataracts in a population based study of persons with diabetes mellitus. Ophthalmology. 1985;92:1191-1196.

35. Appen RE, Chandra SR, Klein R, Myers FL: Diabetic papillopathy. Am J Ophthalmol. 1980;90:203-209.

36. Diabetes Control and Complications Trial Research Group: Early worsening of diabetic retinopathy in the Diabetes Control and Complications Trial. Arch Ophthalmol. 1998;116:874-886.

37. Ferris FL: How effective are treatments for diabetic retinopathy? JAMA. 1993;269:1290-1291.

38. Preferred Practice Pattern: Diabetic Retinopathy. San Francisco: American Academy of Ophthalmology; 1998:11.

CHAPTER 20
DERMATOLOGICAL ISSUES IN A CHILD WITH DIABETES MELLITUS

Pearl C. Kwong MD, PhD
Department of Dermatology
Nemours Children's Clinic, Jacksonville, Fl

INTRODUCTION

It is now a well-recognized fact that diabetes mellitus (DM) is associated with cutaneous manifestations[1-4]. Cutaneous manifestations in DM are estimated to occur at a frequency of at least 30 % to 70 %, but with increasing awareness of the various cutaneous manifestations of DM, it may even approach almost 100%[4]. The spectrum of skin diseases in DM are numerous and diverse. These conditions can range from benign conditions to life threatening conditions with bad consequences. Some are pathognomonic for DM; yet some are weakly associated with diabetes. Others are a result of the complications or treatment of DM. Sometimes the skin condition may precede the diagnosis of DM, but most often appear after the diagnosis of DM. Regardless of all of these, it is important for the clinician to recognize the cutaneous manifestations of DM so that treatment and /or prevention can be instituted appropriately. This chapter will address the dermatological issues that can present in a child with diabetes. Table 1 is an outline of the major skin disorders associated with DM in children and adolescents.

Table 1. Skin Manifestations Associated with Childhood Diabetes

- Skin disorders directly associated with DM
  - Limited joint mobility and waxy skin syndrome
  - Necrobiosis lipoidica diabeticorum
- Skin disorders secondary to metabolic derangements of DM
  - Infections – Bacterial and fungal
  - Eruptive xanthomas
- Skin disorders occurring at a higher frequency but not specific for DM
  - Diabetic dermopathy
  - Granuloma annulare

Skin disorders related to complications of DM
- Microangiopathy
- Neuropathy

Skin disorder related to secondary diabetes
- Acanthosis Nigricans

Skin disorders associated with insulin therapy
- Lipohypertrophy
- Lipoatrophy
- Insulin allergy
- Injection abscesses

LIMITED JOINT MOBILITY AND WAXY SKIN SYNDROME

Limited joint mobility (LJM) is one of the most common cutaneous manifestations associated with childhood diabetes. It occurs in about 30% of type I diabetics in the first two decades[5,6]. This syndrome has also been referred to as diabetic cheiroarthropathy[7] or digital sclerosis[8] and is has also been included in the spectrum of Dupuytren's contracture[9] and scleroderma-like syndromes[10].

Clinically, there is a painless contracture of the fingers affecting most commonly the 4th and 5th fingers. The flexion contracture can be subtle or diffuse. The skin overlying the flexion contracture is usually stiff and waxy in appearance. The presence of LJM can be demonstrated by the "prayer" test in which the patient is unable to completely extend the affected fingers when asked to oppose the fingers together as if in prayer. Sometimes one can also notice thickening of the digits with loss of dermatoglyphics. LJM is not limited to the hands. Other areas that can also be involved are the wrists, ankles, toes, elbows, knees, and cervical and thoracolumbar spines. Occasionally, LJM have been found to be associated with short stature, hepatosplenomegaly, as well as restrictive pulmonary disease[10]. Other organs including the heart and the aorta may also be involved[11,12].

Histologically, there is an increased deposition of dermal collagen but there are no observed pigmentary or atrophic changes. It is the current belief that the pathogenesis of LJM may be related to increased nonenzymatic glycosylation of the skin collagen[13].

A correlation between the occurrence of LJM and the duration or severity of DM remains controversial. Nevertheless, it is strongly recommended that DM patients with LJM should have tighter control of their blood sugars as it is believed that children with LJM are at higher risk for developing retinopathy and nephropathy[14]. Furthermore, patients with

LJM may experience improvement of their joint mobility after improved control of their blood sugars[15,1].

NECROBIOSIS LIPOIDICA DIABETICORUM

Necrobiosis lipoidica diabeticorum (NLD) can be regarded as a cutaneous marker almost specific for DM. Despite the high prevalence of DM in patients with NLD, only 0.3 % of patients with DM will have NLD lesions[16]. Sixty percent of patients with NLD were found to have DM. Another 30% have glucose intolerance or a family history of DM[17]. NLD usually follows the diagnosis of DM, but occasionally may precede the diagnosis of DM. Hemoglobin A1C can be normal in patients who develop NLD, indicating that hyperglycemia is not a prerequisite for the development of NLD[17].

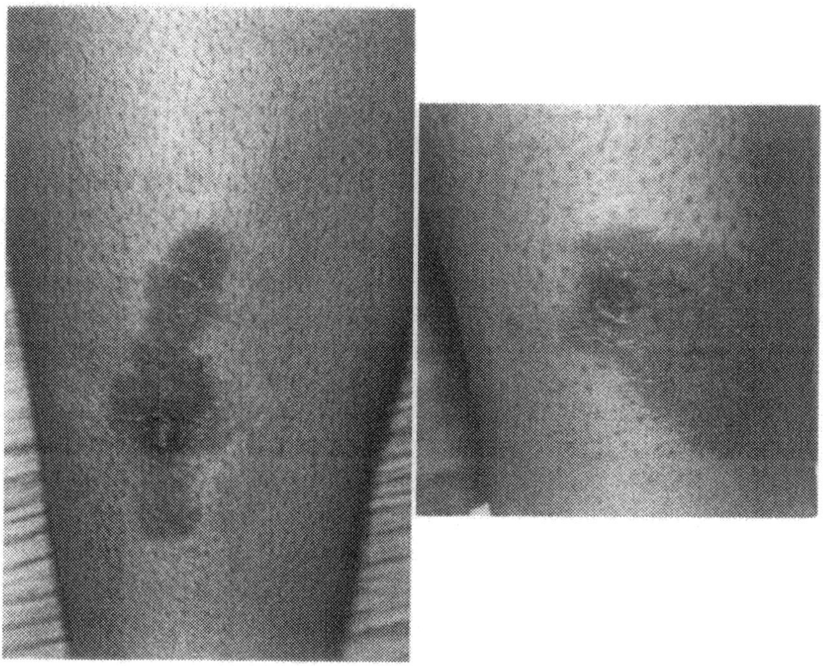

Figure 1. Necrobiosis lipoidica in a patient with a family history of diabetes. The patient was subsequently diagnosed with diabetes after the skin lesion was diagnosed. Note the atrophic shiny center and the superficial telangiectasias.

Clinically, NLD begins as a well-demarcated round plaque, which starts as a red papule, or nodule that expands with time. It is raised peripherally and is atrophic centrally. The indurated edges may be smooth, or sometimes scaly. The depressed center has a waxy yellowish to orange appearance. Superficial telangiectasias and scattered hyperkeratotic plugs are often noted. Occasionally the atrophic part can ulcerate in about 16% of patients and this is often precipitated by minor trauma[3]. The area is often slow to heal. NLD can be solitary or multiple and the sizes can vary from a few centimeters to involving the entire length of the whole anterior tibia. Besides the anterior shins, NLD had also been reported in other sites such as the upper extremities, trunk, face and scalp[17].

Histologically, the changes are generally seen in the dermis. Degenerated irregular collagen fibers are surrounded by pallisading arrangement of histiocytes and lymphocytes, as well as foreign body giant cells. There is accumulation of mucin between the collagen fibers. The histological picture resembles that of granuloma annulare and rheumatoid nodule[18].

There is no effective treatment for NLD. High potency steroids with occlusion and intralesional steroids had been tried with limited success[17]. Antiplatelet agents such as aspirin and dipyridamole did not seem to make any difference in controlled studies[19]. When ulceration occurs, prevention of infection with topical and systemic antibiotics should be considered. Conservative treatment with hydrocolloid dressings may also prove helpful in noninfected ulcers. If this fails, then surgical treatments such as grafting had been attempted with some success[20].

In general, patients with NLD should be advised to protect the lower legs from trauma. They should avoid traumatic situations such as certain sports and should wear knee length stockings and shin pads for protection.

Spontaneous remission of NLD lesions had been reported to occur in 13-19% of patients who had NLD between 1 to 34 years. However, residual scarring and atrophy still remain[21].

DIABETIC DERMOPATHY

Also called pretibial papules or shin spots, this is one of the most common cutaneous manifestations of DM seen in adults[21]. However, it is uncommonly reported in children[22]. This condition is not always specific for diabetes; it has been shown to occur in 20% of patients with normal glucose tolerance tests[23]. The genesis of diabetic dermopathy (DD) is unknown; it is believed that DD may be an exaggerated response to mechanical trauma[21]. DD can precede the diagnosis of DM and should alert the physician to look for DM in nondiagnosed diabetics. Present in about 50% of known diabetic patients, shin spots are always disregarded and overlooked by both the patients and their physicians because they are asymptomatic. Since multiple DD are found to be significantly related to microangiopathy and neuropathy[23,24], its presence in a diabetic should also prompt a search for these systemic complications.

Clinically, the lesions are multiple, well circumscribed, round to oval pink patches measuring 0.5 to 1 cm in diameter, typically bilateral and asymmetrical in distribution over the anterior tibia or lateral calf. It may also occur on the side of the foot or over bony prominences. The lesions have also been observed to evolve into atrophic hyperpigmented red brown patches with fine scales.

Histopathologically, there is epidermal atrophy with superficial perivascular lymphocytic infiltrate and associated extravasation of red blood cells with hemosiderin deposits[25,26]. Since the lesions are asymptomatic and since they typically undergo spontaneous resolution after a year or two, treatment is generally not recommended.

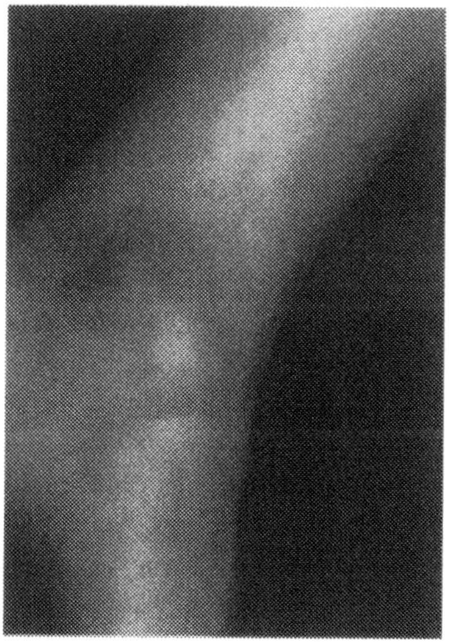

Figure 2. A typical lesion of granuloma annulare overlying a joint area. This patient was screened for diabetes and did not have diabetes.

GRANULOMA ANNULARE

Granuloma annulare (GA) is a common disorder seen in children and is poorly correlated with diabetes[27]. Clinically these patients have annular plaques, mostly involving the joint areas of the hands, elbows and knees. They can be solitary or can occur in multiple numbers. Histologically, granuloma annulare resembles NLD with localized necrobiosis of collagen with abundant mucin and infiltration with histiocytes and lymphocytes. GA lesions tend to be longstanding but their usual natural course is spontaneous regression. Patients with typical GA lesions do not need to be checked for the presence of diabetes or glucose intolerance. It is still not well established whether the disseminated form of GA is correlated with the presence of diabetes[28]. The significance of disseminated GA in children is even less as thus far, this has not been reported to be associated with DM in children[1].

INFECTIONS ASSOCIATED WITH DM

At the present time there are conflicting opinions as to whether cutaneous infections are more prevalent in the diabetic patient than in the nondiabetic population[29]. However there is consensus that cutaneous infections are more severe and harder to treat in the diabetic patient[30]. It is believed that infections are more severe in diabetics because of poor microcirculation, decreased phagocytic activity in the monocytes, decreased cell mediated immunity, diminished response to phytohemagglutinin and delayed chemotaxis[31]. The infectious lesions seen in diabetics are generally divided into fungal and bacterial infections.

Fungal Infections

Candidal infection of the mouths (oral thrush), corners of the mouth (angular cheilitis), nail folds (paronychia), nails (onychomycosis), genitals (vaginitis or balanitis), between the finger and toewebs (blastomycosis erosio interdigitalis), and flexural surfaces (intertrigo) can present frequently in the diabetic patient.

Candidal vulvovaginitis is the most common fungal infection encountered in girls with DM[32]. Candidal vulvovaginitis is always pruritic and pruritus seems to be worse when there is poor glucose control. The vulva is erythematous and excoriated. There is white curdly material seen on the labia and the introitus. Satellite lesions are rarely seen. Treatment includes topical clotrimazole. Recurrences usually occur if diabetic control is poor.

Increased concentration of glucose in the saliva accounts for the overgrowth of Candida in the mouths of DM patients. Candidal angular cheilitis is a classic common lesion seen in children with DM. This is characterized by the presence of white curdlike materials on a fissured erythematous base. Diagnosis is confirmed by performing a potassium hydroxide (KOH) preparation on the curdlike material. Sometimes the cheilitis can be accompanied by oral thrush. The treatment is usually accomplished by the use of topical nystatin suspension in addition to good glycemic control. Oral antifungals such as diflucan may be indicated for recalcitrant lesions[33].

Candida paronychia commonly involves the proximal nailfolds. It starts as erythema, swelling and separation of the nailfold from the lateral margin of the nail. Occasionally, pus can be expressed from the site of involvement. Sometimes the purulent drainage is misdiagnosed as a primary bacterial infection and as a result, antibiotics are instituted. However, this could worsen the condition. It is important to confirm the presence of both the candida and bacterial infection by performing both potassium hydroxide (KOH) and gram stain preparations. Usually, treatment can be accomplished by the use of clotrimazole or miconazole, applied twice daily. Treatment includes keeping the hands, draining the abscesses, application of topical antifungals and maintenance of good glycemic control. Although it can be easily treated, recurrences can be common, especially if glycemic control is poor.

Infections of the interdigital web spaces are less common, occurring more commonly between the third and fourth fingers. Intertriginous candida often responds to antifungal creams and drying.

The incidence of dermatophyte infections of the toenails and toewebs are not reported to be higher in patients with DM[34]. However, if these infections do occur in a patient with DM, they may cause inflammation and fissuring which could serve as a portal of entry for bacterial infection. When detected in patients in DM, management with oral antifungals is recommended.

In debilitated patients with diabetic ketoacidosis, opportunistic deep mycotic infections such as mucormycosis can occur. The predisposition is not related to the duration of the diabetes, but rather secondary to poor glycemic control[29]. Overwhelming fatal mucormycosis had been reported in patients following trauma[35], surgery, burns or even dental extractions[36,37].

Clinically, a black eschar with pus can be seen in the nasal turbinates, nasal septum or palate, with infection extending into the maxillary and ethmoid sinuses. Palatal ulcers can be present. When they are present, they are large ranging from 3 to 5 cm in size and often covered with cheesy brownish substance. The breath is foul. Nodules can occur beneath the eyes. Cerebral involvement may occur in about two thirds of the cases[29].

Pansinusitis and cavernous sinus as well as lateral sinus thrombosis are common complications.

The diagnosis of mucormycosis requires a biopsy, which documents the presence of non-septate branching hyphae with H and E stains. The tissue should also be cultured in Saboraud agar. Therapy includes aggressive debridement of all necrotic tissues, intravenous amphotericin, correction of acidosis and hyperglycemia. Severe infection extending to the sinuses can lead to disfiguring perforating consequences and can be fatal.

Bacterial Infections

Recurrent staphylococcal furunculosis and/or folliculitis are common in patients with DM[38]. Chronic or intermittent systemic antibiotics in conjunction with antibacterial cleansers and intranasal topical antibiotics is the usual mode of treatment.

Although rare, malignant otitis externa secondary to *Pseudomonas* is a severe potentially fatal infection reported in diabetic children[39]. The patient presents with pain and discharge. Polypoid granulation tissue can be seen in the external ear canal. Extension of the infection can lead to mastoiditis, 7th to 12th cranial nerve involvement and even meningitis[40]. Topical therapy is not adequate. Intravenous antipseudomonas drugs are the treatment of choice. Sometimes surgical debridement and mastoidectomy may be required in severe cases.

Periodontal disease is also seen commonly in children with DM. Abscesses with gingivitis require prompt attention[41]. Regular dental hygiene and check ups should be maintained in children with diabetes.

Erythrasma is seen uncommonly in children, but is reported more commonly in adults with DM[42]. This seems to occur more in obese individuals. Scaly red plaques can be seen in intertriginous areas. These lesions exhibit a coral red fluorescence when viewed with a Wood's lamp. The lesions are caused by *Corynebacterium Minutissimum.* Topical erythromycin is effective. If left untreated, the lesions can fissure and can be a portal of entry for other potentially pathogenic organisms. This condition should not be confused with candidal intertrigo, which was discussed under the fungal infection section.

Necrotizing soft tissue deep infections and fasciitis are rarely seen in children[1].

ERUPTIVE XANTHOMAS

Poor glycemic control may result in elevation of circulating concentrations of triglycerides[1]. The hypertriglyceridemia may result in the sudden eruption of diffuse xanthomatous lesions. These lesions appear as crops of discrete papules or nodules with yellow waxy centers on an erythematous base. The lesions develop rapidly over the buttocks, elbows and knee and are often pruritic and painful. These lesions resolve upon resolution of the hypertriglyceridemia.

ACANTHOSIS NIGRICANS

Acanthosis nigricans (AN) has long been well recognized to be correlated with insulin resistance and an indicator of high risk for DM[43, 44]. In syndromes associated with insulin resistance, it is believed that the primary abnormalities may lie in the insulin receptor or the post receptor apparatus. This results in excessive circulating insulin which can stimulate the receptors for insulin-like growth factors[45]. The development of AN is believed to be mediated through the stimulation of these receptors.

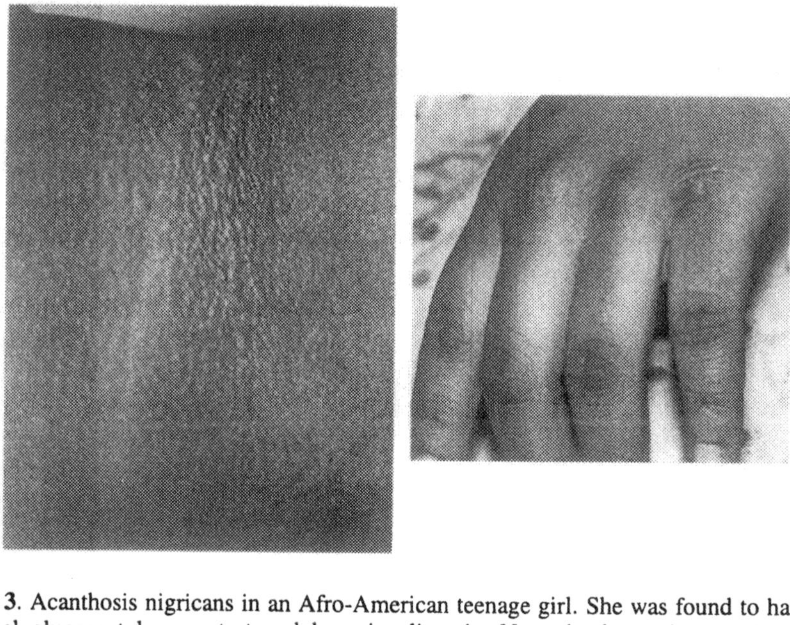

Figure 3. Acanthosis nigricans in an Afro-American teenage girl. She was found to have an abnormal glucose tolerance test and hyperinsulinemia. Note the hyperpigmented velvety plaques over the neck and the dorsum of the hand and fingers.

Kahn[43] had defined two broad categories of insulin resistant syndromes. Type A syndrome occurs in girls 8 to 16 years of age with severe insulin resistance, fasting hyperglycemia and ovarian dysfunction.

These patients are not obese. There may be associated virilizing symptoms such as hirsutism, clitoromegaly and amenorrhea. There are associated skin tags and accelerated early growth. Most of the physical findings may be related to ovarian hyperandrogenism such as acne, hirsutism, male pattern hair loss and muscular hypertrophy. Type B syndromes occur in the 12-60 yr old females and occasionally males. Anti-insulin receptor antibodies are responsible for the insulin resistance. It is frequently associated with systemic lupus erythematosus, Sjogren's syndrome, ataxia telangiectasia, immune complex nephritis, and rheumatoid arthritis. Associated arthralgias, vitiligo, alopecia, mumps-like parotid pain and enlargement are common. These patients can also present with some symptoms associated with polycystic ovarian syndrome.

Other genetic syndromes associated with insulin resistance such as Donovan's (Leprechaunism) syndrome[46] and congenital localized or generalized lipodystrophy[47] may also have dermatological manifestations. In leprechaunism, the patients have elfin facies and are small for gestational age, with diminished subcutaneous fat, hypertrichosis, pachyderma and acanthosis nigricans. Their genitals appear enlarged. The lips are thick and the gingiva hypertrophied. The skin is dry, hyperpigmented and wrinkled.

Partial upper body or total loss of subcutaneous fat, hepatomegaly, apparent genital enlargement and acanthosis nigricans characterizes the syndrome of lipoatrophic diabetes or congenital generalized lipodystrophy. These syndromes are described in detail in the Chapter on Lipoatrophy and Lipodystrophy Syndromes.

AN does not always have to be associated with insulin resistance[48]. Obesity per se without significant insulin resistance has been highly associated with AN. AN have also been reported in patients with other endocrinopathies such as Cushings, acromegaly, Addison's disease, congenital adrenal hyperplasia, hypothyroidism and hyperandrogenic syndromes with or without obesity. Malignancies associated with AN had been reported in adults, but not in children[1].

MICROANGIOPATHY AND NEUROPATHY

Complications related to microangiopathy and neuropathy are usually not seen in the prepubertal child with diabetes and are rare in patients within five years of the diagnosis of DM[1,49]. Skin changes in the feet such as coolness, mottling, atrophy and loss of hair over the toes and shins are uncommon manifestations. Dystrophic thickened nails due to lack of blood flow is not usually observed in children.

Poor healing of traumatic skin lesions may be the result of vascular insufficiency and neuropathy. Occasionally, these are seen in the older adolescent. Although severe motor and sensory neuropathies are rarely seen in the young diabetics, it is not too early to recommend that all patients with DM should be instructed to test the temperature of the water before immersing their extremities in heated water.

Gangrene and mal perforans, a circular punched out lesion associated with foot calluses is complications of neuropathy rarely seen in the pediatric diabetic population.

Although foot problems are rare in children, foot skin care should be stressed from the start, with meticulous hygiene, straight cutting of the nails, emollients for dry feet and early detection and treatment of fungal and bacterial infections, to prevent the progression to severe systemic infections.

SKIN LESIONS RELATED TO THERAPY OF DIABETES

Insulin Allergy

Insulin allergy can be local or systemic. The reaction can be immediate or delayed. There may be burning, stinging, or pruritus at the site of injection. Sometimes the site can be warm, red and indurated. There is usually a strong personal or family history of allergy. Systemic reactions such as serum sickness, angiodedema, urticaria or anaphylaxis are rare[50]. They usually occur two to three weeks after the reintroduction of insulin. The reactions may be related to the impurities of the insulin preparations, zinc additive, and the use of animal insulin or to the protamine. Insulin resistance and insulin allergy may coexist in 25 to 35% of the patients[51]. IgE is elevated in the allergic state and IgG is elevated in the resistant state[52]. Diagnosis of insulin allergy is confirmed by the presence of anti-insulin IgE antibody. Intradermal injections of insulin give a positive reaction. The newer monocomponent porcine insulins and purified human insulins have made these side effects very rare with an incidence of 0.1- 0.2%[4].

Insulin Lipohypertrophy and Lipoatrophy

Lipohypertrophy rather than lipoatrophy is more common in children[1,53]. The lesions of lipohypertrophy resemble lipomas. They are firm, tender and skin colored nodules with ill-defined borders, usually seen under the needle marks of the insulin injection sites. Histologically, these regions consist of fat and fibrous tissues. These lesions are believed to be the result of lipogenic effects of insulin that is chronically injected at the same site. Lesions resolve by avoiding these areas as injection sites and rotating the injection sites.

Lipoatrophy on the other hand occur at sites remote from the injection sites such as the face, neck and chest[54]. This is reported to be more common in females than males. They are seen as depressed but not hyperpigmented areas. This can occur in about 25% of patients after 6 months to two years of insulin use. The cause is unknown; it may be due to a local immune response to injected insulin. The incidence is noted to be decreasing and this may be attributed to the use of more purified forms of insulin[55].

Insulin Abscesses

Poor sterile technique of injection can lead to infected abscesses[4]. These abscesses can be solitary or generalized. They can be identified by ultrasound or gallium scans. The infecting organisms are usually Staphylococcus and Streptococcus. These nodules are usually warm, tender and erythematous, beginning as firm lesions and progressing to being fluctuant. Abscesses may also complicate continuous subcutaneous insulin infusions delivered by insulin pumps.

SUMMARY AND CONCLUSIONS

The skin is one of the major organs affected in children and adolescents with DM. The myriad dermatological manifestations of DM range from benign lesions to lesions that are potentially life threatening. Hence it is important for the clinician to be cognizant of these manifestations of DM and to incorporate this knowledge into the schema for evaluation and management of children and adolescents with DM.

REFERENCES

1. Edidin, D.V. Cutaneous manifestations of diabetes mellitus in children. Pediatr Dermatol 1985; 2, 161-179.
2. Jelinek, J.E. Cutaneous manifestations of diabetes mellitus. Int J Derm 1994; 33, 605-617.
3. Perez, M.I., and Kohn, S.R. Cutaneous manifestations of diabetes mellitus. J Am Acad Dermatol 1994; 30, 519-529.
4. Sibbald, R.G., Landolt, S.J., and Toth, D. Skin and Diabetes. Endocrino Metab Clin North Am 1996; 25, 463-472.

5. Rosenbloom, A.L., and Frias, J.L. Diabetes, short stature and joint stiffness – a new syndrome. Clin Res 1974; 22, 92A.
6. Starkman, H. , and Brink, S. Limited joint mobility of the hand in type I diabetes mellitus. Diabetes Care 1982; 5, 534-536.
7. Grgic, A., Rosenbloom, A.L., Weber, F.T., Giordano, B., Malone, J.I., and Shuster, J.J. Joint contracture-common manifestation of childhood diabetes mellitus. J Pediatr 1976; 88, 584-588.
8. Seibold, J.R. Digital sclerosis in children with insulin dependent diabetes mellitus. Arthritis Rheum 1982; 25, 1357-1361.
9. Heathcote, J.G., Cohen, H., and Noble, J. Dupuytren's disease and diabetes mellitus. Lancet 1981; 1; 1420.
10. Buckingham, B.A., Uitto, J., Sandborg, C., Keens, T. , Kaugman, F., and Landing, B. Scleroderma-like syndrome and the non-enzymatic glycosylation of collagen in children with poorly controlled insulin-dependent diabetes (IDDM). Pediatr Res 1981; 15, 626.
11. Friedman, N.E., Levitsky, L.L., Edidin, D.V., Vitullo, D.A., Lascina, J.J., and Chiemming-Kottip, P. Echocardiographic evidence for impaired myocardial performance in children with type I diabetes mellitus. Am J. Med 1982; 173, 846-850.
12. Savin, J.A. Bacterial infections in diabetes mellitus. Br J Dermatol 1974; 91, 481-487.
13. Lyons, T.J., and Kennedy, L. Non-enzymatic glycosylation of skin collagen in patients with type I (insulin-dependent) diabetes mellitus and limited joint mobility. Diabetologia 1985; 28(2-5).
14. Rosenbloom, A.L., Silverstein, J.H., Lezotte, D.C., Richardson, K., and McCallum, M. Limited joint mobility in childhood diabetes mellitus indicates increased risk for microvascular disease. N Engl J Med 1981; 305, 191-194.
15. Lieberman, L.A., Rosenbloom, A.L., Riley, W.J., and Silverstein, J.H. Correlated changes in skin thickness and glycosylated hemoglobin with pump administration of insulin. Clin Res 1980; 28, 866A.
16. Muller, S.A., and Winkelmann, R.K. Necrobiosis lipoidica diabeticorum. Results of glucose tolerance tests in nondiabetic patients. JAMA 1961; 119; 139-142.
17. Lowitt, M.H., and Dover, J.S. Necrobiosis lipoidica. J Am Acad Dermatol 1991; 25, 735-748.
18. Boulton, A.J.M., Cutfield, R.G., Abouganem, D. et al. Necrobiosis lipoidica diabeticorum: A clinicopathologic study. J Am Acad Dermatol 1988; 18, 530-537.

19. Stratham, B., Finlay, A.Y., and Marks, R. A randomized double-blind comparison of aspirin-dipyramidole combination vs placebo in the treatment of necrobiosis lipoidica. Acta Dermatol Venereol 1981; 61; 270-271.
20. Dubin, B.J., and Kaplan, E.N. The surgical treatment of necrobiosis lipoidica diabeticorum. Plast Reconstr Surg 1977; 60, 421-427.
21. Huntley, A.C. The cutaneous manifestations of diabetes mellitus. J Am Acad Dermatol 1982; 7, 427-455.
22 Boyd, S.G., Innes, S.M., and Campbell, I.W. Skin manifestations of diabetes mellitus. Practitioner 1982; 226, 253-264.
23 Binkley, G.W. Dermopathy in diabetes mellitus. Arch Dermatol 1965; 92, 106-107.
24. Danowski, T.S., Sabeh, G., Sarver, M.E., Shelkrot, J. and Fisher, E.R. Shin spots and diabetes mellitus. Am J Med Sci 1966; 251, 570-575.
25. Binkley, G.W., Giraldo, B., and Stoughton, K.B. Diabetic dermopathy – A clinical study. Cutis 1967; 3, 955-958.
26. Fisher, E.R., and Danowski, T.S. Histologic histochemical and electron microscopic features of the shin spots of diabetes mellitus. Am J Clin Path 1968; 50, 547-554.
27. Haim, S., Friedman-Birnbaum, R., Shafir, A. Generalized granuloma annulare:relationshipto diabetes mellitus as revealed in 8 cases. Br J Dermatol 1970; 83, 302-305.
28. Dicken, C.H., Carrington, S.G., and Winkelmann, R.K. Generalized granuloma annulare. Arch Dermatol 1969; 99, 556-563.
29. Edwards, J.E., Tillman, D.B., Miller, M.E. et al. Infection and diabetes mellitus. West J Med 1979; 130, 515-521.
30. Kimmerly, S.A. Dermatologic manifestations of infections in diabetics. Infect Dis Clin of North Am 1994; 8, 523-532.
31. Moutschen, M.P., Scheen, A.J., and Lefevre, P.J. Impaired immune responses in diabetes mellitus: analysis of the factors and mechanisms involved. Relevance to the increased susceptibility of diabetic patients to specific infections. Diabet Metab 1992; 18, 187-201.
32. Sonck, C.E., and Somersalo, O. The yeast flora of the anogenital region in diabetic girls. Arch Dermatol 1963; 88, 846-852.
33. Knight, L., and Fletcher, J. Growth of candida albicans in saliva: Stimulation by glucose associated with antibiotics, corticosteroids, and diabetes mellitus. J Infect Dis 1971; 123, 371-377.
34. Alteras, I., and Saryt, E. Prevalence of pathogenic fungi in the toewebs and toenails of diabetic patients. Mycopathologia 1979; 67, 157-159.

35. Ryan-Poirier, K., Eiseman, R.M., Beaty, J.H., Hunt, P.G., Burghen, G.A., and Leggidro, R.J. Post-traumatic cutaneous mucormycosis in diabetes mellitus. Clin Pediatr 1988; 27, 609-612.
36. Tomford, J.W., Whittlesey, D., Ellner, J.J., Tomashefski, J.F. Invasive primary cutaneous phycomycosis in diabetic leg ulcers. Arch Surg 1980; 115, 770-771.
37. Limongelli, W.A., Clark, M.S., Jaglimbene, R., Baden, E., Washington, J.A., and Williams, A.C. Successful treatment of mucocutaneous mucormycosis after dental extraction in a patient with uncontrolled diabetes. J Oral Surg 1975; 33, 705-712.
38. Lipsky, B.A., Pecoraro, R.E., Chen, M.S. et al. Factors affecting staphylococcal colonization among NIDDM outpatients. Diabetes Care 1987; 10, 483-486.
39. Merritt, W.T., Bass, J.W., and Bruhn, F.W. Malignant external otitis in an adolescent with diabetes. J Pediatr 1980; 96, 872-873.
40. Joachims, H.Z. Malignant external otitis in children. Arch Otolaryngol 1976; 102, 236-237.
41. Haroon, T.S. Diabetes and skin – a review. Scot Med J 1974; 19, 257-267.
42. Montes, L.F., Dobson, H., Dodge, B.G., and Knowles, W.R. Erythrasma and diabetes mellitus. Arch Dermatol 1969; 99, 674-680.
43. Kahn, C.R. The syndromes of insulin resistance and acanthosis nigricans: insulin receptor disorders in man. N Engl J Med 1976; 294, 736-745.
44. Stuart, C.A., Smith, M.M., Gilkison, C.R., Shaheb, S., and Stahn, R.M. Acanthosis Nigricans among native americans: an indicator of high diabetes risk. Am J Public Health 1994; 84, 1839-1842.
45. Cruz, P.D. Excess insulin binding to insulin-like growth factor receptors: Proposed mechanism for acanthosis nigricans. J Invest Dermatol 1992; 98 (suppl), 82S-85S.
46. Rosenberg, A.M., Haworth, J.C., Degroot, G.W., Trevenen, C.L., and Rechler, M.M. A case if leprechaunism with severe hyperinsulinemia. Am J Dis Child 1980; 134, 170-175.
47. Lawrence, R.D. Lipodystrophy and hepatosplenomegaly with diabetes, lipaemia, and other metabolic disturbances. A case throwing new light on the action of insulin. Lancet 1946; 1, 724-731.
48. Hogan, P.A. "Cutaneous manifestations of endocrine diseases". In Textbook of Pediatric Dermatology, Harper, J., Oranje, A., Prose, N., eds. Malden, MA: Blackwell Science, Inc., 2000.

49. Torigoe, K., Numata, O., Yazaki, S., Hasegawa, S., Boku, N., Hiura, M., Ino, H., and Matsunaga, M. Sympathetic skin response in diabetic children: Do diabetic children have diabetic neuropathy? Pediatrics international 1999; 41, 631-636.
50. Palcy, R.G., and Turnbridge, R.E. Dermal reaction in insulin therapy. Diabetes 1952; 1, 22-27.
51. Kahn, C.R., and Rosenthal, A.S. Immunologic reactions to insulin, insulin allergy, insulin resistance and the autoimmune insulin syndrome. Diabetes Care 1979; 2, 283-295.
52. Patterson, R,, Mellies, C.J., and Roberts, M. Immunologic reactions against insulin. II. IgE anti-insulin, insulin allergy and combined IgE and IgG immunologic insulin resistance. J Immunol 1973; 110, 1135-1145.
53. Johnson, D.A. , and Parlette, H.Z. Insulin-induced hypertrophic lipodystrophy. Cutis 1983; 32, 273-275.
54. Reeves, W.G., Allen, B.R., and Tattersall, R.B. Insulin induced lipoatrophy: evidence for an immune pathogenesis. Br Med J 1980; 280, 1500-1503.
55. Wright, A.D., Walsh, C.H., Fitzgerald, M.G., et al. Very pure porcine insulin in clinical practice. BMJ 1979; 1, 25-27.

Chapter 21
PSYCHOLOGICAL ISSUES IN CHILDHOOD DIABETES MELLITUS

Alan M. Delamater, Ph.D.
University of Miami School of Medicine, Department of Pediatrics

Diabetes imposes considerable demands on children and their families. As they are coping with normal developmental challenges, the additional burden of diabetes may be difficult for many children and families to deal with effectively. Especially challenging may be the demands of intensive management. With children as patients, families play a significant role in diabetes management, and are instrumental in the implementation of interventions. The quality of life of all family members is potentially affected by diabetes.

The chapter provides a summary of key findings from the behavioral science literature focusing on psychological, social, and behavioral issues in children with type 1 diabetes. The review considers specific issues such as psychosocial adjustment and psychiatric disorders, stress and coping, family functioning, sociodemographic factors, neurocognitive functioning, quality of life, and psychosocial and behavioral interventions. Implications for clinical practice will also be discussed.

Psychosocial and Behavioral Factors

A considerable literature exists on psychosocial and behavioral factors related to diabetes management in children and adolescents[1,2]. While most of this research has focused on the relationship of behavioral and psychosocial factors to diabetes-related outcomes such as regimen adherence and metabolic control, some studies have specifically focused on the impact of diabetes on behavioral and psychosocial functioning. This section will highlight some of the most important findings related to psychosocial functioning.

PSYCHOLOGICAL ADJUSTMENT

Adjustment after Diagnosis.

The diagnosis of diabetes poses considerable challenges and stress for children and families. Several longitudinal studies have been conducted.

Kovacs and colleagues[3] found 36% of newly diagnosed children had diagnosable psychiatric disorders soon after diabetes onset, most commonly being adjustment disorders. However, the majority of these cases had resolved within the first year after diagnosis. Jacobson and colleagues[4] also investigated the psychosocial outcomes of children with newly diagnosed diabetes. Evaluations conducted within the first five months after diagnosis showed no differences between the group of diabetic children and a medical control group on a variety of behavioral and psychological measures, with the exception of decreased school-related competence in children with diabetes. In a more recent study, Grey and colleagues[5] found that mild adjustment problems had dissipated by the end of the first year, but some problems reappeared by the end of the second year. While the majority of children's adjustment problems appear to resolve within the first year, children who do not may be at risk for poor adaptation to diabetes, including regimen adherence problems, poor metabolic control, and continued psychosocial difficulties[5-7].

Long-term Adjustment

Earlier studies comparing children with established diabetes to other groups on psychological variables generally did not reveal significant differences[2], although one report found boys with later onset of diabetes to have more behavioral problems[8]. However, more recent findings indicate that children with diabetes, like children with various chronic diseases, may be at increased risk for psychological problems[9]. Blanz, Rensch-Riemann, Fritz-Sigmund, & Schmidt[10] found that one-third of their sample of 93 diabetic adolescents had psychiatric disorders (mostly internalizing symptoms), compared with 10% of the subjects in a control group. In a ten-year follow-up study of newly diagnosed youth, Kovacs and colleagues[11] found that nearly half of the study sample had a psychiatric diagnosis, the most frequent being major depression, conduct disorder, and generalized anxiety disorder. In another 10-year follow-up study of newly-diagnosed children and adolescents, Jacobson and colleagues[12] found that as young adults, patients reported lower self-esteem relative to control participants. As shown in a study by Wysocki, Hough, Ward, & Green[13], poorer adjustment to diabetes during adolescence may persist into early adulthood. In a recent longitudinal study of 76 adolescents, Bryden et al.[14] found that patients with behavioral problems during their teen years had significantly poorer glycemic control as young adults.

Psychological factors have been related to glycemic control within samples of children with diabetes. For example, Anderson et al.[15] found that youths in poor glycemic control had increased anxiety and lower self-concept. La Greca et al.[16] found that girls were more likely than boys to be depressed, and that depression was associated with poorer glycemic control.

Eating Disorders

There is also evidence that diabetic youths, particularly females, are at increased risk for eating disorders, and that eating disorders are associated with poor metabolic control[17]. Both eating disorders and sub-clinically disordered eating attitudes and behaviors (e.g., severe dietary indiscretion and repeated insulin omissions) have been observed in adolescent girls with diabetes, and have been associated with worse metabolic control[18-20]. At least 10% of adolescent girls with type 1 diabetes may meet diagnostic criteria for an eating disorder, a rate twice as common as in girls without diabetes[19]. Without intervention, disordered eating and insulin manipulation may worsen over time and increase the risk of health complications[21]. Results from recent studies suggest that disordered eating in girls with diabetes is associated with problems in the mother-daughter relationship[22] and less perceived control[23]. Although not all studies have found increased rates of diagnosable eating disorders in samples of adolescent with diabetes, it is clear that with increasing numbers of symptoms of eating disorder, glycemic control worsens[24,25].

Stress and Coping

Research findings have shown that children with high life stress tend to have worse metabolic control[26-28]. Studies of attributional and coping styles suggest youths in poor metabolic control are more likely to use the learned helplessness style[29] and engage in avoidance and wishful thinking in response to stress[30], while youths in good metabolic control have high levels of self-efficacy[31]. Maladaptive coping has also been associated with poor regimen adherence[32].

Specific health beliefs related to the serious of diabetes, personal vulnerability to complications, costs of regimen adherence, and beliefs in the efficacy of treatment, have also been associated with both regimen adherence and glycemic control in studies of adolescents[33-35]. In another study of adolescents, Skinner and Hampson[36] showed that personal models of diabetes, i.e., specific illness beliefs, were associated with psychological adjustment and regimen adherence. These investigators found that greater impact of diabetes was related to increased anxiety, while beliefs about the effectiveness of treatment predicted better dietary self care. In a large study of adolescents and young adults, Skinner et al.[37] recently found that personal model beliefs about diabetes mediated the relationship between personality variables (emotional stability and conscientiousness) and self care behaviors. Studies with younger children have also shown the importance of health beliefs in diabetes management. Charron-Prochownick et al.[30] found that beliefs regarding barriers and self efficacy were related with adherence, and beliefs regarding severity of diabetes were related to glycemic control.

Family Functioning

Research findings have shown that families of youths in poor metabolic control have more conflict and financial problems, and less cohesion and stability than those of youths in good metabolic control[15,26]. Improved levels of metabolic control have been associated with better family communication and conflict resolution skills[39], agreement about family responsibilities and appropriate involvement in diabetes management tasks[40,41] and more structured and controlling family environments[42]. Clinical studies of adolescents selected for chronically poor metabolic control have revealed significant family dysfunction for the majority of families[43,44].

There is also evidence that family relations are linked with regimen adherence. Adherence levels of youths have been associated with both general and regimen-specific family support[45,46] as well as communication skills[47] and conflict[48]. A recent study of parenting styles in relation to regimen adherence of young children with diabetes found that parental warmth was predictive of better adherence[49]. While youths receive instrumental support from their families, they also receive considerable emotional support from their friends[46].

Studies indicate that many mothers of newly diagnosed children are at risk for psychological adjustment problems, with clinically significant depression noted in approximately one-third of mothers; however, most of these adjustment problems are resolved within the first year after the child's diagnosis[50]. Few studies have addressed the role of fathers in diabetes management. A recent study by Landolt et al.[51] found 24% of mothers and 22% of fathers met diagnostic criteria for post-traumatic stress disorder six weeks after their child had been diagnosed with diabetes. Other recent studies indicate that fathers have relatively little involvement in diabetes management tasks[52], and suggests that psychological maladjustment of fathers predicts poor glycemic control in children five years after diagnosis[53].

Sociodemographic Factors

Research has shown that regimen adherence declines over time, and is especially poor among some adolescents[54,55]. Studies also indicate that metabolic control tends to be worse in children from single-parent families, both in the United States[56,57], and in studies from Sweden[58]. The role of ethnicity has also been examined in relation to regimen adherence and metabolic control. Studies have consistently shown that African American youths exhibit poorer metabolic control than Caucasian youths[59-61]. Such findings may be explained in part by the greater prevalence of single parent families and lower adherence to diet and glucose testing among African Americans[59].

Neurocognitive Functioning

A number of studies have examined neurocognitive functioning in children with diabetes. Children with early onset of diabetes and a history of hypoglycemic episodes have been shown to have significantly poorer cognitive performance, particularly for visual-spatial functioning[62,63]. Other research findings suggest that children who develop diabetes early in life may be at increased risk for later neurocognitive deficits, both verbal and visual-spatial[64,65]. Ryan, Longstreet, & Morrow[66] found that children with diabetes missed twice as much school as their peers who did not have diabetes, and lower reading achievement was associated with more school absences. A study by Holmes et al.[67] found diabetic youths were more likely to have learning problems, with such problems more likely among boys than girls: 40% of boys and 16% of girls had learning problems. Rovet and Alvarez[68] found poorer attentional functioning and lower verbal intelligence in diabetic children and adolescents, which was related to history of hypoglycemic seizures. However, a recent study found no differences in processing speed between diabetic and control children.

In a neuropsychological study of newly diagnosed children, Kovacs, Goldston, and Iyengar[69] found that verbal intelligence and school grades were average shortly after diagnosis, but declined significantly over time. This decline in verbal skill was predicted in part by memory dysfunction[70]. In a recent prospective study of newly-diagnosed children, mild neuropsychological deficits were observed two years after diagnosis, with reduced speed of information processing and decrements in conceptual reasoning and acquisition of new knowledge[71]. Predictors of these changes in neurocognitive function included onset of diabetes prior to age four years, related to poorer visuospatial functioning, and both recurrent severe hypoglycemia and hyperglycemia, related to decreased memory and learning capacity[72]. These same investigators evaluated neuropsychological functioning six years after diagnosis and found that, compared to controls, children with diabetes performed more poorly on various measures of intelligence, attention, processing speed, and long-term memory. Children diagnosed before age four years showed weaknesses in attention, processing speed, and executive functioning, while those with recurrent severe hypoglycemia had lower intellectual abilities[73].

Quality of Life

Diabetes management imposes considerable demands that may potentially interfere with children's ability to negotiate important developmental tasks and achieve good psychosocial adjustment. This is especially the case in the post-DCCT era when the expectation is to initiate intensive insulin regimens in order to attain and maintain optimal levels of glycemic control and reduce the risk of later health complications[74]. Diabetes-related quality of life (DQOL) refers to those aspects of child and adolescent functioning that are directly affected by diabetes and its treatment. This construct includes disease state and physical symptoms, functional status, psychological functioning, and social functioning[75].

The first study to report on DQOL in youths was done by Ingersoll and Marrero[76]. These investigators modified the QOL measure used in the DCCT so that it would be better suited for use by youths. The demographic and clinical correlates of DQOL were evaluated in a study of 74 children and adolescents from culturally and socially diverse backgrounds. Age was not associated with DQOL, but shorter diabetes duration was associated with greater disease impact. Girls reported more disease worries than boys. None of the DQOL scales was related with glycemic control as measured by glycohemoglobin.

Several recent studies have examined DQOL using the measure developed by Ingersoll and Marrero[76]. Grey and colleagues[77] studied the personal and family correlates of DQOL in 52 adolescents, primarily a Caucasian sample from middle to upper socioeconomic status. Youths who reported greater disease impact and less satisfaction felt that diabetes was more upsetting and diabetes management was more difficult. Similarly, those who reported more disease-related worries felt that diabetes was more upsetting and diabetes management more difficult. Additionally, more disease-related worries was associated with lower levels of self-efficacy, higher levels of depression, and less family support. Multiple regression analyses revealed that DQOL was bested predicted by depression, and to a lesser extent, difficulty coping with diabetes. Glycohemoglobin levels were not associated with any aspect of DQOL.

Guttmann-Bauman, Flaherty, Sturgger, and McEvoy[78] evaluated the relationship between metabolic control and DQOL in a sample of 69 youths. One-third of the study sample was comprised of minority youth (Hispanic and African American), but the socioeconomic status (SES) of the sample was not reported. Metabolic control was assessed both by glycohemoglobin and by the frequency of acute events such as diabetes-related emergency room visits or hospital admissions. Significant correlations were obtained between DQOL and glycohemoglobin, as well as between DQOL and acute events, such that youths who reported better DQOL had lower levels of glycohemoglobin and fewer acute events. Analyses of the three DQOL scales revealed significant associations of glycohemoglobin with satisfaction and disease impact, but not with worries; acute events were significantly related to impact and worries.

It is important to focus on DQOL in minority patients because they are at increased risk for metabolic control problems[59-61]. Such findings suggest the potential for lower DQOL in poor and minority youth over other social groups. Delamater and colleagues[79] studied DQOL in a culturally diverse sample of 96 youths comprising the full range of SES. Participants included Caucasian, African American, and Hispanic youths. The findings revealed significantly lower DQOL (i.e., greater impact and worries) in youths from single parent families and those with lower SES status. African American youths reported more disease worries than did Caucasian youths, but when SES was controlled for, this effect was attenuated. A number of psychosocial factors were significantly related with lower DQOL, including maladaptive coping, increased diabetes-related stress, more behavior problems, and greater levels of non-supportive family behavior. Multivariate analyses identified SES and diabetes-related stress to be the best predictors of DQOL impact and worry scores. Age, diabetes duration, gender, and glycohemoglobin were unrelated with DQOL.

In a recent study of over 2000 adolescents using the DQOL measure modified by Ingersoll and Marrero[76], Hoey and colleagues from the Hvidore Study Group on Childhood Diabetes[80] found that lower glycosylated hemoglobin A1c was associated with lower impact, fewer worries, and greater satisfaction. In addition, girls reported more worries and less satisfaction than boys, and patients from ethnic minority groups had more impact and worries.

SUMMARY

Research findings indicate diabetic youths are at risk for adjustment problems during the initial period of adaptation after diagnosis, and to the degree that there are such problems, the risks for continued difficulties related to adjustment appear to be increased. In particular, diabetic youths, especially girls, seem to have a greater incidence of depression and eating disorders, and when present are associated with poor glycemic control. Psychosocial problems including anxiety, depression, poor self-esteem, high levels of stress, and maladaptive coping styles, have all been associated with poorer metabolic control. In addition, family conflict, poor communication, and lack of appropriate parental involvement and support for diabetes care, are also linked with poor metabolic control and regimen adherence. Studies of neuropsychological functioning and school performance indicate that diabetic youths are also at risk for learning problems, especially with early diabetes onset and chronic poor metabolic control.

All of these factors are important aspects of quality of life and indicate the challenges that diabetic youths face in simultaneously facing the expected tasks of development and daily management of diabetes. Research findings suggest that DQOL is lower among youths from single-parent families, ethnic minority and lower SES groups, as well as girls, and in youths with shorter disease duration. Poorer DQOL also appears to be associated with youths' perceptions that diabetes is upsetting, difficult to manage, and stressful, and is related to higher levels of self-reported depression. There is some evidence that better DQOL is associated with good metabolic control.

PSYCHOSOCIAL & BEHAVIORAL INTERVENTIONS

A number of controlled studies have examined the efficacy of psychosocial and behavioral interventions for children and adolescents with diabetes[1]. A recent systematic review of these studies indicates that the effects of these interventions are positive, although generally modest in effect size[81]. Most of these interventions have included the family as an integral part of treatment. It is essential to involve the family in diabetes management, as studies have shown that when parents allow older children and adolescents to have self-care autonomy without sufficient cognitive and social maturity, youths are more likely to have problems with diabetes management[82,83].

The results of controlled intervention studies indicate that family-based behavioral procedures such as goal-setting, self-monitoring, positive reinforcement, behavioral contracts, supportive parental communications, and appropriately shared responsibility for diabetes management have improved regimen adherence and glycemic control[84,85]. In addition, such interventions can improve the parent-adolescent relationship[84,86]. For example, Wysocki and colleagues[87] demonstrated that improvements in parent-teen relationships were maintained for one year, and that the family intervention had positive, delayed effects on regimen adherence. Psychoeducational interventions with children and their families that promote problem-solving skills and increase parental support early in the disease course have been shown to improve long-term glycemic control of children[88].

The efficacy of group interventions for diabetic youth has also been evaluated. For example, research findings have shown that peer group support and problem-solving have improved short-term glycemic control[89,90]. Grey and colleagues[91,92] evaluated the effect of group coping skills training, and found that it improved glycemic control and quality of life for adolescents involved in intensive insulin regimens, effects which were maintained after the intervention was completed[93]. In a peer group intervention study targeting problem-solving, Cook et al.[94] showed that problem-solving and glucose monitoring increased, while HbA1c decreased for treated youths. In addition, stress management and coping skills training delivered in small groups of youths has reduced diabetes-related stress[95,96] and improved social interaction[97].

A recent uncontrolled study by Greco et al.[98] examined the effects of an intervention involving diabetic youths and their best friends who did not have diabetes. The intervention, focused on increasing diabetes knowledge, problem solving, and self-management, was delivered in small groups of patients and their friends in four weekly sessions. Results showed increased knowledge and peer support for diabetes management, although measures of glycemic control were not reported. Although this study is limited by the lack of a control group and the small sample size, it is noteworthy for the innovation approach.

Another example of an innovative intervention approach was recently reported by Couper and colleagues[99]. In this randomized study, adolescents in poor glycemic control received either usual care or usual care plus a home based intervention targeting knowledge and goal-setting, consisting of six monthly sessions with telephone contact between home sessions. Results showed gains in knowledge and improved glycemic control after six months, but lack of maintenance over the following year. Other innovative intervention studies have shown the potential benefits of computer-assisted approaches[100,101] and telecommunication technology[102] to improve diabetes management.

Although not much recent research has addressed the role of physical activity in diabetes management, studies conducted during the 1980's demonstrated that increasing the physical activity of diabetic children and adolescents through structured exercise programs (conducted three times per week) improved glycemic control[103,104]; however, less frequent exercise (once per week) did not achieve improved glycemic control[105].

Implications for Clinical Practice

The goals of diabetes management for diabetic youths, besides the attainment and maintenance of good metabolic control, are to ensure that youth develop optimally in all areas of their life: psychologically, socially, academically, and physically. Clinicians should therefore routinely utilize standardized measures to assess youths' developmental progress in these areas, as well as disease-related skills, regimen adherence, and metabolic control. It is critical to maintain consistent contact with families, as studies have shown children who have infrequent and irregular visits with the health care team are more likely to have significant problems with metabolic control[106,107]. Efforts to intensify regimens with insulin pumps, multiple daily injections, and more frequent glucose monitoring are important, but many youths and their families may be unable to commit to and succeed with this type of regimen. A recent report revealed that only 57% of adolescents agreed to participate in a trial of intensive therapy, with the major reasons for refusal being not wanting to have more frequent clinic visits, injections, and glucose monitoring[108]. Psychological and family factors are essential in the success of optimal diabetes management for children and adolescents.

Given the fact that research has shown quality of life is associated with stress related to diabetes management and depression, interventions to reduce stress and depression through improvement in coping abilities are clinically indicated. As described earlier in this chapter, empirical support for such clinical approaches have been demonstrated[95,92,93,97]. Because research has shown that youths who do not manage diabetes well are more likely to have psychological problems, eating disorders, family conflict, and less than optimal parental involvement and support for diabetes tasks, interventions must also consider these psychosocial factors. Many children are given self-care autonomy without sufficient cognitive and emotional maturity. Interventions to appropriately involve parents are essential. A study by Weissberg-Benchell et al.[109] showed that 25% of youths admitted to missing insulin injections, 29% fabricated blood glucose test results, and 81% ate inappropriately.

Parental involvement in children's diabetes care should be assessed routinely, and interventions to promote teamwork initiated to ensure good control of diabetes. Empirical support for these approaches has been demonstrated. For example, interventions to improve parent-adolescent teamwork in diabetes management resulted in less conflict[84], and family-based behavioral intervention utilizing communication skills, goal-setting with behavioral contracts, and problem-solving strategies resulted in improvements in adherence and parent-teen relationships[86,110]. Interventions to improve these kinds of psychosocial factors are also likely to improve the quality of life of children and adolescents with diabetes.

SUMMARY AND CONCLUSIONS

Studies have shown that type 1 diabetes is a risk factor for the development of psychiatric disorders in children and adolescents. Many children show adjustment problems after diagnosis, and if they do, they are at risk for continued problems of adjustment as well as difficulties with diabetes management. Diabetic children's risk for depression and eating disorders is increased, and likely to be associated with poor metabolic control. Increasing evidence indicates that the neurocognitive development of children may be adversely impacted by poor glycemic control, particularly among children with early onset and recurrent severe hypoglycemia. Research findings indicate that better quality of life in youths is associated with increased self-efficacy and less depression, but not necessarily improved metabolic control.

Studies have also examined the role of stress and coping in relation to diabetes management. Children who have less life stress and who cope well with diabetes management are likely to have fewer problems with regimen adherence and glycemic control. High levels of self-efficacy and low levels of learned helplessness have been associated with good glycemic control. Specific health beliefs related to the seriousness of diabetes, personal vulnerability to complications, costs of regimen adherence, and beliefs in the efficacy of treatment, have also been associated with both regimen adherence and glycemic control.

Research has demonstrated that regimen adherence and metabolic control typically decline over time, and that the risk of metabolic control problems is higher among single-parent, lower-income, African American youths. Family factors are reliably associated with regimen adherence and metabolic control: high levels of cohesion and organization, low levels of family conflict and stress, good communication skills, and appropriate involvement of both parents and children in diabetes management, have been associated with higher levels of regimen adherence and better metabolic control. When parents allow adolescents to have self care autonomy without sufficient cognitive and social maturity, they are likely to have more problems with diabetes management.

A number of controlled studies have examined the efficacy of psychosocial interventions for children and adolescents with diabetes. Research findings indicate that family-based behavioral procedures such as goal-setting, self-monitoring, positive reinforcement, behavioral contracts, supportive parental communications, and appropriately shared responsibility for diabetes management have improved regimen adherence and glycemic control, as well as the parent-adolescent relationship. Interventions with children and their families that promote problem-solving skills and increase parental support early in the disease course have improved long-term glycemic control of children. Research findings have also shown that interventions focusing on peer group support and problem-solving have improved glycemic control. In addition, stress management and coping skills training has reduced diabetes-related stress, and improved social interaction and quality of life in adolescents.

In conclusion, a significant amount of behavioral science research has demonstrated that psychological, social, and behavioral factors play an integral role in the management of diabetes in children. Quality of life in youths with diabetes is a very important, yet understudied, issue in diabetes management Research has shown the efficacy of a number of psychosocial therapies that can improve self care behaviors, glycemic control, and psychosocial functioning and quality of life. More research is needed to develop psychosocial intervention programs for specific patient populations, and to demonstrate the cost-effectiveness of these approaches.

REFERENCES

1. Delamater, A.M., Jacobson, A.M., Anderson, B., Cox, D., Fisher, L., Lustman, P., Rubin, R. & Wysocki, T.: Psychosocial therapies in diabetes: Report of the Psychosocial Therapies Working Group. Diabetes Care 24: 1286-1292, 2001.
2. Johnson, S.B.: Insulin-dependent diabetes mellitus in childhood. In Handbook of pediatric psychology (pp. 263-285). Roberts, M.C. (Ed.). New York, Guilford, 1995.
3. Kovacs, M., Feinberg, T.L., Paulauskas, S., Finkelstein, R., Pollock, M. & Crouse-Novak, M.: Initial coping responses and psychosocial characteristics of children with insulin-dependent diabetes mellitus. Journal of Pediatrics 106: 827-834, 1985.
4. Jacobson, A.M., Hauser, S.T., Wertlieb, D., Woldsdorf, J., Orleans, J. & Viegra, M.: Psychological adjustment of children with recently diagnosed diabetes mellitus. Diabetes Care 9: 323-329, 1986.
5. Grey, M., Cameron, M., Lipman, T., & Thurber, F.: Psychosocial status of children with diabetes in the first 2 years after diagnosis. Diabetes Care 18: 1330-1336, 1995.
6. Jacobson, A.M., Hauser, S.T., Lavori, P., et al.: Family environment and glycemic control: a four-year prospective study of children and adolescents with insulin-dependent diabetes mellitus. Psychosom Med 56: 401-409, 1994.
7. Kovacs, M., Ho, V., & Pollock, M.H.: Criterion and predictive validity of the diagnosis of adjustment disorder: a prospective study of youths with new-onset insulin-dependent diabetes mellitus. Am J Psychiatry 152: 523-528, 1995.
8. Rovet, J, Ehrlich, R. & Hoppe, M.: Behavior problems in children with diabetes as a function of sex and age of onset of disease.

Journal of Child Psychology and Psychiatry 28: 477-491, 1987.
9. Lavigne, J., & Faier-Routman, J.: Psychological adjustment to pediatric physical disorders: A meta-analytic review. Journal of Pediatric Psychology 17: 133-157, 1992.
10. Blanz, B., Rensch-Riemann, B., Fritz-Sigmund, D., & Schmidt, M.: IDDM is a risk factor for adolescent psychiatric disorders. Diabetes Care 16: 1579-1587, 1993.
11. Kovacs, M., Goldston, D., Obrosky, D., & Bonar, L.: Psychiatric disorders in youths with IDDM: Rates and risk factors. Diabetes Care 20: 36-44, 1997.
12. Jacobson, A.M., Hauser, S.T., Willett, J., Wolfsdorf, J.I., Herman, L., & de Groot, M.: Psychological adjustment to IDDM: 10-year follow-up of an onset cohort of child and adolescent patients. Diabetes Care 20: 811-818, 1997.
13. Wysocki, T., Hough, B.S., Ward, K. M., & Green, L.B.: Diabetes mellitus in the transition to adulthood: Adjustment, self-care, and health status. Journal of Developmental and Behavioral Pediatrics 13: 194-201, 1992.
14. Bryden, K.S., Peveler, R.C., Stein, A., Neil, A., Mayou, R.A., Dunger, D.B.: Clinical and psychological course of diabetes from adolescence to young adulthood: A longitudinal cohort study. Diabetes Care 24: 1536-1540, 2001.
15. Anderson, B. J., Miller, J. P., Auslander, W. F., & Santiago, J. V.: Family characteristics of diabetic adolescents: Relationship to metabolic control. Diabetes Care 4: 586-594, 1981.
16. La Greca, A. M., Swales, T., Klemp, S., Madigan, S., & Skyler, J.: Adolescents with diabetes: Gender differences in psychosocial functioning and glycemic control. Children's Health Care 24: 61-78, 1995.
17. Rodin, F., & Daneman, D.: Eating disorders and IDDM. Diabetes Care 15: 1402-1412, 1992.
18. Daneman D, Olmsted M, Rydall A, Maharaj S, Rodin G: Eating disorders in young women with type 1 diabetes: Prevalence, problems and prevention. Hormone Research 50 (Suppl 1): 79-86, 1998.
19. Jones, J.M., Lawson, M.L., Daneman, D., Olmsted, M.P., Rodin, G.: Eating disorders in adolescent females with and without type 1 diabetes: Cross sectional study. British Medical Journal 320:1563-1566, 2000.

20. Neumark-Sztainer, D., Patterson, J., Mellin, A., Ackard, D., Utter, J., Story, M., & Sockalosky, J.: Weight control practices and disordered eating behaviors among adolescent females and males with type 1 diabetes: Associations with sociodemographics, weight concerns, familial factors, and metabolic outcomes. Diabetes Care 25: 1289-1296, 2002.
21. Rydall, A.C., Rodin, G.M., Olmsted, M.P., Devenyi, R.G., Daneman, D.: Disordered eating behavior and microvascular complications in young women with insulin-dependent diabetes mellitus. New England Journal of Medicine 336:1849-1854, 1997.
22. Maharag, S., Rodini, G., Olmsted, M., Connolly, J., Daneman, D.: Eating problems and the observed quality of mother-daughter interactions among girls with type 1 diabetes. Journal of Consulting and Clinical Psychology 69: 950-958, 2001.
23. Schwartz, S.A., Weissberg-Benchell, J., & Perlmuter, L.C.: Personal control and disordered eating in female adolescents with type 1 diabetes. Diabetes Care 25: 1987-1991, 2001.
24. Kuttner, M.J., Delamater, A.M., & Santiago, J.V.: Learned helplessness in diabetic youths. Journal of Pediatric Psychology 15: 581-594, 1990.
25. Meltzer, L.J., Johnson, S.B., Prine, J.M., Banks, R.A., Desrosiers, P.M., & Silverstein, J.H.: Disordered eating, body mass, and glycemic control in adolescents with type 1 diabetes. Diabetes Care 24: 678-682, 2001.
26. Bryden, K.S., Neil, A., Mayou, R.A., Peveler, R.C., Fairburn, C.G., & Dunger, D.B.: Eating habits, body weight, and insulin misuse: A longitudinal study of teenagers and young adults with type 1 diabetes. Diabetes Care 22: 1956-1960, 1999.
26. Hanson, C.L., Henggeler, S.W., & Burghen, G.A.: Model of associations between psychosocial variables and health-outcome measures of adolescents with IDDM. Diabetes Care 10: 752-758, 1987.
27. Hanson, S.L., & Pichert, J.W.: Perceived stress and diabetes control in adolescents. Health Psychology 5: 439-452, 1986.
28. Kager, V. & Holden, W.: Preliminary investigation of the direct and moderating effects of family and individual variables on the adjustment of children and adolescents with diabetes. Journal of Pediatric Psychology 17: 491-502, 1992

29. Holmes, C., Dunlap, W., Chen, R., & Cornwell, J.: Gender differences in the learning status of diabetic children. Journal of Consulting and Clinical Psychology 60: 698-704, 1992.
30. Delamater, A. M., Kurtz, S. M., Bubb, J., White, N. H., & Santiago, J. V.: Stress and coping in relation to metabolic control of adolescents with type I diabetes. Journal of Developmental and Behavioral Pediatrics 8: 136-140, 1987.
31. Grossman, H.Y., Brink, S., & Hauser, S.T.: Self-efficacy in adolescent girls and boys with insulin-dependent diabetes mellitus. Diabetes Care 10: 324-329, 1987.
32. Hanson, C.L., Cigrant, JA, Harris, M, Carle, DL, Relyea, G., Burghen, GA: Coping styles in youths with insulin-dependent diabetes mellitus. Journal of Consulting and Clinical Psychology 57: 644-651, 1989.
33. Bond, G.G., Aiken, L.S., & Somerville, S.C.: The health belief model and adolescents with insulin-dependent diabetes mellitus. Health Psychology 11: 190-198, 1992.
34. Brownlee-Duffeck, M., Peterson, L., Simonds, J.F., Goldstein, D., Kilo, C. & Hoette, S.: The role of health beliefs in the regimen adherence and metabolic control of adolescents and adults with diabetes mellitus. Journal of Consulting and Clinical Psychology 55: 139-144, 1987.
35. Palardy, N., Greening, L., Ott, J., Holderby, A., & Atchison, J.: Adolescents' health attitudes and adherence to treatment for insulin-dependent diabetes mellitus. Developmental and Behavioral Pediatrics 19: 31-37, 1998.
36. Skinner, T.C., & Hampson, S.E.: Personal models of diabetes in relation to self-care, well-being, and glycemic control: A prospective study in adolescence. Diabetes Care 24: 828-833, 2001.
37. Skinner, T.C., Hampson, S.E., & Fife-Schaw, C.: Personality, personal model beliefs, and self-care in adolescents and young adults with type 1 diabetes. Health Psychology 21: 61-70, 2002.
38. Charron-Prochownik, D., Becker, M.H., Brown, M.B., Liang, W., & Bennett, S.: Understanding young children's health beliefs and diabetes regimen adherence. The Diabetes Educator 19: 409-418, 1993.
39. Wysocki, T.: Associations among teen-parent relationships, metabolic control, and adjustment to diabetes in adolescents. Journal of

Pediatric Psychology 18: 441-452, 1993.

40. Anderson, B.J., Auslander, W F., Jung, K.C., Miller, J.P., & Santiago, J.V.: Assessing family sharing of diabetes responsibility. Journal of Pediatric Psychology 15: 477-492, 1990.

41. Anderson, B.J., Ho, J., Brackett, J., Finkelstein, D., & Laffel, L.: Parental involvement in diabetes management tasks: Relationships to blood glucose monitoring adherence and metabolic control in young adolescents with insulin-dependent diabetes mellitus. Journal of Pediatrics 130: 257-265, 1997.

42. Weist, M., Finney, J., Barnard, M., Davis, C., & Ollendick, T.: Empirical selection of psychosocial treatment targets for children and adolescents with diabetes. Journal of Pediatric Psychology 18: 11-28, 1993.

43. Orr, D., Golden, M.P., Myers, G., & Marrero, D.G.: Characteristics of adolescents with poorly controlled diabetes referred to a tertiary care center. Diabetes Care 6: 170-175, 1983.

44. White, K., Kolman, M., Wexler, P., Polin, G., & Winter, R.J.: Unstable diabetes and unstable families: A psychosocial evaluation of diabetic children with recurrent ketoacidosis. Pediatrics 73: 749-755, 1984.

45. Schafer, L.C., Glasgow, R.E., McCaul, K.D., & Dreher, M.: Adherence to IDDM regimens: Relationship to psychosocial variables and metabolic control. Diabetes Care 6: 493-498, 1983.

46. La Greca, A.M., Auslander, W.F., Greco, P., Spetter, D., Fisher, E.B., & Santiago, J.V.: I get by with a little help from my family and friends: Adolescents' support for diabetes care. Journal of Pediatric Psychology 20: 449-476, 1995.

47. Bobrow, E.S., AvRuskin, T.W., & Siller, J.: Mother-daughter interaction and adherence to diabetes regimens. Diabetes Care 8: 146-151, 1985.

48. Miller-Johnson, S., Emery, R., Marvin, R., Clarke, W., Lovinger, R., & Martin, M.: Parent-child relationships and the management of insulin-dependent diabetes mellitus. Journal of Consulting and Clinical Psychology 62: 603-610, 1994.

49. Davis, C.L., Delamater, A.M., Shaw, K.H., La Greca, A.M., Eidson, M.S., Pewrez-Rodriguez, J.E., & Nemery, R.: Parenting styles, regimen adherence, and glycemic control in 4- to 10-year-old children with diabetes. Journal of Pediatric Psychology 26: 123-129, 2001.

50. Wysocki, T., Miller, K., Greco, P., Harris, M.A., Harvey, L., Taylor, A., Elder Danda, C., McDonell, K., & White, N.H.: Behavior therapy for families of adolescents with diabetes: Effects on directly observed family interactions. Behavior Therapy 30: 507-525, 1999.

51. Landolt, M.A., Ribi, K., Laimbacher, J., Vollrath, M., Gnehm, H.E., & Sennhauser, F.H.: Posttraumatic stress disorder in parents of children with newly diagnosed type 1 diabetes. Journal of Pediatric Psychology 27: 647-652, 2002.

52. Seiffge-Krenke, I.: "Come on, say something, Dad!": Communication and coping in fathers of diabeteic adolescents. Journal of Pediatric Psychology 27: 439-450, 2002.

53. Forsander, G.A., Persson, B., Sundelin, J., Berglund, E., Snellman, K., & Hellstrom, R.: Metabolic control in children with insulin-dependent diabetes mellitus 5 y after diagnosis: Early detection of patients at risk for poor metabolic control. Acta Paediatr 87: 857-864, 1998.

54. Jacobson, A.M., Hauser, S.T., Lavori, P., Wolfsdorf, J., Herskowitz, R., Milley, J., Bliss, R., Gelfand, E., Wertlieb, D., Stein, J: Adherence among children and adolescents with insulin-dependent diabetes mellitus over a four-year longitudinal follow-up: I. The influence of patient coping and adjustment. Journal of Pediatric Psychology, 15, 511-526, 1990.

55. Johnson SB, Kelly M, Henretta JC, Cunningham WR, Tomer A, Silverstein JH: A longitudinal analysis of adherence and health status in childhood diabetes. Journal of Pediatric Psychology 17:537-553, 1992.

56. Overstreet, S., Goins, J., Chen, R.S., Holmes, C.S., Greer, T., Dunlap, W.P., & Frentz, J.: Family environment and the interrelation of family structure, child behavior, and metabolic control for children with diabetes. Journal of Pediatric Psychology 20: 435-447, 1995.

57. Thompson, S.J., Auslander, W.F., & White, N.H.: Comparison of single-mother and two-parent families on metabolic control of children with diabetes. Diabetes Care 24: 234-238, 2001.

58. Forsander, G.A., Sundelin, J., & Persson, B.: Influence of the initial management regimen and family social situation on glycemic control and medical care in children with type 1 diabetes mellitus. Acta Paediatr 89: 1462-1468, 2000.

59. Auslander, W.F., Thompson, S., Dreitzer, D., White, N.H., & Santiago, J.V.: Disparity in glycemic control and adherence between African-American and Caucasian youths with diabetes: Family and Community Contexts. Diabetes Care 20: 1569-1575, 1997.
60. Delamater, A. M., Albrecht, D. R., Postellon, D. C., & Gutai, J. P.: Racial differences in metabolic control of children and adolescents with Type I diabetes mellitus. Diabetes Care 14: 20-25, 1991.
61. Delamater, A.M., Shaw, K., Applegate, B., Pratt, I., Eidson, M., Lancelotta, G., Gonzalez-Mendoza, L., & Richton, S.: Risk for metabolic control problems in minority youth with diabetes. Diabetes Care 22: 700-705, 1999.
62. Rovet, J, Ehrlich, R. & Hoppe, M.: Specific intellectual deficits associated with the early onset of insulin-dependent diabetes mellitus in children. Child Development 59: 226-234, 1988.
63. Ryan, C., Vega, A. & Drash, A.: Cognitive deficits in adolescents who developed diabetes early in life. Pediatrics 75: 921-927, 1985.
64. Holmes, C. & Richman, L.: Cognitive profiles of children with insulin-dependent diabetes. Developmental and Behavioral Pediatrics 6: 323-326, 1985.
65. Ryan, C., Vega, A., Longstreet, C. & Drash, A.: Neuropsychological changes in adolescents with insulin-dependent diabetes. Journal of Consulting and Clinical Psychology 52: 335-342, 1984.
66. Ryan, C., Longstreet, C. & Morrow, L.: The effects of diabetes mellitus on the school attendance and school achievement of adolescents. Child: Care, Health and Development 11: 229-240, 1985.
67. Kovacs, M., Ryan, C. & Obrosky, D.S.: Verbal intellectual and verbal memory performance of youths with childhood-onset insulin-dependent diabetes mellitus. Journal of Pediatric Psychology 19: 475-483, 1994.
68. Rovet, J., & Alvarez, M.: Attentional functioning in children and adolescents with IDDM. Diabetes Care 20: 803-810, 1997.
69. Kovacs, M., Goldston, D. & Iyengar, S.: Intellectual development and academic performance of children with insulin-dependent diabetes mellitus: A longitudinal study. Developmental Psychology 28: 676-684, 1992.
70. Kovacs, M., Finkelstein, R., Feinberg, T.L., Crouse-Novak, M., Paulauskas, S., Pollock, M: Initial psychologic responses of parents to

the diagnosis of insulin dependent diabetes mellitus in their children. Diabetes Care 8: 568-575, 1985.
71. Northam, E., Anderson, P., Werther, G., Warne, G., Adler, R., & Andrewes, D.: Neuropsychological complications of IDDM in children 2 years after disease onset. Diabetes Care 21: 379-384, 1998.
72. Northam, E., Anderson, P., Werther, G., Warne, G., Adler, R., & Andrewes, D.: Predictors of change in the neuropsychological profiles of children with type 1 diabetes 2 years after disease onset. Diabetes Care 22: 1438-1444, 1999.
73. Northam, E.A., Anderson, P.J., Jacobs, R., Hughes, M., Warne, G.L., Werther, G.A.: Neuropsychological profiles of children with type 1 diabetes 6 years after disease onset. Diabetes Care 24: 1541-1546, 2001.
74. Diabetes Control and Complications Trial Research Group: Effect of intensive diabetes treatment on the development and progression of long-term complications in adolescents with insulin-dependent diabetes mellitus, Diabetes Control and Complications Trial. Journal of Pediatrics 125: 177-188, 1994.
75. Spieth, L.E., & Harris, C.V.: Assessment of health-related quality of life in children and adolescents: An integrative review. Journal of Pediatric Psychology 21: 175-193, 1996.
76. Ingersoll, G.M., & Marrero, D.G.: A modified quality-of-life measure for youths: Psychometric properties. The Diabetes Educator 17: 114-120, 1991.
77. Grey, M., Boland, E. A., Yu, C., Sullivan-Bolyai, S., & Tamborlane, W.V.: Personal and family factors associated with quality of life in adolescents with diabetes. Diabetes Care 21: 909-914, 1998.
78. Guttmann-Bauman, I., Flaherty, B.P., Strugger, M., & McEvoy, R.C.: Metabolic control and quality-of-life self-assessment in adolescents with IDDM. Diabetes Care 21: 915-918, 1998.
79. Delamater, A.M., Tercyak, K., Applegate, B., Eidson, M., & Nemery, R.: Quality of life in minority youths with diabetes. Manuscript submitted for publication, 2002.
80. Hoey, H., Aanstoot, H., Chiarelli, F., Daneman, D., Danne, et al. for the Hvidore Study Group on Childhood Diabetes. Good metabolic control is associated with better quality of life in 2,101 adolescents with type 1 diabetes. Diabetes Care 24: 1923-1928, 2001.

81. Hampson, S.E., Skinner, R.C., Hart, J., Storey L., Gage, H., Foxcroft, D., Kimber, A., Cradock, S., McEvilly, E.A.: Behavioral interventions for adolescents with type 1 diabetes: How effective are they? Diabetes Care 23: 1416-1422, 2000.
82. Ingersoll, G.M., Orr, D., Herrold, A., & Golden, M. Cognitive maturity and self-management among adolescents with insulin-dependent diabetes mellitus. Journal of Pediatrics 108: 620-623, 1986.
83. Wysocki, T., Taylor, A., Hough, B., Linscheid, T., Yeates, K., Naglieri, J.: Deviation from developmentally appropriate self-care autonomy: Association with diabetes outcomes. Diabetes Care 19: 119-125, 1996.
84. Anderson, B.J., Wolf, R.M., Burkhart, M.T., Cornell, R.G. & Bacon, G.E. (1989). Effects of peer-group intervention on metabolic control of adolescents with IDDM: Randomized outpatient study. Diabetes Care, 12, 179-183.
85. Anderson, B.J., Brackett, J., Ho, J., & Laffel, L.: An office-based intervention to maintain parent-adolescent teamwork in diabetes management: Impact on parent involvement, family conflict, and subsequent glycemic control. Diabetes Care 22: 713-721, 1999.
86. Satin, W., La Greca, A., Zigo, M., & Skyler, J.: Diabetes in adolescence: Effects of multifamily group intervention and parent simulation of diabetes. Journal of Pediatric Psychology 14: 259-276, 1989.
87. Delamater, A.M., Smith, J., Bubb, J., Davis, S., Gamble, T., White, N., & Santiago, J.: Family-based behavior therapy for diabetic adolescents. In Advances in child health psychology: Proceedings of the Florida Conference. Johnson, J., & Johnson, S.B., Eds. Gainesville, FL, University of Florida Press, 1991.
88. Wysocki, T., Greco, P., Harris, M. A., Bubb, J., & White, N. H.: Behavior therapy for families of adolescents with diabetes: Maintenance of treatment effects. Diabetes Care 24: 441-446, 2001.
89. Delamater, A.M., Bubb, J., Davis, S., Smith, J., Schmidt, L., White, N., & Santiago, J.V. Randomized, prospective study of self-management training with newly diagnosed diabetic children. Diabetes Care 13: 492-498, 1990.
90. Kaplan, R.M., Chadwick, M.W., & Schimmel, L.E. (1985). Social

learning intervention to promote metabolic control in Type I diabetes mellitus: Pilot experimental results. Diabetes Care, 8, 152-155.

91. Boland, E.A., Grey, M., Oesterle, Al., Fredrickson, L., & Tamborlane, W.V.: Continuous subcutaneous insuli infusion: A new way to lower risk of severe hypoglycemia, improve metabolic control, and enhance coping in adolescents with type 1 diabetes. Diabetes Care 22: 1779-1784, 1999.

92. Grey, M., Boland, E. A., Davidson, M., Yu, C., Sullivan-Bolyai, S., & Tamborlane, W.V.: Short-term effects of coping skills training as adjunct to intensive therapy in adolescents. Diabetes Care 21: 902-908, 1998.

93. Grey, M., Boland, E., Davidson, M., Yu, C., & Tamborlance, W.: Coping skills training for youth on intensive therapy has long-lasting effects on metabolic control and quality of life. Journal of Pediatrics 137: 107-113, 2000.

94. Cook, S., Herold, K., Edidin, D.V., & Briars, R.: Increasing problem solving in adolescents with type 1 diabetes: The Choices Diabetes Program. The Diabetes Educator 28: 115-124, 2002.

95. Boardway, R.H., Delamater, A.M., Tomakowsky, J., & Gutai, J.P.: Stress management training for adolescents with diabetes. Journal of Pediatric Psychology 18: 29-45, 1993.

96. Hains, A.A., Davies, W.H., Parton, E., Totka, J., & Amoroso-Camarata, J.: A stress management intervention for adolescents with type 1 diabetes. The Diabetes Educator 26: 417-424, 2000.

97. Mendez, F., & Belendez, M.: Effects of a behavioral intervention on treatment adherence and stress management in adolescents with IDDM. Diabetes Care 20: 1370-1375, 1997.

98. Greco, P., Shroff Pendley, J., McDonell, K., & Reeves, G.: A peer group intervention for adolescents with type 1 diabetes and their best friends. Journal of Pediatric Psychology 26: 485-490, 2001.

99. Couper, J.J., Taylor, J., Fotheringham, M.J., & Sawyer, M.: Failure to maintain the benefits of home-based intervention in adolescents with poorly controlled type 1 diabetes. Diabetes Care 22: 1933-1937, 1999.

100. Marrero, D.G., Kronz, K.K., Golden, M.P., Wright, J.C., Orr, D.P. & Fineberg, N.S.: Clinical evaluation of computer-assisted self-monitoring of blood glucose system.Diabetes Care 12:345-350, 1989.

101. Horan, P., Yarborough, M., Besigel, G., & Carlson, D. Computer-

assisted self-control of diabetes by adolescents. The Diabetes Educator, 16, 205-211, 1990.
102. Marrero, D.G., Vandagriff, J., Kronz, K., Fineberg, N., Golden, M., Bray, D., Orr, D., Wright, J., & Johnson, N.: Using telecommunication technology to manage children with diabetes: The Computer-Linked Outpatient Clinic (CLOC) Study. The Diabetes Educator 21: 313-319, 1995.
103. Campaigne, B.N., Gilliam, T.B., Spencer, M.L., Lampman, R.M. & Schork, M.A.: Effects of a physical activity program on metabolic control and cardiovascular fitness in children with IDDM. Diabetes Care 7: 57-62, 1984.
104. Stratton, R., Wilson, D.P., Endres, R.K. & Goldstein, D.E.: Improved glycemic control after supervised 8-week exercise program in insulin-dependent diabetic adolescents. Diabetes Care 10: 589-593, 1987.
105. Huttunen, N.P., Lankelaa, S.L., Knip, M., Lautala, P., Kaar, M.L., Laasonen, K. & Puukka, R.: Effect of once-a-week training program on physical fitness and metabolic control in children with IDDM. Diabetes Care, 12: 737-739, 1989.
106. Jacobson, A.M., Hauser, S.T., Willett, J., Wolfsdor, J., & Herman, L.: Consequences of irregular versus continuous medical follow-up in children and adolescents with insulin-dependent diabetes mellitus. Journal of Pediatrics 131: 727-733, 1997.
107. Kaufman, F.R., Halvorson, M., & Carpenter, S.: Association between diabetes control and visits to a multidisciplinary pediatric diabetes clinic. Pediatrics 103: 948-951, 1999.
108. Tercyak, K.P., Johnson, S.B., Kirkpatrick, K.A., & Silverstein, J.H.: Offering a randomized trial of intensive therapy for IDDM to adolescents: Reasons for refusal, patient characteristics, and recruiter efforts. Diabetes Care 21: 213-215, 1998.
109. Weissberg-Benchell, J., Glasgow, A.M., Tynan, W.D., Wirtz, P., Turek, J., & Ward, J.: Adolescent management and mismanagement. Diabetes Care 18: 77-82, 1995.
110. Wysocki, T., Harris, M. A., Greco, P., Bubb, J., Danda, C.E., Harvey, L.M., McDonell, K., Taylor, A., & White, N.H.: Randomized, controlled trial of behavior therapy for families of adolescents with insulin-dependent diabetes mellitus. Journal of Pediatric Psychology 25: 23-33, 2000.

Index

GPSR Compliance
The European Union's (EU) General Product Safety Regulation (GPSR) is a set of rules that requires consumer products to be safe and our obligations to ensure this.

If you have any concerns about our products, you can contact us on

ProductSafety@springernature.com

In case Publisher is established outside the EU, the EU authorized representative is:

Springer Nature Customer Service Center GmbH
Europaplatz 3
69115 Heidelberg, Germany

www.ingramcontent.com/pod-product-compliance
Ingram Content Group UK Ltd.
Pitfield, Milton Keynes, MK11 3LW, UK
UKHW021828170926
475607UK00007B/28
9781402075575